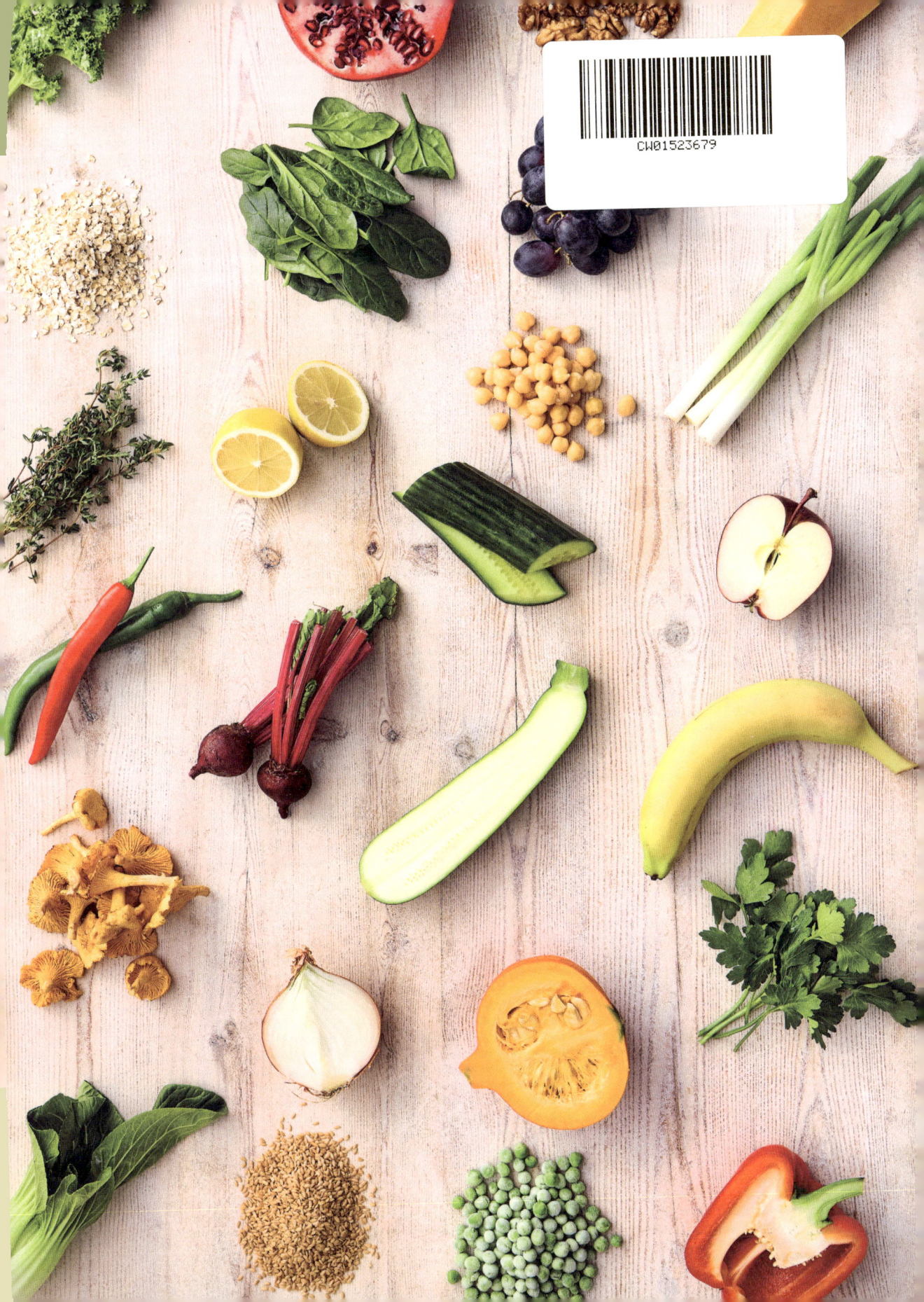

Eat Yourself Healthy

Food photography DAVID LOFTUS

Design JAMES VERITY

MICHAEL JOSEPH

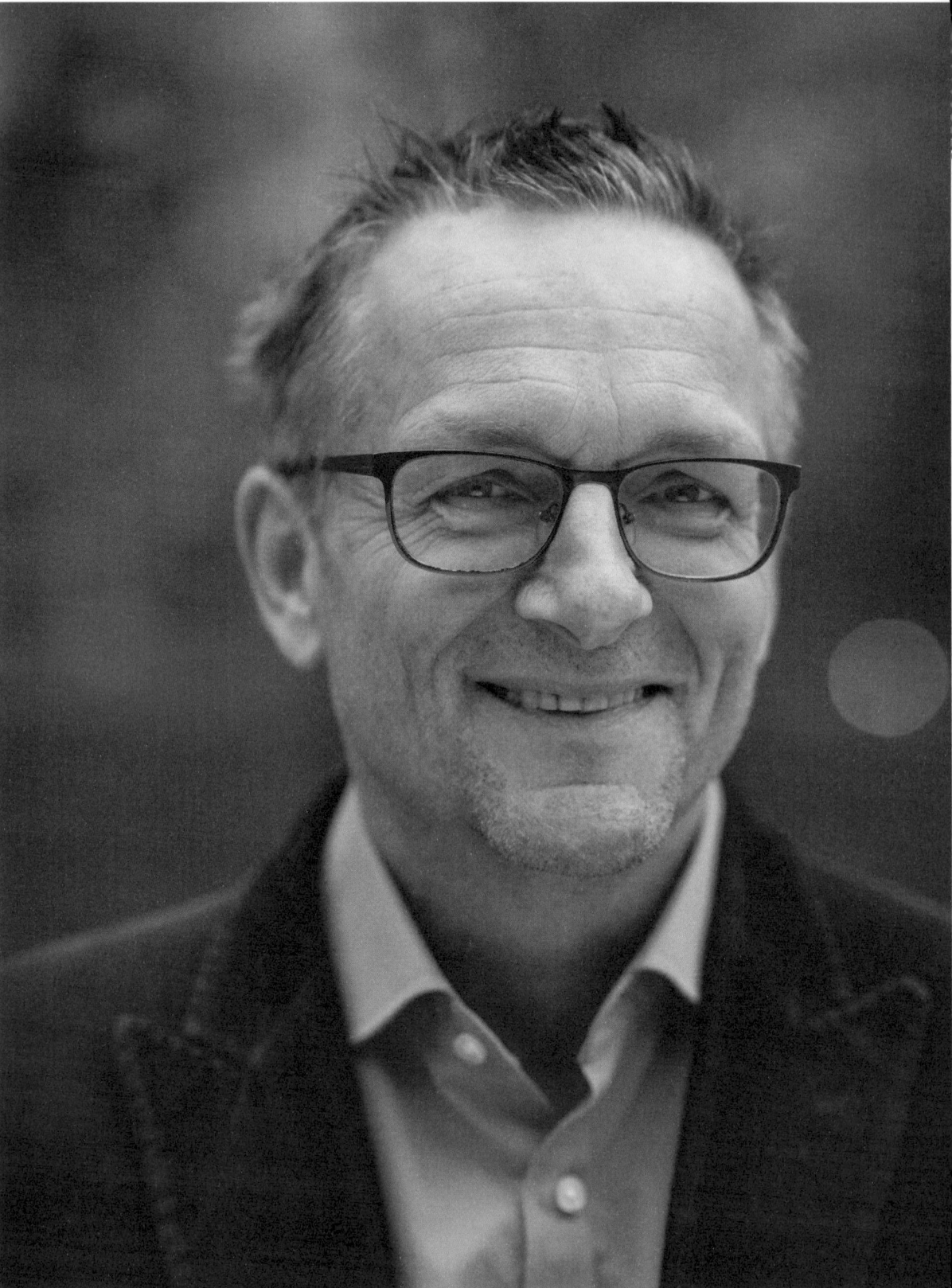

DEDICATED TO

Michael Mosley

1957 — 2024

It felt only right to dedicate this book to Michael Mosley. I was lucky enough to meet Michael a number of times, and the legacy of work he leaves behind when it comes to public health will live on for many years. In his unique, inquisitive, approachable style, he brought important health conversations into the spotlight, serving the public and giving us all food for thought. A kind, sweet, gentle man, Michael will be missed by all. Sending much love to his dear wife Clare, and their four children.

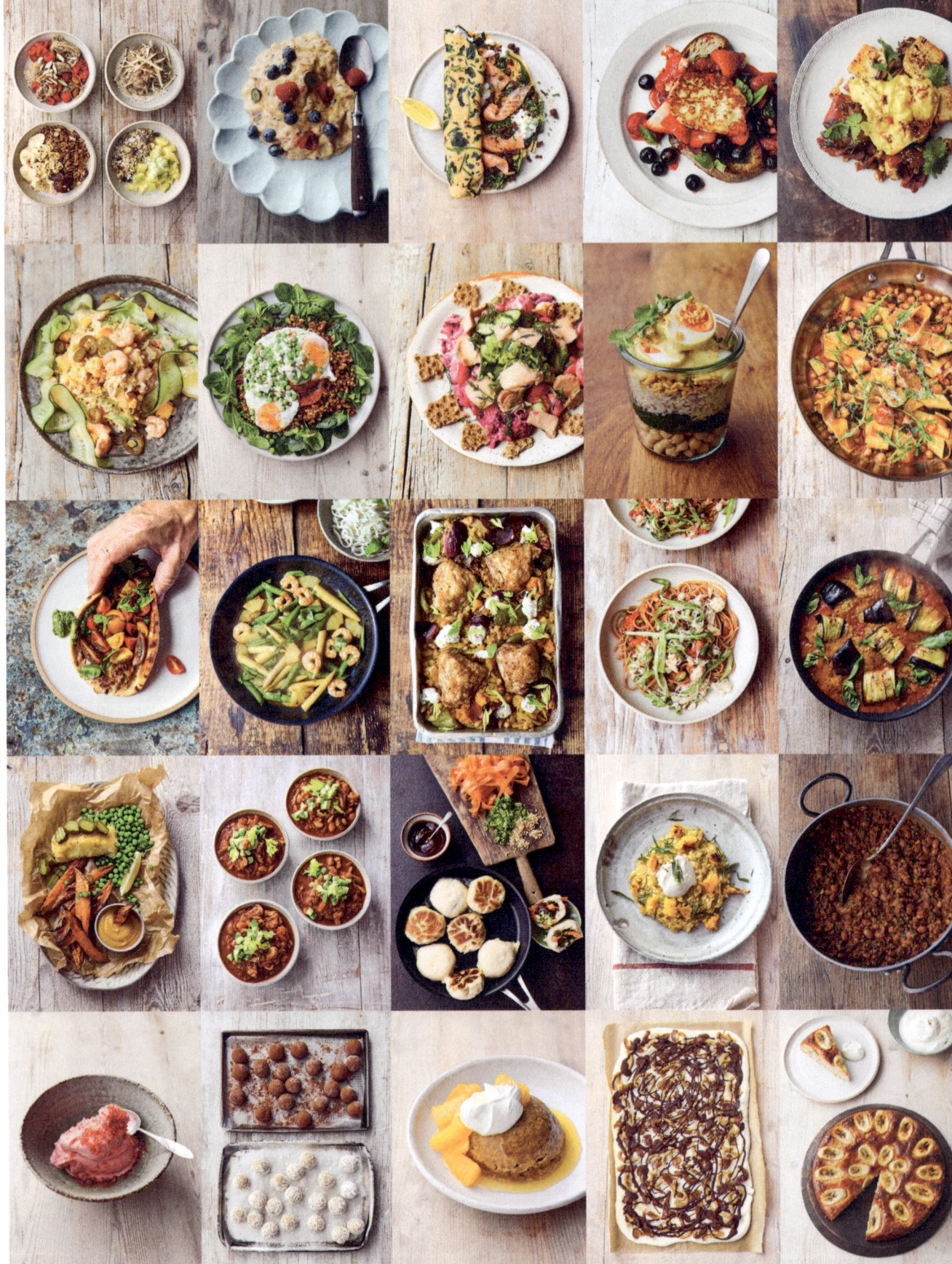

Contents

Introduction — 7

Pantry & kit — 11

50 healthy hacks — 13

The 2-week kickstarter — 20

How to balance your plate — 26

Getting your 7-a-day — 29

Breakfast — 33

Lunch — 71

Dinner — 129

Weekend — 217

Healthier sweet treats — 257

Drinks — 283

Cooking sustainably & kitchen notes — 294

Nutrition — 296

Index — 306

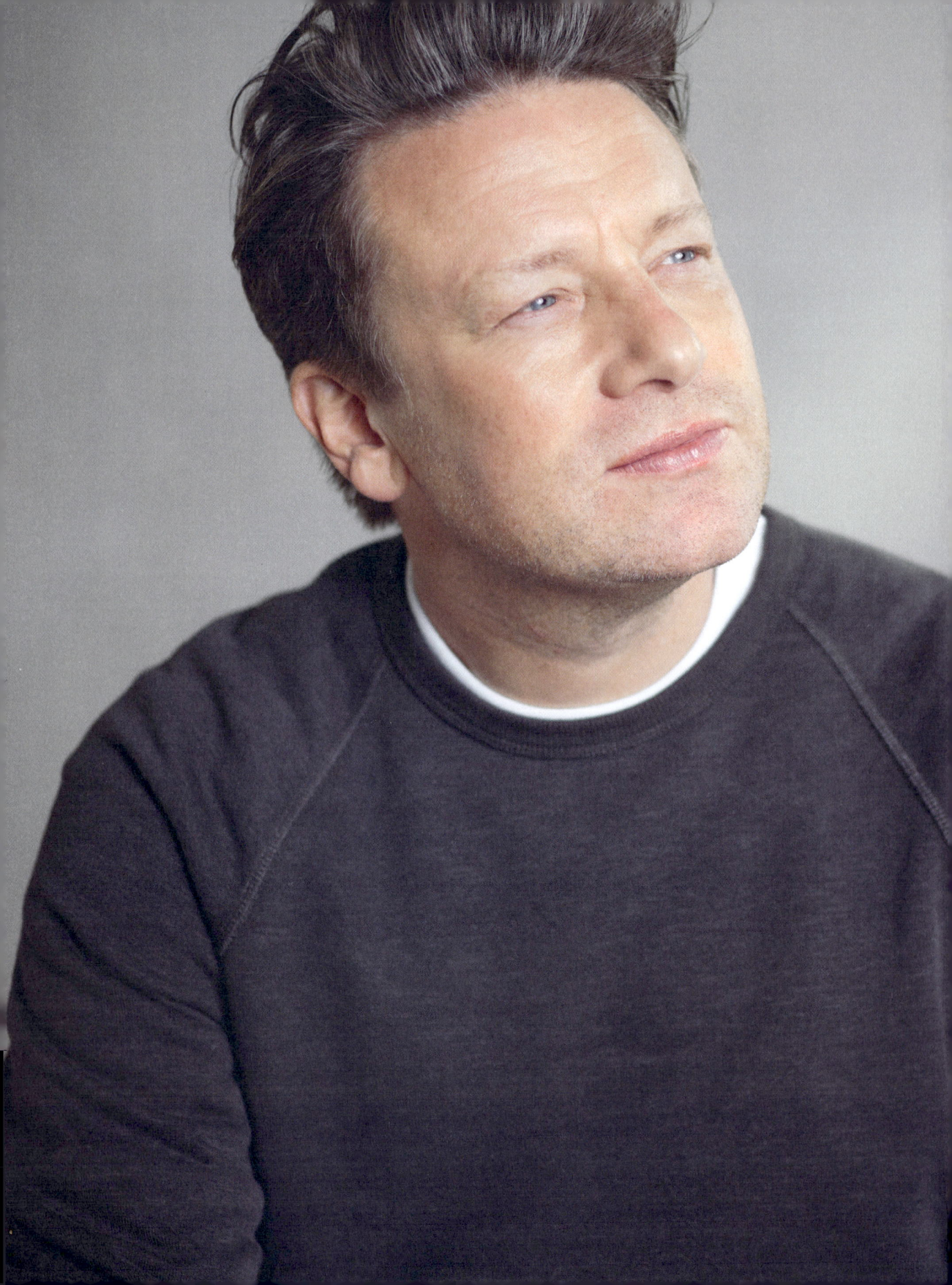

Do you want to feel better?

I truly believe that our health is the most important thing we have, and I'm sure you're asking yourself the same questions that I am. How do we help our bodies be the best they can be? How do we maintain a healthy weight? How do we sleep better? How do we support our immune systems so they can protect us from common illnesses? And, ultimately, how do we feel healthier and happier in a world designed to make us unhealthy?

I turned 50 this year, and that shift from one decade to another really gave me a moment to pause and reflect on my own health, to think about what I need to do to get myself in the best shape for the future.

In turn, it inspired me to write this book, to share all the knowledge and insights I've garnered over the years, and to help you on your own health journey in the most authentic way I can, which is through delicious, abundant, joyous, beautiful food. Because, let's face it, we've all got to eat!

I've been immersed in this wonderful world of food for over 40 years now, and have more than 25 years of publishing under my belt, which I feel ever so grateful for. About 10 years ago, I had the honour of studying for a Royal Society of Public Health Level 4 Award in Nutrition at St Mary's Twickenham University under Professor Ann Kennedy. I gained a deeper understanding of our bodies' relationship with food, how what we eat affects us, and the impact it can have.

Creating this book, and pouring everything I've learnt into these pages, has been a helpful and cathartic process and, I'll be honest, a fantastic reminder for me of the power of food to make us feel good. What I've come out with is this trusted companion that can be used for life. Whether that's every day of the week, or simply dipping in and out of it as you choose, you can be confident that you're doing something positive for your health. Within a week of delicious eating there's more than enough space to indulge in the things we all love – we don't have to eat healthily 100% of the time – but this book will help you build a celebratory relationship with food, safe in the knowledge that every time you cook from it, you're making a good choice. In a world of misinformation, it exists to give you a place of truth, certainty and balance.

Food to change your life

What I've really valued in writing these recipes is that feeling of taking back control of my health. And I hope that you'll use the book to have that impact in your own life. *Eat Yourself Healthy* is about everything that you *can* have on the food front, not about taking things away. It's about boosting your meals with colour, excitement, nutrients and, of course, bags of flavour. It's about abundant, generous platefuls that will energize, satisfy, nourish and revitalize you. It's a reliable, happy, safe space packed with ideas, hacks and helpful hints, all of which will set you up on the food front to be on top of your health. This is about arming you with ideas and inspiration.

When it comes to nutrition, you can be confident that I've covered all the bases. I've worked within a simple framework of nutritional parameters for each meal, meaning you can go ahead and choose any recipe in the book, knowing that the thinking has been done for you.

Breakfast Every recipe here gives you at least 1 portion of your 7-a-day (pages 28 to 31), and comes in at under 400 calories, under 6g of saturated fat, and under 1.8g of salt.

Lunch / Dinner / Weekend Everything in these chapters will give you at least 2 portions of your 7-a-day, often a lot more, and is sitting at under 600 calories, under 6g of saturated fat, and under 1.8g of salt. Feel free to mix and match within the chapters!

Healthier sweet treats This lovely little bunch of recipes are all under 250 calories and under 2.5g of saturated fat – now it doesn't get much better than that.

You'll find the full nutritional breakdown for each recipe at the back of the book, should you need it (pages 298 to 303). And, within each chapter, I've ordered the recipes starting with the fastest options, so it's super-easy to find a meal that will fit into the time you have available to you. Knowing how important it is to have quick options, I've made sure I'm giving you plenty of convenient choices here. The breakfasts start from just 3 minutes, the 27 lunch recipes range from just 6 to 20 minutes in length, and within the bumper dinner chapter, 17 of the recipes take 15 minutes or less. I want to prove that you can cook healthily, even when you're short on time.

Before the recipes, I'm kicking you off with 50 healthy hacks (pages 13 to 19). These are easy little swaps to help you get more consistency in your life, and set you on the path to a healthier, happier you. Straight after that you'll find my 2-week kickstarter (pages 20 to 25), which is a helpful meal plan focused on two weeks of solid nutrition, bags of veg and fruit and, ultimately, delicious eating, hopefully giving you a great health boost if you want to go all in.

Each hack you follow, every recipe you make, adds up to a much greater whole. There's no silver bullet when it comes to our health, but what we can have is consistency, and embracing the power of food to make us healthier and happier is a really doable thing. I want to make it easier than ever to make healthy choices, which, in turn, will help you to truly thrive.

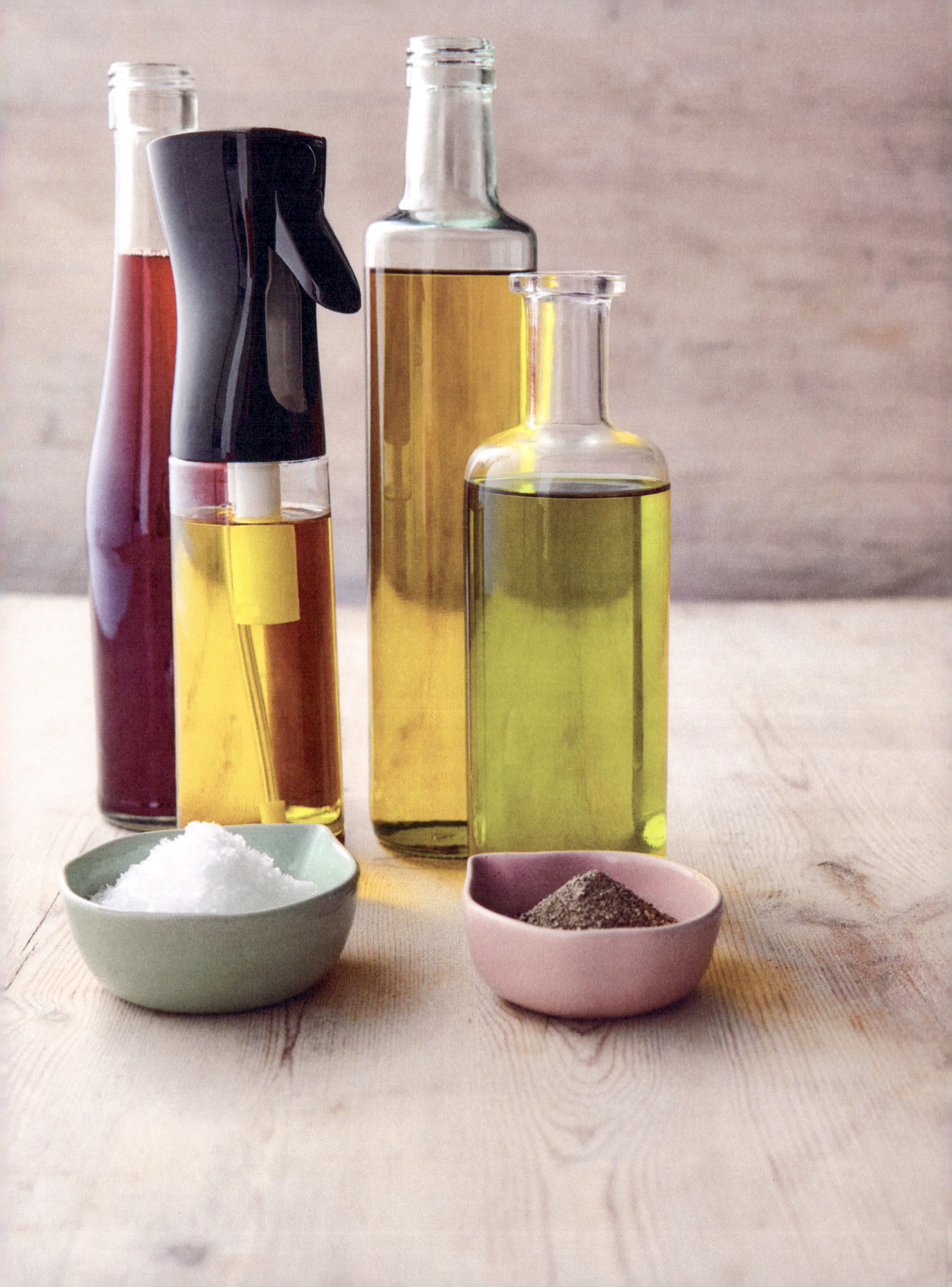

Pantry & kit

There are five staple ingredients that I presume you will have in stock before you start cooking – and I couldn't recommend these kitchen heroes enough. They pop up regularly throughout this book and aren't included in each individual ingredients list. They are olive oil for cooking; extra virgin olive oil for dressing and finishing dishes; red wine vinegar as a good all-rounder when it comes to acidity and balancing marinades, sauces and dressings; and, of course, sea salt and black pepper for seasoning to perfection. I use an olive oil spritzer a lot in these recipes – and in all my cooking at home these days. It makes it much easier to control your oil use, giving more even coverage and meaning you can often get away with less oil, thus helping you to be healthier, too. I'd recommend investing in a decent empty spritz bottle, and decanting your own oil (like you see in the picture on the left), so you know exactly what you're using.

When it comes to equipment, I tend to use a small range of kit on repeat, so please don't feel like you need to spend a fortune to get set up in the kitchen. Some frying pans, a couple of casserole pans (one shallow and one deep) and a few roasting trays are your key cooking vessels. A chopping board and decent knife is a given for nearly every recipe. When it comes to making your life easier, a speed-peeler, box grater, and pestle and mortar are all fantastic for creating texture and boosting flavour. A blender or stick blender and a food processor will always be a bonus, too, especially if you're short on time, and you'll find these items handy for this book.

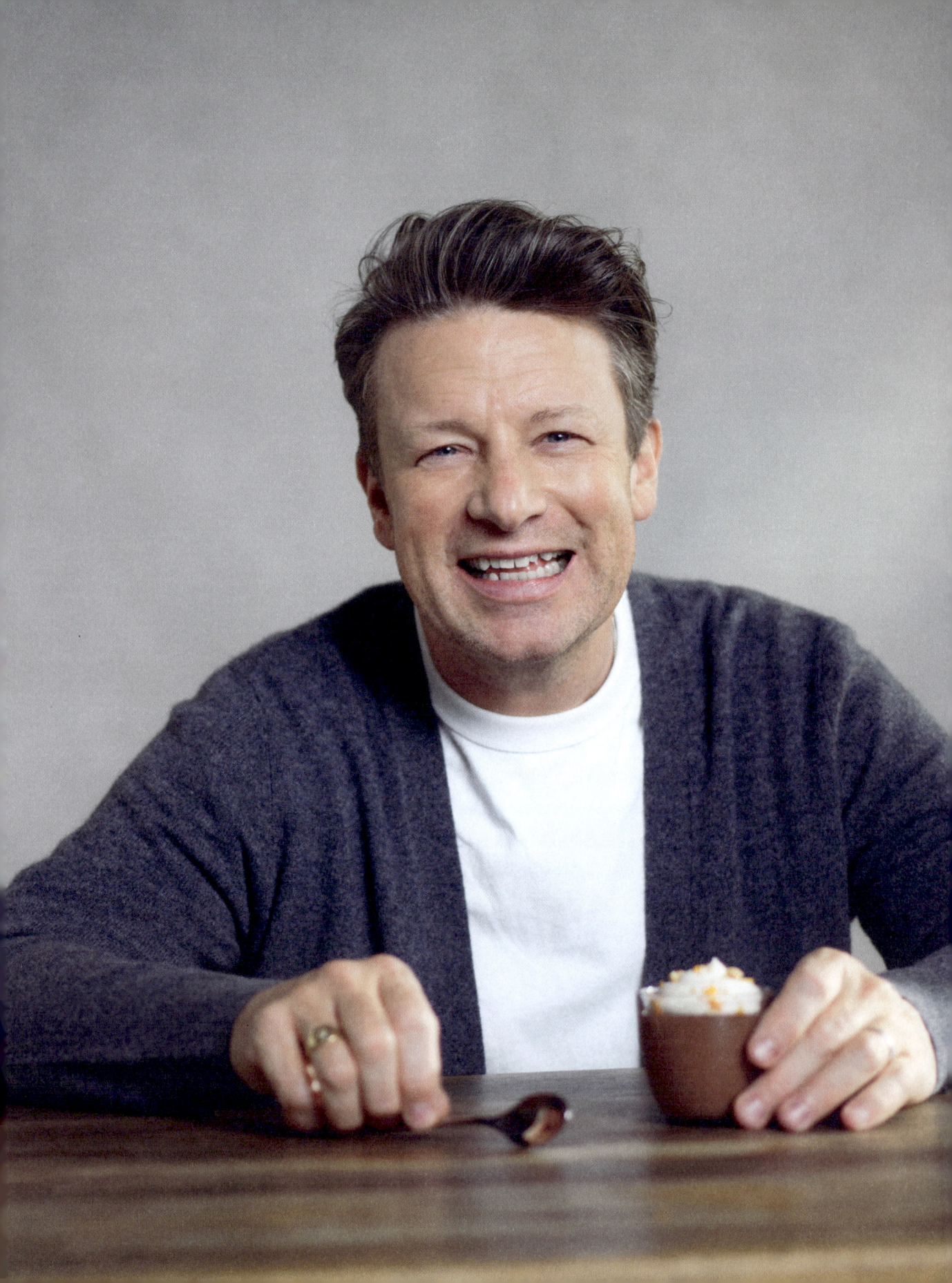

50 healthy hacks

Our bodies are extraordinary. When you break it down, we're essentially made up of trillions of cells that work together to mean we can breathe, communicate, move, sleep and generally go about our daily lives. Each of us is like an individual factory of energy and repair, and when you look at it that way, you realize that every single day we – knowingly or unknowingly – make a lot of choices that directly impact our bodies.

So, the hacks on the pages that follow exist to help you take positive steps towards healing, fuelling and protecting your own body. These are small, sometimes obvious, but powerful hacks that you can easily work into your life. You may already be able to tick a bunch off and feel confident that you're on the right track.

As good as our intentions might be, the reality is that we need to take a step back from the kitchen and look at how we shop for food. I don't believe our choices have drastically changed, but the way that food is processed has. We're also creatures of habit. Most of us buy the same stuff, week in, week out, with very little variation. Why? Because the biggest motivator for all of us is convenience, then price, then health down at number three. Convenience trumps all. But convenience only wins if you don't know how to cook. Even when you're short on time and energy, if you can knock out something better, quicker, cheaper or tastier, then you're in the driving seat. By buying this book, you're arming yourself with knowledge, which means choice, which means you'll have the tools to get it right most of the time. You're taking back control of your health!

First up, I've got a whole host of easy hacks and helpful little swaps that will help you get more consistency in your shopping basket. Then we're on to tips for shopping, eating, living and sleeping. These are simple, achievable things that most of us can slot naturally and effortlessly into our weekly routines. And it's all about the bigger picture – lots of little changes add up and will have a positive impact on your health. Let's get started!

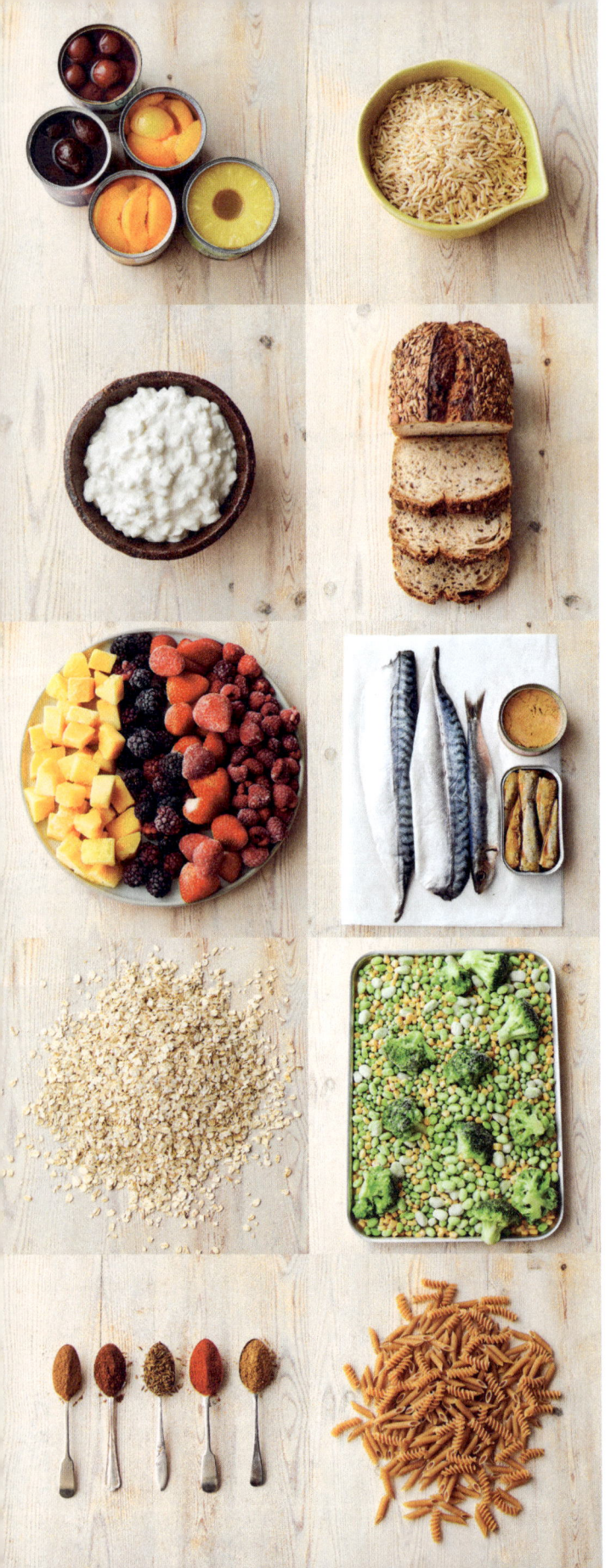

Shopping

☐ Write a shopping list

Sounds simple, but having a list means you can be more intentional about what you want to buy. Our bodies like variation, so it gives you the chance to add a few different veg and fruits each week. You're less likely to impulse buy – and you might save a bit of money, too.

☐ Embrace frozen fruit

It's amazing, often cheaper than buying fresh, and frozen at its optimum and most nutritious, meaning it's ready to be added to everything from Cheat's soft-serve ice cream (page 258) to Choccy fro-yo sandwiches (page 270) at a moment's notice.

☐ ... And frozen veg

Likewise, veg are a great thing to have in your freezer. Simply grab a handful of what you need, when you need it, meaning less waste. Quick freezing after harvesting means veg retain their nutritional value very efficiently.

☐ Switch up your bread

Going from white, highly processed bread to wholemeal, mixed-seed or naturally fermented sourdough is a really good step in the right direction. Think more fibre, more flavour and more nutrients. Slice and freeze any excess bread so it's ready to toast from frozen, to avoid waste.

☐ Celebrate seasonal

Always aim to buy seasonally – things taste better and are much more nutritious and affordable, too.

☐ Big up wholegrain rice

Switching from white to wholegrain rice means you get more fibre. Wholegrain rice is also packed with B-vitamins, which help keep our metabolisms going so we can break down the food we eat to create energy. I know sometimes only white rice will do, but when it's appropriate to swap to wholegrain, like a stew or pan-fried dish, it's well worth it. Try black and wild rice, too.

☐ Tinned fruit is a win

Not just for your nan, choose tinned fruit in juice, and that'll rack up towards your 7-a-day (pages 28 to 31). A handy and convenient choice to stash in the cupboard.

☐ Try cool cottage cheese

Protein-rich and a good source of calcium chloride, which helps to keep our digestive systems healthy, cottage cheese is lower in saturated fat than any other cheese so it's a great way to get some dairy in your diet.

☐ Dried fruit counts!

You can count one 30g portion of dried fruit as one of your 7-a-day, so from mango to apricots, apples to dates, get your fill! I particularly love finely chopping it to transform salads (see pages 76 and 90).

☐ Freeze your fish

We should all be eating two portions of fish a week. Seeking out your local fishmonger, buying more than you need and freezing it is a great hack to ensure you're getting the freshest fish, exactly when you want it. Read more in my bonus hack on page 173.

☐ Include oily fish

One of our weekly portions of fish should be oily, like trout, mackerel or sardines. Whether it's fresh, jarred or tinned, cover your bases and try to get those portions in. Omega-3s in oily fish are essential for both our brain function and development.

☐ Buy white fish

It's one of the few foods that's super-high in iodine, the mineral our thyroid glands depend on in order to function properly, in turn helping to control our metabolism. Frozen fillets can be very handy, and the quality tends to be very consistent. Try them in my Thai-style fish curry (page 140).

☐ Don't shop hungry

A classic, but helpful. If you shop when you're hungry, you're more likely to stray from your list and end up with extra, often less healthy, bits you don't need.

☐ Try wholewheat pasta

It's a super-easy way to up your fibre intake, and has a lovely nutty flavour. Try swapping it in sometimes for a bit of variation – it works particularly well with tomato-based sauces, like in my Crab spaghetti (page 184).

☐ Put eggs in your weekly shop

As well as being a source of protein, the mighty egg contains 10 other micronutrients that our bodies need to keep healthy and happy. We love eggs!

☐ Buy black beans

Not only are they delicious, but they're higher in protein than any other bean or pulse, so a great choice post exercise, helping your muscles to recover and repair. Try popping them in a dry pan (page 122), throwing them in a salad (page 146) or even using them for a quick houmous (page 98).

☐ Stock up on oats

Packed with fibre, helping to keep our guts healthy and happy, and keep us regular, whole rolled porridge oats keep us fuller for longer. Plus, they're one of the only ingredients proven to help lower cholesterol. Try my Overnight oats (page 46) or Frosty porridge (page 40).

☐ Try some tofu

Nearly half of the calories in tofu come from protein, so it's a great ingredient for vegetarians, and is low in sat fat. It's also a great source of calcium and phosphorus, both of which make for strong and healthy bones!

☐ Get some wholemeal flour

It's a super-easy swap and much higher in fibre than plain flour, so well worth it. Use it in my One-cup pancakes (page 58). Or, you could meet halfway and make yourself a 50/50 mix of plain and wholemeal, which is quite a nice compromise to start with.

☐ Spice up the flavour

Dried spices are super-nutritious, and a clever way to lower salt intake as they add big flavour, so you can get away with less seasoning. A great cupboard staple.

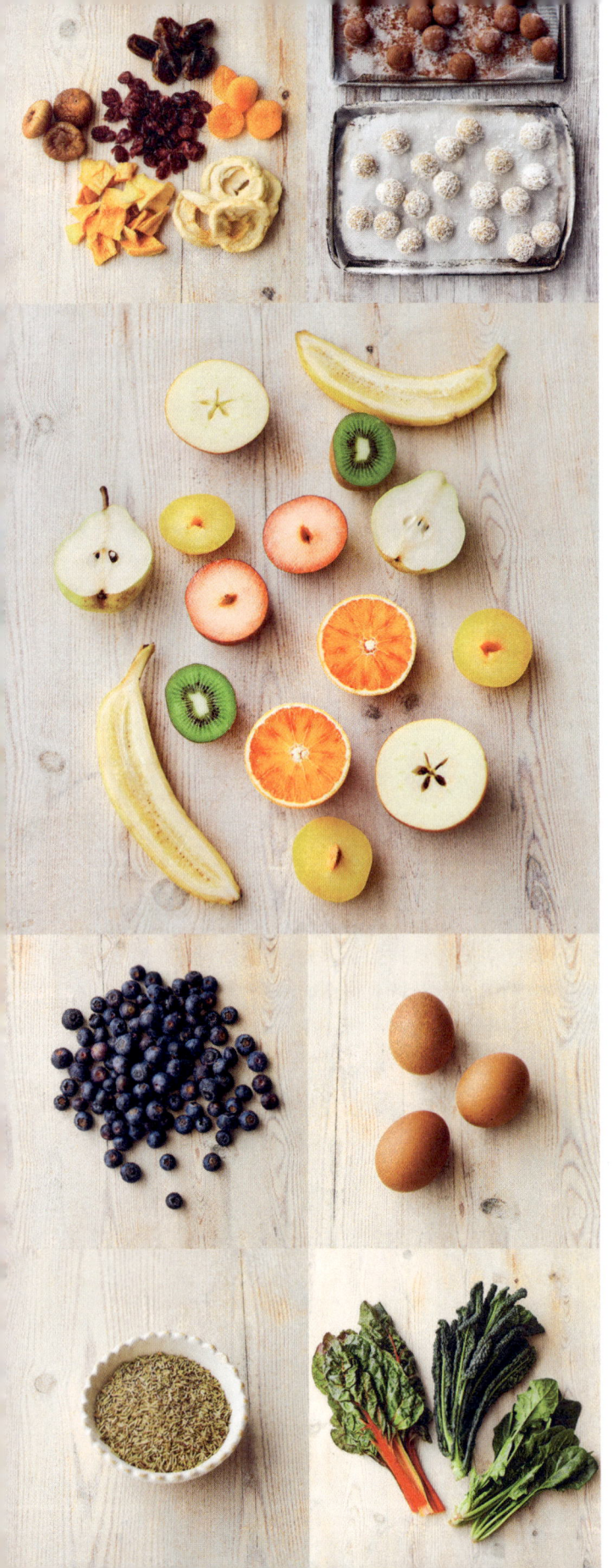

Eating

☐ Eat the rainbow

Most of us are creatures of habit, but each veg and fruit has a different nutritional make-up, so do your body a favour and mix things up. It'll be a treat for the tastebuds, and make for a happier gut.

☐ Try a meat-free meal

And not just on a Monday! Aiming for two or three meat-free days a week is a great start and, believe me, I'm a big meat lover! Choosing a plant-based meal might just save you a few pennies, allowing you to trade up on the days you do eat meat. Plus, embracing plant-based proteins like tinned beans and pulses is a win as they're high in fibre and lower in saturated fat, so it's a double whammy for your tummy.

☐ Embrace fresh herbs

Packed with lots of brilliant qualities on the nutritional front, fresh herbs mean you can add single-minded flavour to your cooking. Most are easy to grow and ready to pick as and when you need them, so why not get a pot on your windowsill? Read more on page 295.

☐ Dried herbs rock too

When herbs are dried, happily they still retain a lot of their nutritional value, plus they undergo a wonderfully dramatic change in flavour (see page 295).

☐ Big up blueberries

Adding a vibrant pop of colour to food, blueberries give us vitamin C and antioxidants, and are high in manganese, protecting our cells from damage. Whether fresh or frozen, what's not to love? Enjoy 80g as a snack, go sweet with Blueberry muffins (page 276) or savoury with my Chicken & berry grain bowl (page 182).

☐ Try a meal plan

If you want a helping hand to get in the healthy mindset, and you've got time to prioritize cooking, try my 2-week kickstarter (pages 20 to 25) to get you in the zone.

☐ Fill your fruit bowl!

I like to think of fruit as nature's sweet shop – it's pretty much the simplest snack there is. I tend to leave a little chopping board and knife next to the bowl, then you can have a quarter or half of something when you want it. Just squeeze a little lemon on to the rest to prevent it going brown, and pop in the fridge till you want it.

☐ Snack smart

As well as fresh fruit, a small handful of dried fruit (up to 30g), unsalted nuts or seeds, a handful of popcorn, or some veg sticks are all great fibre-rich options, too. Just be mindful not to snack on dried fruit throughout the day; you're better off sticking to one 30g portion once a day, to help protect your teeth.

☐ Know your 5-a-day

Once you get your head around what an 80g portion of fresh, frozen or tinned veg or fruit looks like, you'll find it easier to work out how to get more portions into your life. And in this book we're aiming for at least 7-a-day, so welcome to the upgrade! Read more and get a visual guide on pages 28 to 31.

☐ Focus on your food

We're more distracted than ever. Emails, TV, social media. Being honest with yourself, how often do you just sit and enjoy your food without these distractions? Food is one of life's simplest pleasures and we're much less likely to overeat if our minds aren't elsewhere.

☐ Make your own sweet treats

Reduce temptation by making your own healthier treats, ready to satisfy that sweet tooth. I've got plenty of inspo for you on pages 257 to 281.

☐ Invest in an oil spritzer

Decanting olive oil into a spritz bottle has been a revelation for me. It means you can be more restrained with how much you add to your cooking, gives perfect distribution, and if you want to, you can even flavour your oils with things like herbs, garlic and chillies.

☐ Use smaller plates

Sounds simple, but it can help you with portion control and might help prevent you from overeating, too.

☐ Boil some eggs

They're a great protein-rich snack or addition to a meal, and you can have fun with colour and flavour (page 101).

☐ Know when you're full

Instead of finishing everything on your plate, try to listen to your body and stop when you're no longer hungry, saving any leftovers for another meal. In the Blue Zone of Okinawa in Japan they have a saying, 'Hara hachi bu', which means to eat until you're 80% full. The Okinawans are one of the healthiest communities on the planet, so they must be on to something!

☐ Start with veg

A great habit to get into is always having a simple salad or little crudités on the table before a meal. It helps you get your veg count up, and is a particularly useful tactic for introducing the good stuff to kids in a habitual way. Let them fill up on veg, not unhealthy snacks.

☐ Embrace batch cooking

If you've got a bit of time at the weekend, batch cooking is a great ritual to get into, stashing good meals in the freezer ready for an easy win another day, like my Beef & borlotti bean ragù (page 252). It could even be as simple as making a meal for four, for two, and keeping the leftovers. It means you're armed with a freezer full of healthy choices for those ever-busy weekday nights.

☐ Embrace the greens

Spinach might not make us Popeye-strong but it's packed with vitamin A, which helps us see properly, especially in the dark. Leafy greens like cabbage, chard, kale, and even rocket and watercress, can be quickly steamed and simply dressed, and are utterly delicious. Other great greens, like broccoli and peas, are packed with vitamin C, which our bodies need for pretty much anything and everything. Eat green!

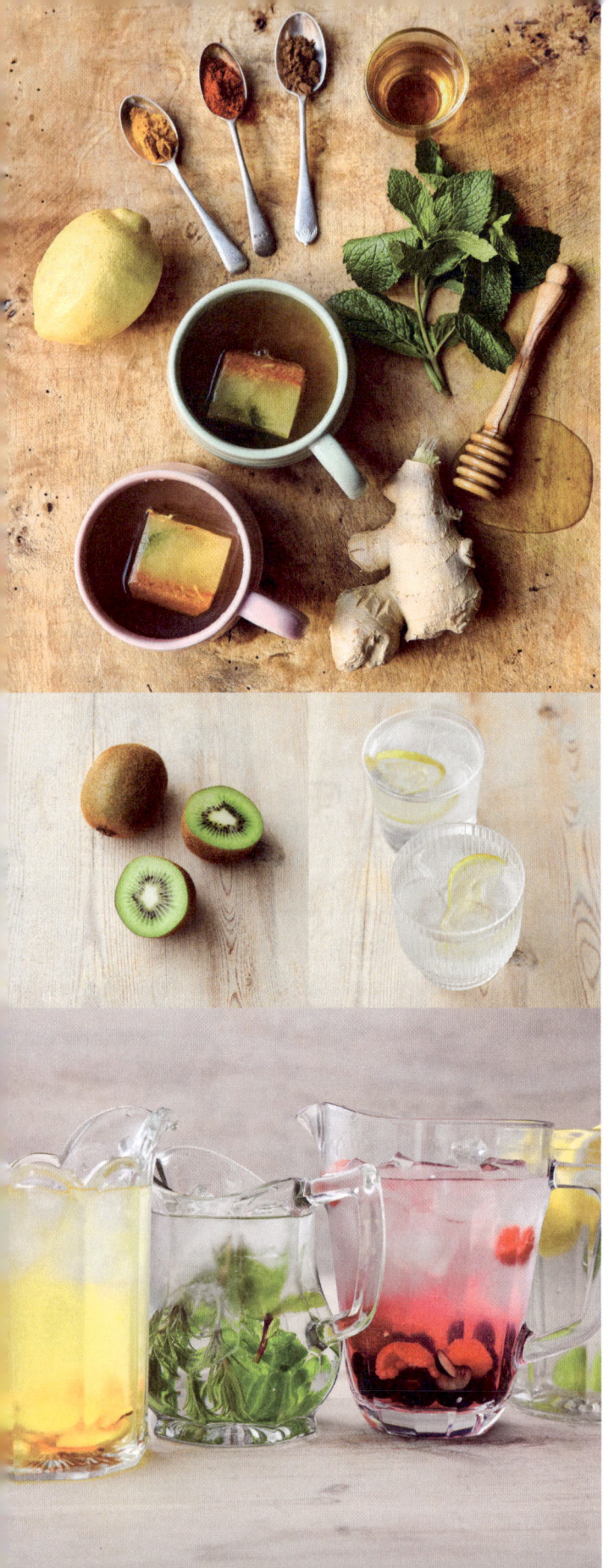

Living

☐ Drink water

The simplest thing you can do for your health is to stay hydrated. Two thirds of the human body is made up of water, and it's integral to every bodily function. It's especially important for our brains, which are more than 70% water! We often mistake thirst for hunger, so staying hydrated can also be helpful in preventing us from overeating. It sounds obvious, but the cheapest way to hydrate is to drink water. So always keep water with you – whether it's a bottle in your bag, a glass at your desk, or a jug on the kitchen table, keep it in sight and keep sipping! If you struggle with that, then try adding a bit of interest with a tasty infusion of fruit, roots or herbs – I've got some of my favourite combos to get you started on pages 284 to 285.

☐ Get moving!

Being active is super-important. And that doesn't mean you have to get a gym membership or massively change your lifestyle. Try to think of easy ways to make your regular day more physical – get off the bus a stop early, take the stairs instead of the lift, work a little walk into your daily routine, do some stretches while watching the TV. If you're just starting out, there's a lot of inspo out there for easy workouts, so see what works for you and have fun with it.

☐ Read cookbooks that inspire you

Soak up that inspiration, and remind yourself just how joyful good food can be. Give new recipes a try, mix up your shopping list, and hopefully you'll be able to expand your regular repertoire.

☐ Morning kickstarter

Give yourself a natural wake-up call with a megamix of ingredients to boost your water and get you going in the morning. Get more info and the recipe on page 286.

Sleeping

☐ Cut down on the booze

I love alcohol and have a little bit here and there like most people, but we all know it's not that good for us, so being a bit mindful about when and how much we drink can only be a good thing. I'd recommend trying to structure it in so you're having a drink socially with family or friends, and if you can have at least a 3-day break every week to give your liver a rest that's a really good approach. When you do drink alcohol, remember to drink water as well – it's an easy habit to get into and very helpful for how your body processes the alcohol.

☐ Give more time to mealtimes

Whether you're with family or friends, or on your own, sit down to eat so you can savour each mouthful and take your time. As well as helping your digestive system, it will give you time to pause, reflect and unwind!

☐ And have a little walk afterwards

Just a 10-minute walk after eating can help your digestion and help to moderate your blood glucose levels. Try to take your post-meal walk within an hour of eating to see more measurable benefits.

☐ Top up your vitamin D

During the summer months, our bodies create vitamin D from sun exposure, but during the winter months it's a good idea to take a daily supplement as we generally don't get enough from our diets. On the food front, vitamin D is found in things like oily fish, eggs and mushrooms grown outdoors.

☐ Prioritize sleep

We spend up to one third of our lives asleep! And sleep is so important, as it gives our bodies and minds time to grow, heal and repair. It's definitely something I've struggled with over the years. I'll be honest, I have to treat sleep like another job now to make sure I give it the focus and attention it needs. Every health expert I've ever spoken to stresses how crucial sleep is for our health. So, as much as you can – and I know there are a lot of factors that can get in the way at different stages of life – try to get into a regular routine, and whenever possible, allow yourself time to get between 7 and 9 hours of sleep a night.

☐ Eat to increase melatonin levels

Melatonin is a natural hormone that helps us get to sleep. It's thought that eating two kiwis in the evening can give your natural levels a boost. Other helpful foods on this front are cherries, walnuts, unripe bananas, raspberries, tomatoes and jasmine rice. Just try to avoid eating in the two hours directly before you go to sleep, so your body has time to digest everything before switching into sleep mode.

☐ Don't clock watch in bed

If you're struggling to get to or stay asleep, having clocks in the bedroom can be distracting, and might mean you're putting unnecessary pressure on yourself. If you need an alarm, keep it far enough away from the bed that it can't be seen during the night.

☐ Take a nap

Naps are great, and if you can get any into your day, good for you. I love a nap when I can. Just try to keep each one to 20 minutes to prevent the body going into a longer sleep cycle, which can mean you wake up groggy, not refreshed.

NOURISH, FUEL & ENERGIZE YOUR BODY

The 2-week kickstarter

If you want to go all in, and prioritize your health in a big way, then my 2-week kickstarter is for you. This is about making a commitment to three delicious meals a day, all of which promote healthy eating and good ingredients. It's about a change of lifestyle, not a diet, a chance to focus on yourself, and put your health first. Now, I know committing to a 2-week plan is a big ask when you're busy, but if you have the time and headspace to work it into your daily life, my hope is that you'll come out of it feeling like you have more energy, you've given your immune system a bit of a boost, and – fingers crossed – you might be sleeping better, too. Having a healthy, balanced approach to the week like this also means, for the average person, you'll be eating in a calorie deficit. So, slowly but surely, it's likely you'll lose a bit of weight, if that's your objective. Or, you can use that deficit for drinks and snacks – read more about our daily energy needs on page 297.

In the very process of cooking from scratch each day, I hope you'll also learn or remind yourself of easy little swaps and tweaks you can make on a regular basis for a healthier outlook. Think of this plan as a loyal friend you can come back to whenever you need a reset and a reboot.

What you'll get from the plan:

— A minimum of 7 portions of veg and fruit every day

— An average of 30g of fibre and 50g of protein per day

— One portion of dairy or dairy alternative each day

— A variety of carbohydrates

Flex the plan for you

I've tried to choose recipes that allow you to get good food on the table quickly and with ease, to make it as achievable as possible. Hopefully you'll find it a useful framework, and adopt some of these meals into your regular repertoire. Of course, feel free to swap out any of the recipes for your own favourites from the book – eating the rainbow and nourishing your body with good food are the main aims here. I've set out to keep the overall costs reasonable, and if you want to make any substitutions to suit your budget, please do.

The plan serves 2

Some of the recipes included are single-serve recipes, so will need to be made twice or doubled. And some serve more than two, in which case I have suggested using the leftovers on another day, or fridge or freezer stashing them for a future week.

Get prepped

It will help you out to have a bit of a prep session on the Sunday before you begin. I would recommend getting ahead with the following three recipes:

Beef & borlotti bean ragù or veggie alternative (page 252)
Portion up and freeze.

Mothership overnight oats (page 46)
Stash in the fridge.

2 x Morning kickstarter (page 286)
Portion up and freeze.

Turbocharge the plan

In order to feel the biggest difference from the two weeks, following the tips below will help you out:

Stay hydrated

Make sure you're getting at least 2 litres (for the average woman over the age of 14) or 2.5 litres (for the average man in the same age bracket) per day.

Get moving!

Whatever you can do will help. See my hack on page 18.

Prioritize sleep

It's one of the biggest contributors to good health and really worth investing in. Read my tips on page 19.

Stay off the booze

Our liver breaks down food, converting it into energy and essential proteins, so giving it a break from processing alcohol is only going to be a good thing.

Reduce your eating window

We naturally have a fast while we're sleeping, and widening that gap from dinner to breakfast a little is an easy step to take. For example, if you generally have 10 hours between dinner and brekkie, try working up to 12 to give your body more of a break from the digestion process. For some people, it can be helpful to reduce your eating window even further, or to temporarily drop down to two meals a day – remember this is a tool, a reboot, so see what works for you. Time-restricted eating won't be appropriate or feasible for everyone, so please consider your own situation, consulting your GP or a dietician for advice, if needed.

MEAL PLAN

Week one

| | BREAKFAST | LUNCH | DINNER |

Monday — WORKING FROM HOME

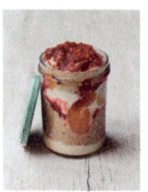

2 x Peach melba overnight oats (page 48)

2 x Morning kickstarter (page 286)

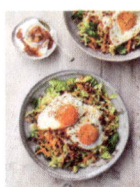

Curried fried eggs & grain salad (page 82)

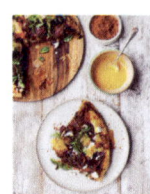

Fragrant veggie filo tart (page 236)

Fridge stash 2 leftover portions for Tuesday's lunch

Tuesday — IN THE OFFICE

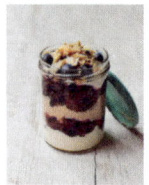

2 x Berry cheesecake overnight oats (page 49)

2 x Matcha & kefir smoothie (page 291)

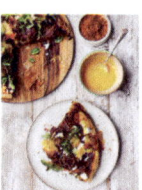

Fragrant veggie filo tart

Leftover from Monday night's dinner

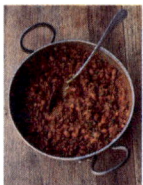

Beef & borlotti bean ragù or veggie alternative (page 252)

Defrost in advance

with Potato gnocchi (page 254)

Wednesday — IN THE OFFICE

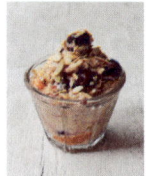

2 x Cherry Bakewell overnight oats (page 48)

2 x Morning kickstarter (page 286)

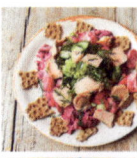

Salmon, beet & potato salad (page 92)

OR

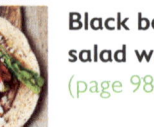 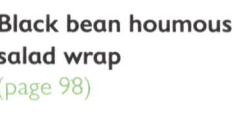

Black bean houmous salad wrap (page 98)

Prep ahead and assemble at work

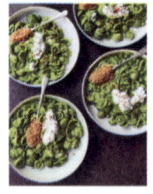

Super-green orecchiette (page 190)

Fridge stash 2 leftover portions for Thursday's lunch

| BREAKFAST | LUNCH | DINNER |

Thursday — IN THE OFFICE

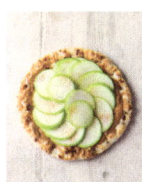
2 x 5-minute tasty topper, with almond butter, apple and cinnamon (page 36)

2 x Merry berry smoothie (page 289)

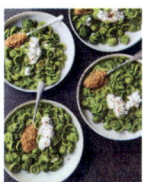
Super-green orecchiette

Leftover from Wednesday night's dinner

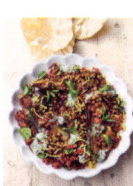
Silky aubergine flavour fest (page 194)

Friday — WORKING FROM HOME

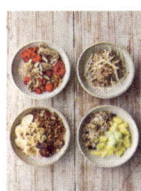
2 x Pink Shredded Wheat, or your favourite Cereal, super-charged (page 34)

2 x Morning kickstarter (page 286)

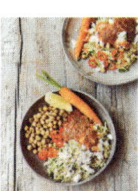
Herby chickpea & feta salad (page 116)

Seared tuna kimchi bowl (page 156)

OR

Silken tofu & black beans (page 152)

Saturday — WEEKEND

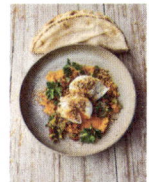
Dukkah poached eggs (page 54)

Whipped coffee (page 292)

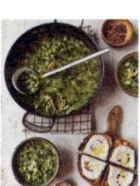
Spring soup & ricotta toasts (page 218)

Freezer stash 2 leftover portions for Tuesday's lunch

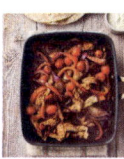
Chicken fajitas (page 154)

OR

Mushroom stew (page 200)

Sunday — WEEKEND

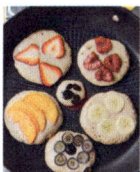
One-cup pancakes (page 58)

Fridge stash 2 leftover batter portions for Monday's breakfast

Gennaro's coffee (page 293)

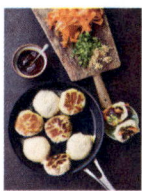
Crispy steamed veggie buns (page 230)

Share with friends or freezer stash 2 leftover portions

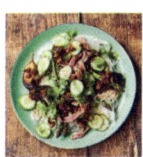
Steak & sticky aubergine salad (page 166)

OR

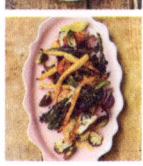
2 x Roasted veg & chickpea smash (page 198)

MEAL PLAN
Week two

| BREAKFAST | LUNCH | DINNER |

Monday —— WORKING FROM HOME

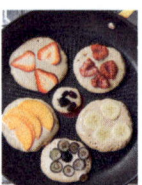

One-cup pancakes

Leftover from Sunday morning week one

2 x Morning kickstarter
(page 286)

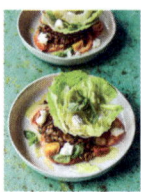

Warm lentil salad
(page 78)

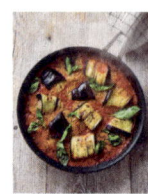

Aubergine involtini
(page 208)

Tuesday —— IN THE OFFICE

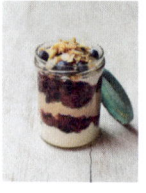

2 x Cheat's bircher muesli or your favourite Cereal, super-charged
(page 34)

2 x Green goddess smoothie
(page 288)

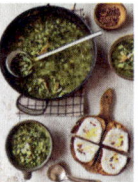

Spring soup & ricotta toasts

Leftover from Saturday lunch week one

Defrost in advance

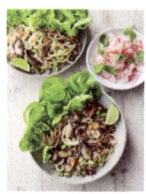

Tahini mushroom noodles
(page 144)

Wednesday —— IN THE OFFICE

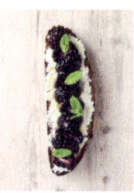

2 x 5-minute tasty toppers, with ricotta, blackberries, mint & honey
(page 36)

2 x Post-workout protein smoothie
(page 290)

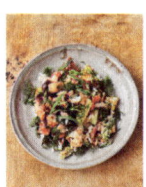

2 x Smashed salad
(page 114)

Make at work or prep ahead and assemble at work

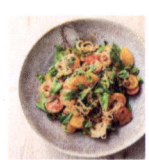

Prawn & noodle salad (page 86)

OR

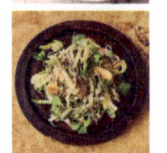

2 x Sesame miso shred salad
(page 96)

	BREAKFAST	LUNCH	DINNER

Thursday — IN THE OFFICE

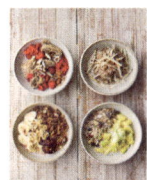 **2 x Piña colada muesli or your favourite Cereal, super-charged** (page 34)

2 x Morning kickstarter (page 286)

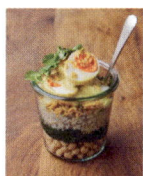 **Curried egg & rice pots** (page 118)

Make ahead

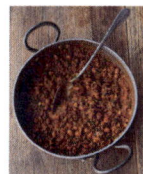 **Beef & borlotti bean ragù or veggie alternative** (page 252)

Defrost in advance

with Bread croutons (page 255)

Friday — WORKING FROM HOME

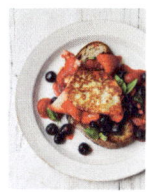 **Golden cheese & jammy berries** (page 52)

Gennaro's coffee (page 293)

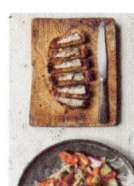 **Sardines on toast & tomato salad or veggie alternative** (page 94)

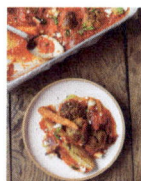 **Meatball traybake or veggie alternative** (page 244)

Share with friends or fridge or freezer stash 2 leftover portions

Saturday — WEEKEND

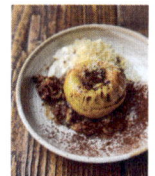 **2 x Speedy stuffed apple** (page 44)

Whipped coffee (page 292)

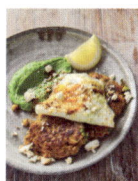 **Carrot & sweet potato fritters** (page 124)

Optional: Chocolate orange pots (page 264)

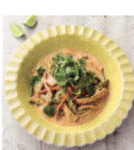 **Creamy peanut chicken** (page 136)

OR

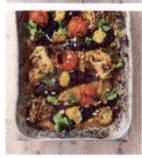 **Veggie curry traybake** (page 212)

Fridge or freezer stash 2 leftover portions

Sunday — WEEKEND

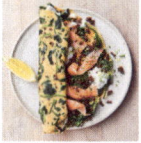 **2 x Smoked salmon & rye omelette** (page 42)

OR

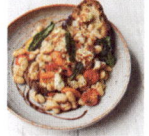 **Cheesy beans on toast** (page 62)

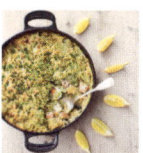 **Happy fish pie** (page 242)

Share with friends

OR

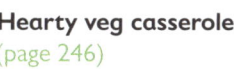 **Hearty veg casserole** (page 246)

Freezer stash 2 leftover portions

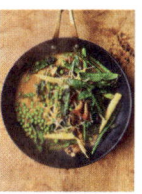 **Super-green stir-fry** (page 132)

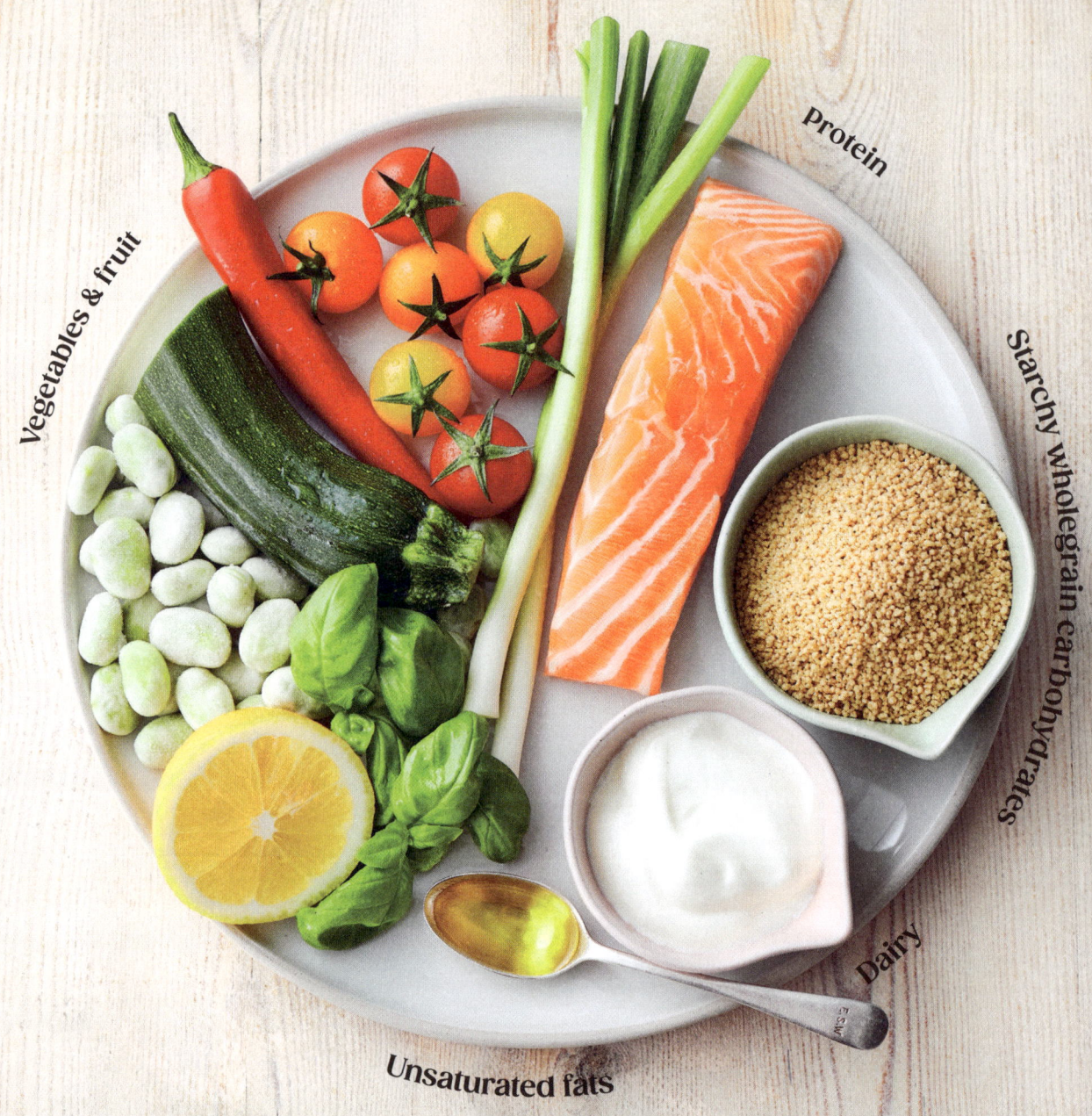

How to balance your plate

Balance is key when it comes to eating well, and we all need a variety of foods to stay healthy. Regardless of the avalanche of specialist diets and misinformation out there, the concept of the 'balanced plate', which echoes the principles of the Mediterranean diet, consistently stands up as an easy-to-follow guide. This is the principle that I use to feed myself, and my family, and it's one backed up by a great body of trusted science.

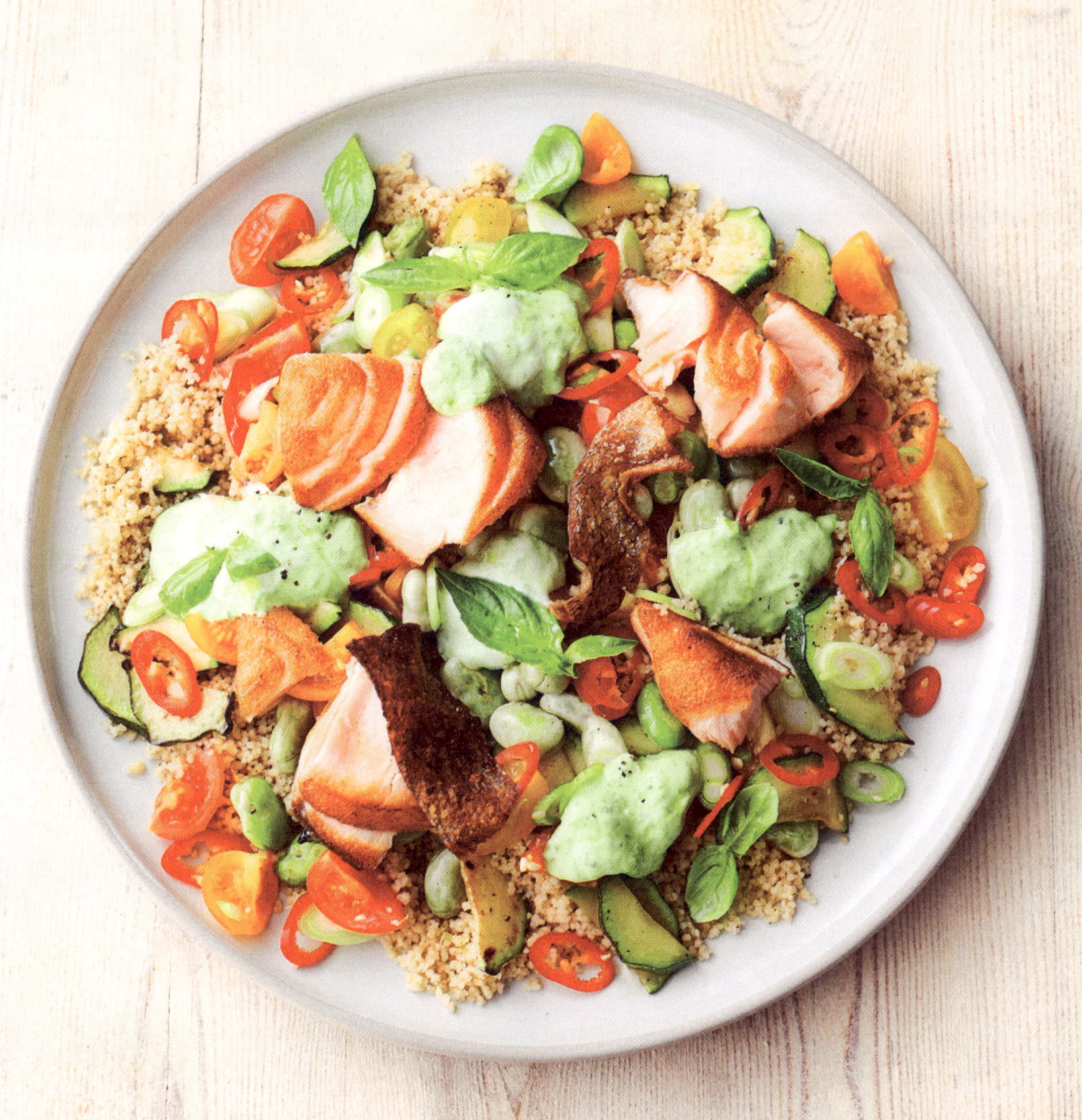

In the image on the left, I've set out to show you visually what to aim for on your plate. Go big on veg and fruit, then wholegrain starchy carbohydrates, bolstered with some protein, a bit of dairy (or dairy alternative) and a small amount of unsaturated fat (see page 296 for the exact breakdown). You can see above how that translates into a plate of food you want to tuck into. You'll soon get into the rhythm of it.

In this book, I've done all the thinking for you. And, where a recipe isn't strictly balanced, I'll give you an idea of how to balance it at the end of the method, by adding a carb like brown rice, or finishing with a dollop of yoghurt to get your dairy in, for example. We don't have to get it right at every meal, but embracing all the food groups across the day and getting our balance right across the week is only going to be a positive thing.

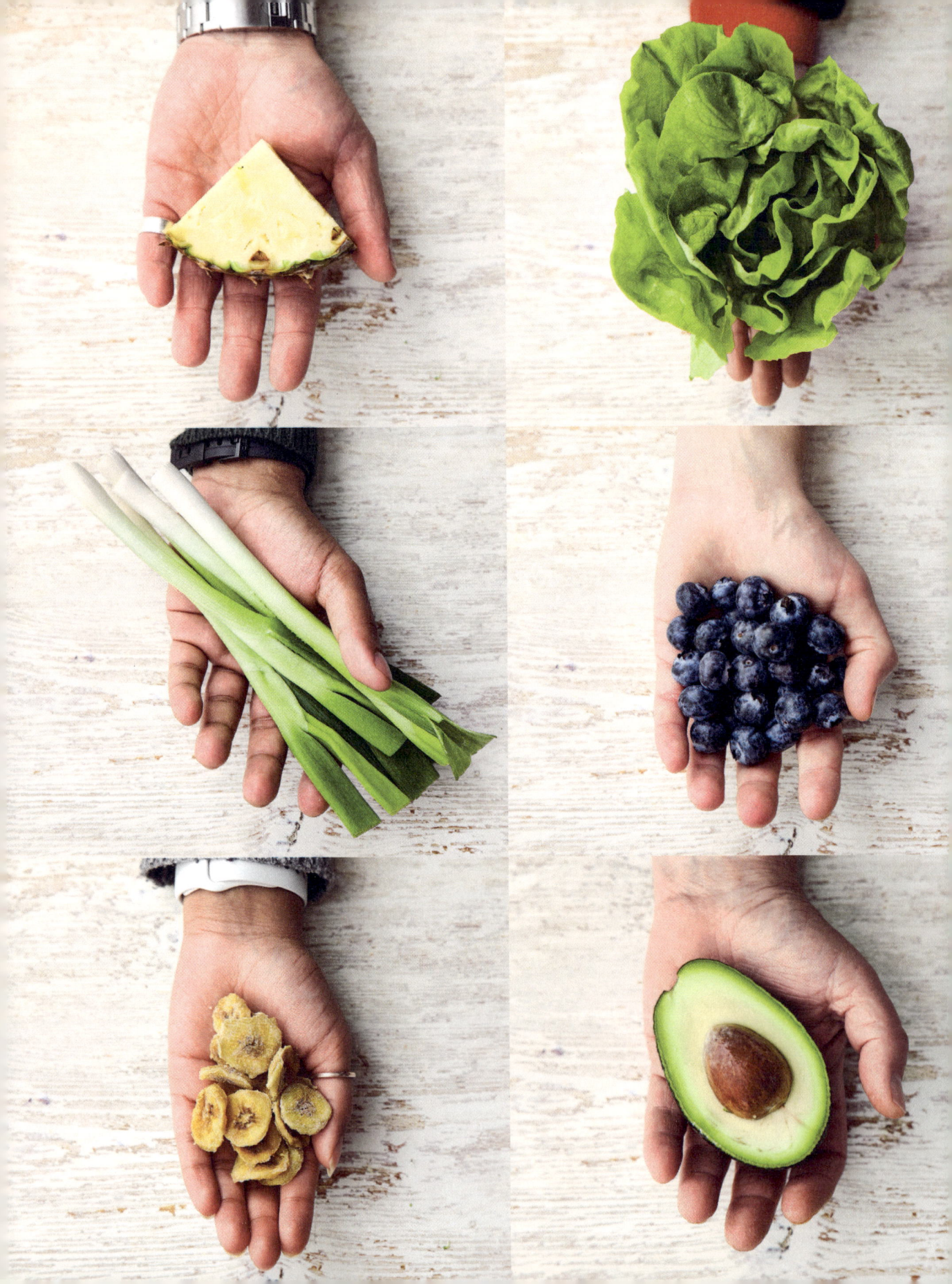

Getting your 7-a-day

Veg and fruit are great, and we all need them in our lives on a daily basis. I'm sure you've heard of 5-a-day, but in this book I'm going to help you reach for 7-a-day, hopefully more. Why? Because that's what will make all the difference when it comes to good health. The average Brit is currently only consuming two or three daily portions of veg and fruit so the UK government has settled on 'at least 5-a-day' because it feels achievable. But surely, when it comes to public health, we should be told the truth? We can take it! The only people paying the price for this mistruth is our already overwhelmed NHS, so it's in everyone's interests to be up front.

Studies show that when you consume 7 to 10 portions of veg and fruit daily, you see a measurable decrease in your risk of developing a diet-related disease. That's a powerful stat. And many countries and communities around the world do it very easily. So, in these pages, I've set out to arm you with inspiration and ideas to get the good stuff in, including some epic salads and veg dishes that include between 5 and 10 portions in just one sitting.

The first step is understanding what a portion of the good stuff looks like, then working out how to get a variety into your diet. You'll see in these pictures that a portion of your 7-a-day will generally fit in the palm of your hand (likewise for kids, a portion fits in their palm). If you can weigh out your portions for a bit, you'll soon get into the groove and be able to do it by eye.

So, what is a portion?

80g (or a large handful) of fresh, frozen or tinned veg and fruit

You can also count one of each of the following per day:

30g of dried fruit

80g of cooked beans or pulses

150ml of unsweetened veg or fruit juice

You'll notice I keep saying veg and fruit, not fruit and veg. I'm putting veg first on purpose, because we want to weight our efforts towards veg, which provide a greater variety of nutrients.

In these recipes I've tried to get you into the habit of getting multiple veg and fruit into every meal, by largely sticking to the portion sizes outlined above. Use these as a guide, and when I say 80g of something in an ingredients list, I mean the peeled or prepped weight, so you're actually eating the full 80g portion. As you'll see from the examples on these pages, the amount is often smaller than you think, so by embracing that portion size, you can get more variety into your meals. Simply stash offcuts and leftovers in your veg drawer or fruit bowl to use another day.

The most important thing to remember is to eat the rainbow, maximizing your nutrients, vitamins and minerals. Plus, you'll be filling your meals with colour, texture and flavour. If the one thing you take away from this book is how to get your 7-a-day, I'll be delighted.

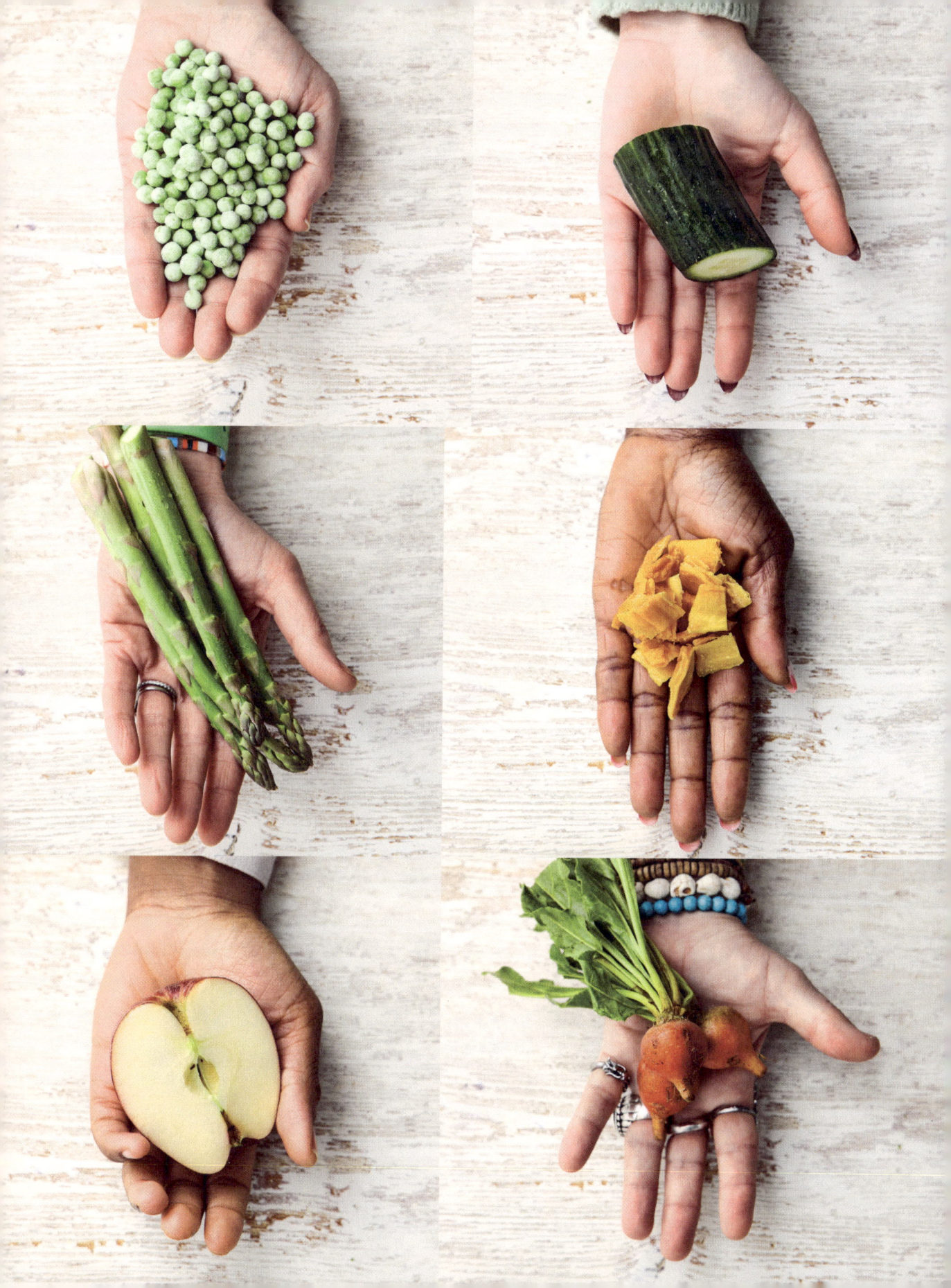

Breakfast

Cereal, super-charged

EACH COMBO SERVES 1 | 3 MINUTES

You're not wrong in thinking most cereals are packed with sugar, meaning they're not a great choice for starting our day. However, if you go for the no-added-sugar options, then Shredded Wheat, Weetabix, puffed oats or rice and muesli are the cream of the crop when it comes to healthier cereal choices. Super-charge your bowl with a portion of fruit, nutrient-packed nuts or seeds, and whichever milk rocks your boat. Try these, then have fun making your own combos!

Pink Shredded Wheat

Put **2 Shredded Wheat (45g)** into a serving bowl. Add **80g of raspberries or ripe strawberries** – I like to crush some with a fork to colour the milk and leave some chunky. Slice and add **30g of skin-on almonds**. Pour over **150ml of your favourite milk – unsweetened, fortified almond plant milk** is a perfect flavour match here. Eat right away.

Cheat's bircher muesli

Put **2 Weetabix (35g)** into a serving bowl with **1 tablespoon of chia seeds** and **1 small pinch of ground cinnamon**. Coarsely grate or matchstick and add **1 crisp eating apple (120g)** and pour over **100ml of your favourite milk – I like good old semi-skimmed** here – fold it all together, then top up with **50ml more milk** and eat right away.

Nutty banana oats

Put **30g of puffed oats or rice** into a serving bowl, sprinkle over **1 pinch of cocoa powder**, then slice and add **1 small ripe banana (80g)** and **2 soft pitted dates (25g)**. Chop and add **1 tablespoon of roasted unsalted peanuts**, pour over **150ml of your favourite milk – unsweetened, fortified cashew plant milk** is nice. Eat right away.

Piña colada muesli

Put **65g of muesli** into a serving bowl. Peel, dice and add **80g of ripe pineapple (or tinned in juice)**, and add the finely grated zest and juice of **1 lime**. Add **½ a teaspoon of desiccated coconut**, pour over **150ml of your favourite milk – unsweetened, fortified coconut plant milk** brings the piña colada vibes. Eat right away.

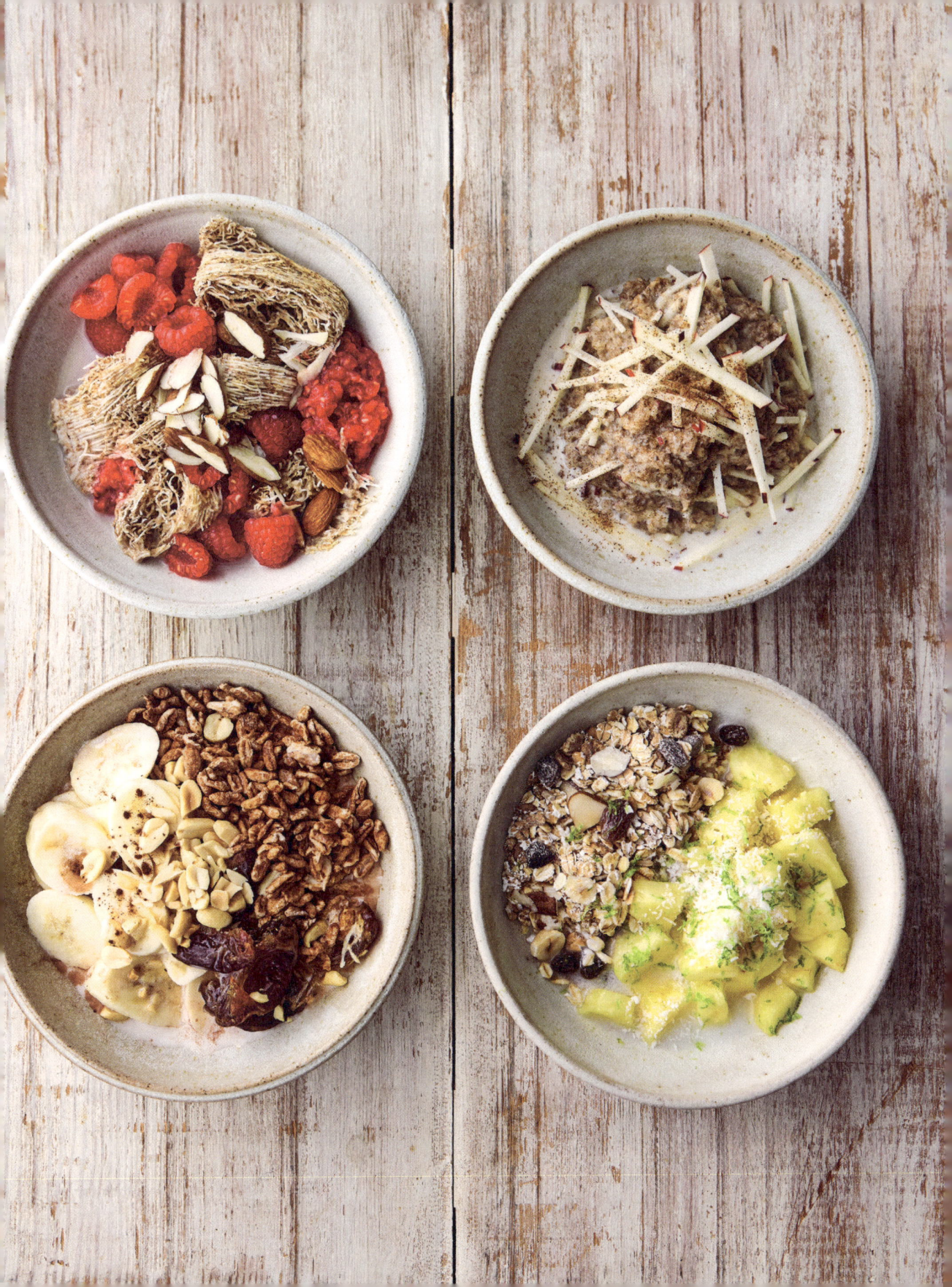

5-minute tasty toppers

EACH COMBO SERVES 1 | 5 MINUTES

The ultimate quick fix, this is all about colourful, nutritious, satisfying combos. Choose your bread – wholemeal, seeded, sourdough, pitta, wrap or flatbread – toast if you desire, and get topping!

A   1 heaped tablespoon crunchy almond butter, 80g finely sliced eating apple, 1 pinch of ground cinnamon.

B   ½ a tin of mackerel in tomato sauce, 80g chopped ripe tomatoes, sliced chilli, a few flat-leaf parsley leaves.

C   1 heaped tablespoon ricotta cheese, 80g blackberries, a few baby mint leaves, a drizzle of runny honey.

D   1 small ripe mashed banana (80g), 80g raspberries, a sprinkling of toasted desiccated coconut.

E   1 heaped tablespoon Greek yoghurt, 80g halved lemon-dressed blueberries, a few chopped pistachio nuts.

F   1 heaped tablespoon houmous, 80g speed-peeled carrot ribbons, a little harissa paste, extra virgin olive oil.

G   1 heaped tablespoon cottage cheese, 80g sliced jarred roasted peppers, a few crumbled walnut halves.

H   ½ a small ripe smashed avocado (80g), 2 marinated anchovy fillets, a little lemon zest and juice.

I   1 heaped tablespoon cream cheese, 80g sliced ripe tomatoes, 1 pinch of dukkah, a kiss of extra virgin olive oil.

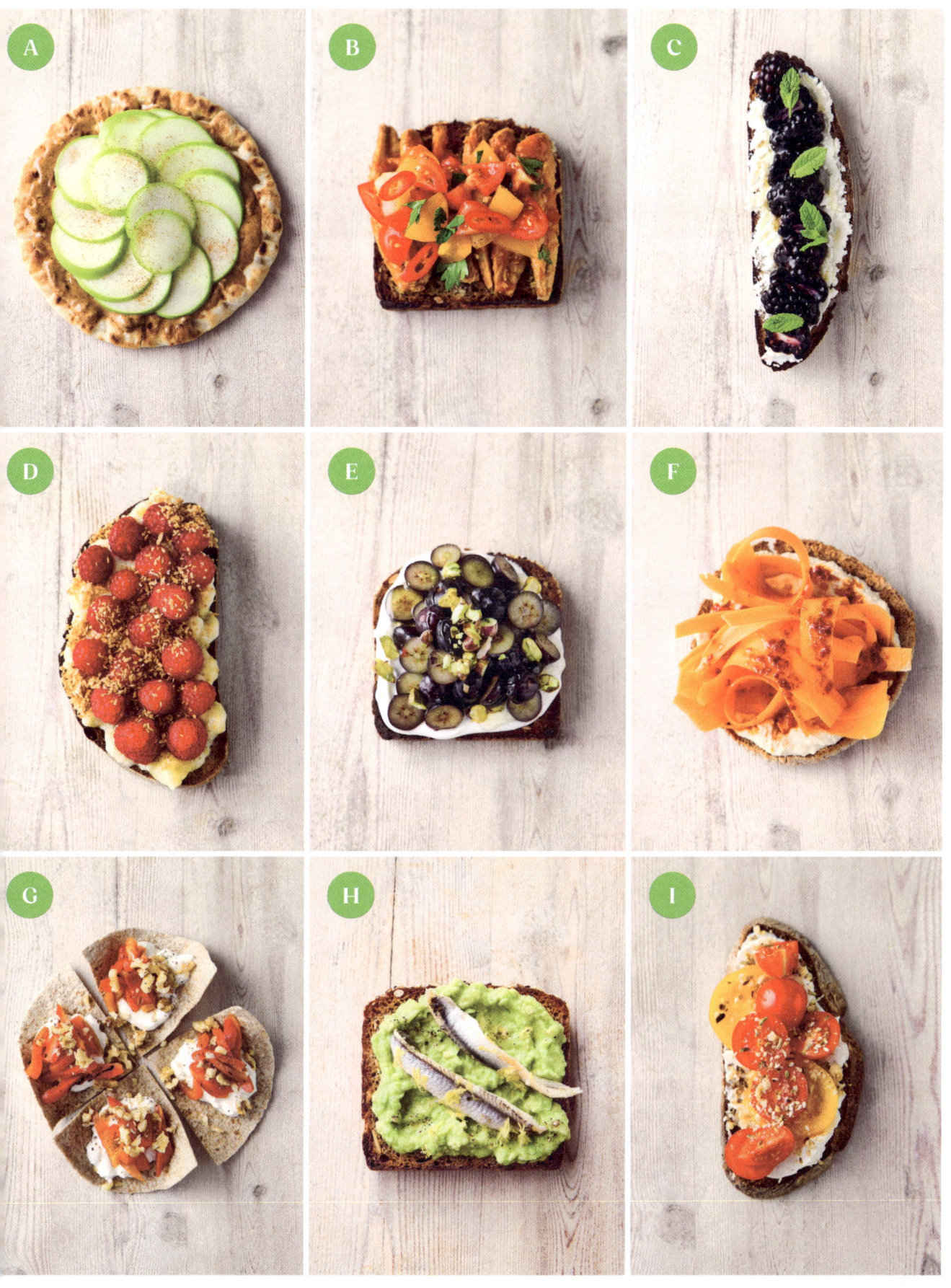

Box grater fruit salad

SERVES 1 | 8 MINUTES

80g each
peach, mango, cantaloupe melon, pear, eating apple, ripe banana

30g soft pitted dates

2 sprigs of mint

1 lime

4 tablespoons Greek yoghurt

1 tablespoon mixed seeds or unsalted nuts

Peel or core the fruit, as needed, then spend a moment coarsely grating or finely chopping each one. Chop the dates, then finely chop the mint leaves and toss it all with a good squeeze of lime juice. Serve over Greek yoghurt, with a scattering of your favourite seeds or nuts, to finish. Nice with toasted oats or crumbled Weetabix, for a more balanced bowlful.

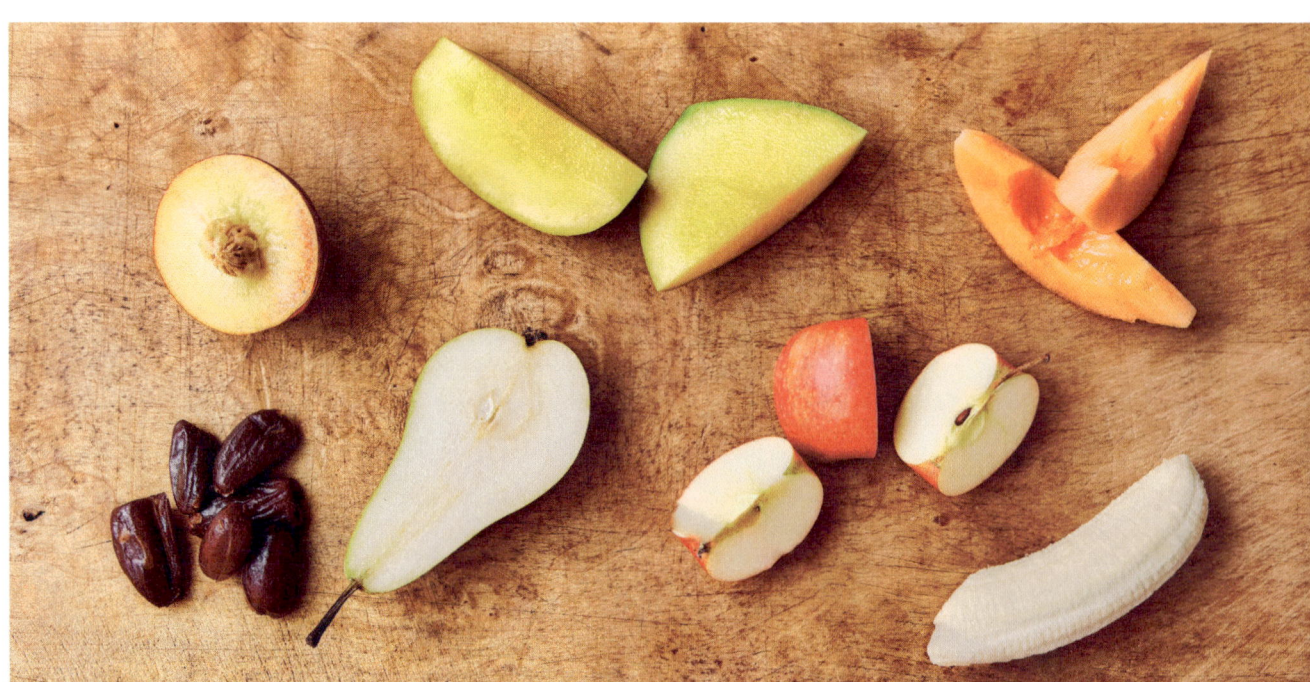

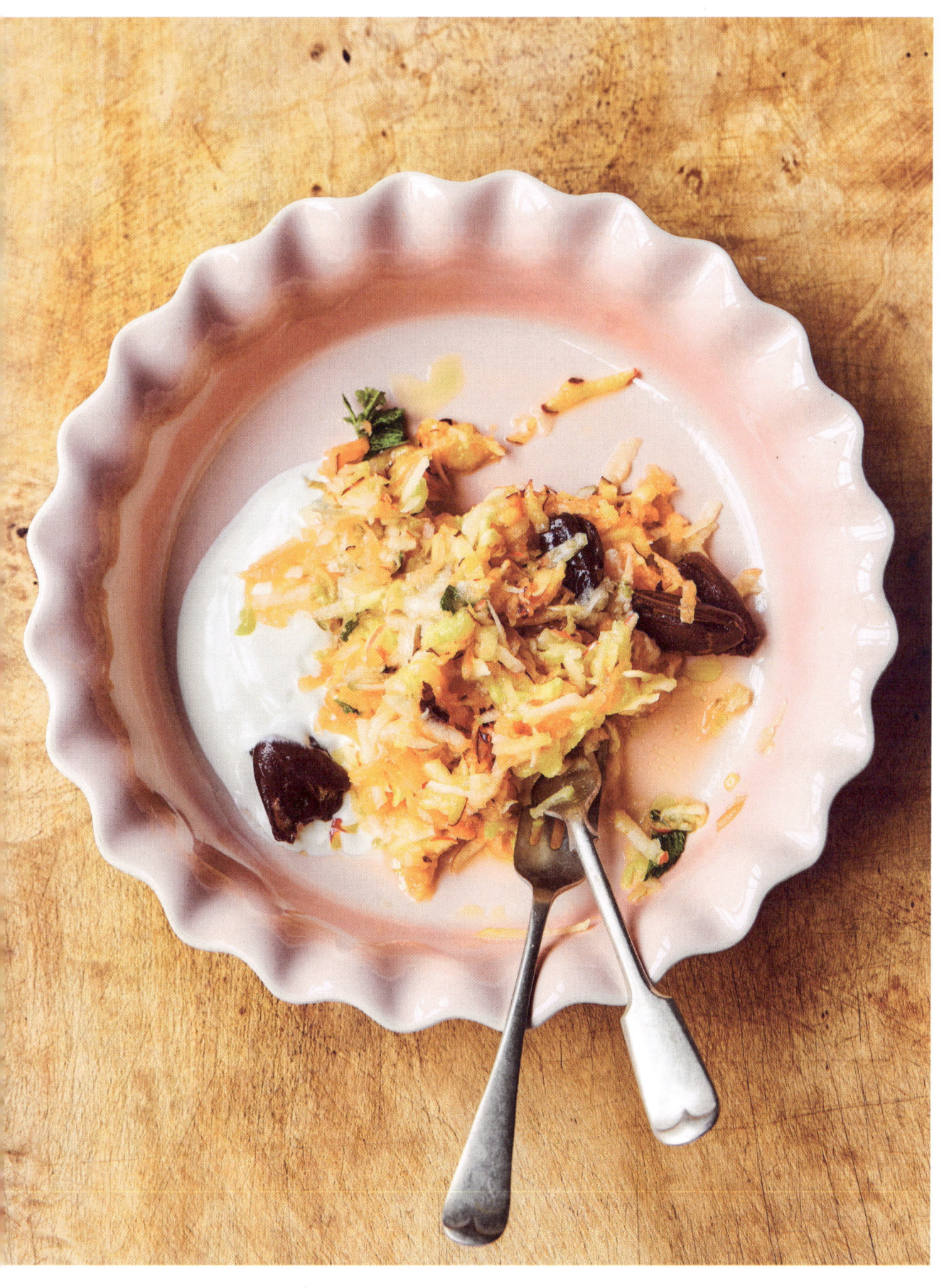

Frosty porridge

Think of this as a frozen smoothie or, if you blitz in the oats at the end, fun frosty porridge

SERVES 4
9 MINUTES

200g porridge oats

40g mixed seeds

1 tablespoon runny honey

320g frozen mango

1 ripe banana (160g)

150g Greek yoghurt

1 teaspoon vanilla bean paste

320g mixed seasonal berries

1. In a non-stick frying pan on a medium heat, cook the oats, seeds and honey with 2 teaspoons of olive oil for 5 minutes, or until golden, stirring regularly.

2. Tip the frozen mango into a food processor, peel and add the banana, along with the yoghurt and vanilla paste, and blitz until smooth and combined.

3. Now, either divide the frozen mango mixture between bowls, scatter over the berries, and serve right away with the hot crunchy oats, or quickly pulse half the hot oats and half the berries into the frozen mango mixture in the processor, then portion up and devour sprinkled with the remaining berries and oats, plus an extra drizzle of honey, if you like.

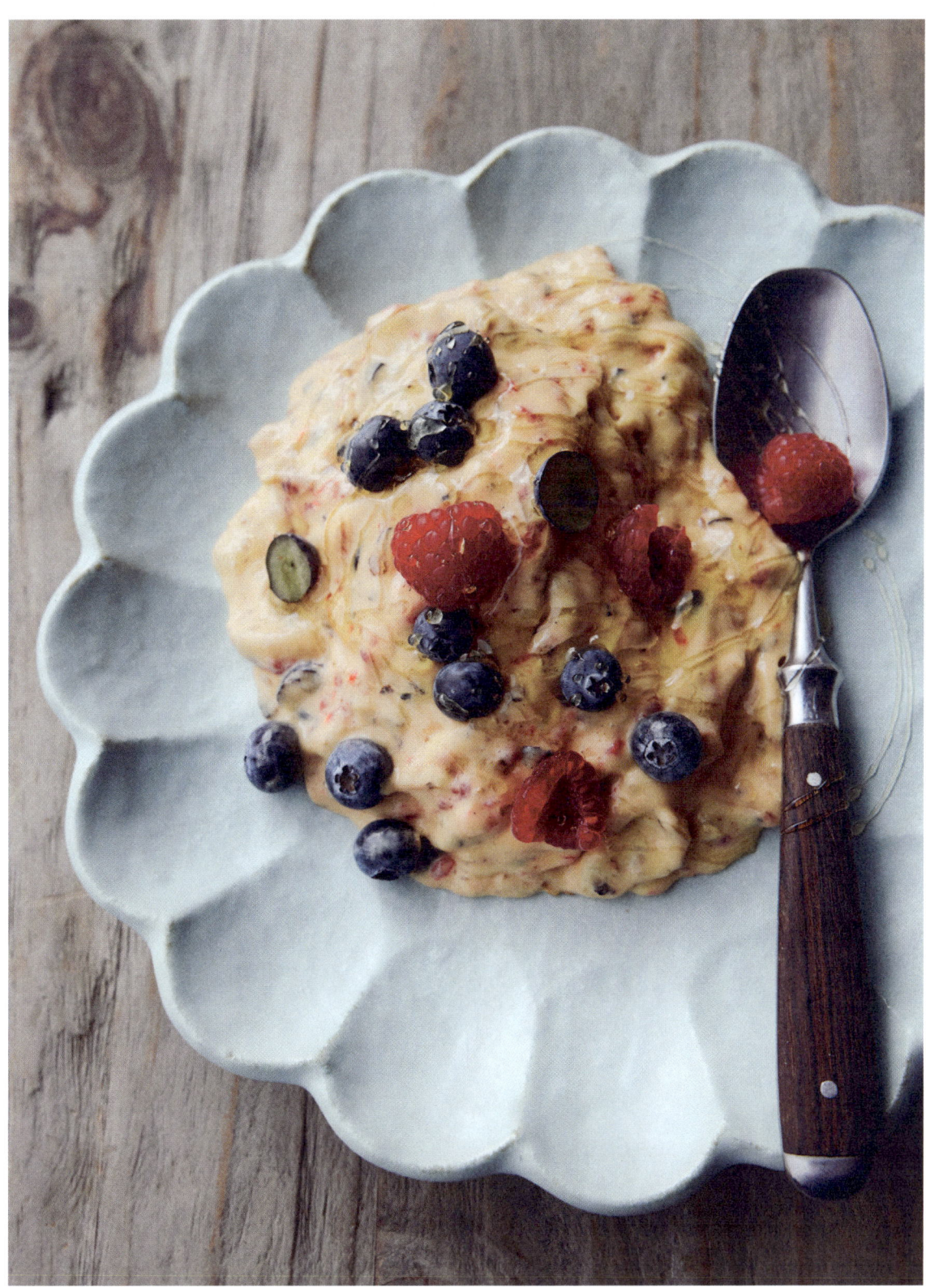

Smoked salmon & rye omelette

A classic combination put together in a completely different way. This omelette rocks!

SERVES 1
9 MINUTES

1 thick slice of rye bread (50g)

2 medium eggs

80g baby spinach

50g smoked salmon

½ a lemon

1 heaped tablespoon cottage cheese (30g)

a few chives

1 Put a large non-stick frying pan on a medium-high heat, finely crumble in the rye bread and spritz with olive oil. Add a sprinkle of black pepper and cook until crispy, while you whisk the eggs together in a bowl. Spoon out half the crispy crumbs for garnish, leaving the rest in the pan.

2 Add the spinach to the pan, stir until wilted, then turn the heat off. Pour in the beaten eggs and gently swirl to cover the base – they'll cook in the residual heat of the pan. Tear over the salmon, finely grate over the lemon zest, sprinkle over the reserved crumbs and dot over the cottage cheese.

3 Finely chop and scatter over the chives, then slide the omelette on to your plate and roll it up. Serve with a wedge of lemon.

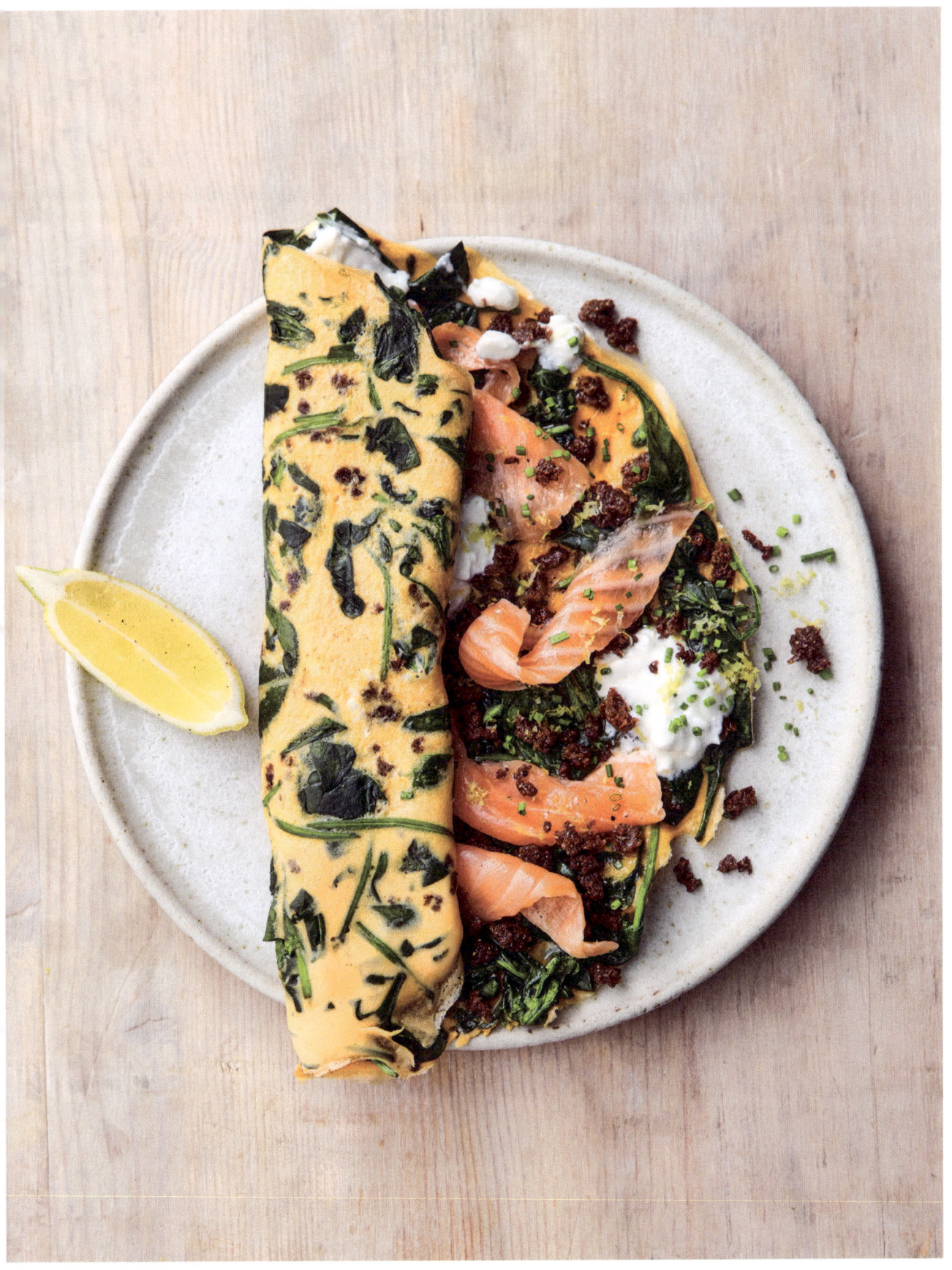

Speedy stuffed apple

Thanks to the microwave, this delicious, unexpected brekkie is ready in no time

SERVES 1
9 MINUTES

1 crisp eating apple (120g)

1 pitted Medjool date

1 small ripe banana (80g)

½ teaspoon cocoa powder, plus extra for dusting

1 pinch of ground allspice

1 teaspoon mixed seeds

6 walnut halves (15g)

2 heaped tablespoons Greek yoghurt

1 Keeping the apple whole, use a corer or small sharp knife to remove and discard the core, then carefully score around the middle of the fruit.

2 Finely chop the date, mash with the peeled banana, then mix in the cocoa, allspice and seeds. Poke in enough mixture to fill the apple core, then spoon the excess into the centre of a heatproof bowl and sit the stuffed apple on top. Microwave at 800W for 5 minutes, or until the apple is soft.

3 Meanwhile, finely grate the walnuts and mix most of them into the yoghurt. When the apple is done, spoon the walnut yoghurt and the rest of the grated walnuts alongside, dust with a little extra cocoa powder, and serve.

BALANCE IT

There are no carbs in this cute dish, so if you want to balance your brekkie, either add some toasted oats to your bowl or follow it up with some wholemeal toast.

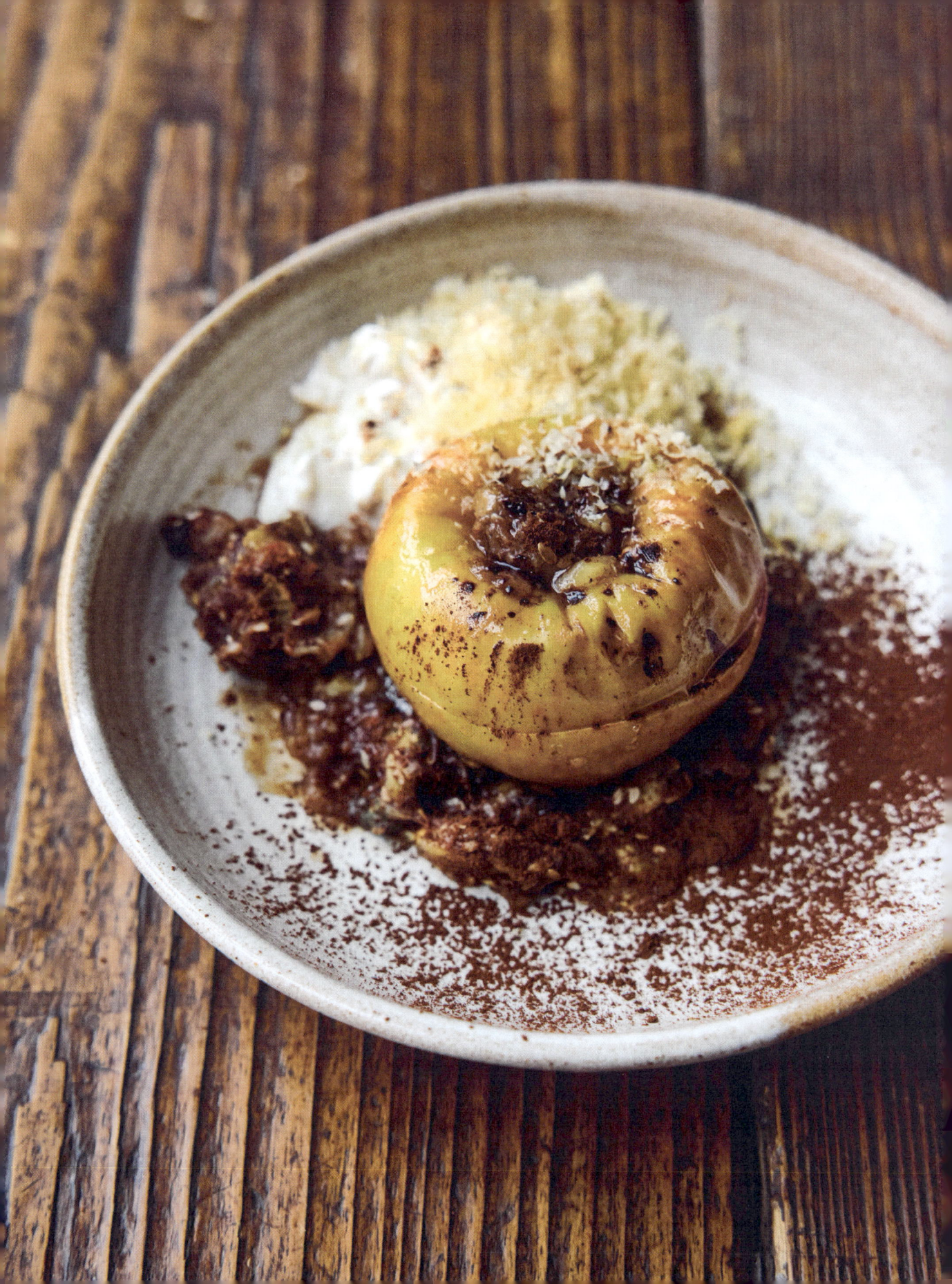

Mothership overnight oats

Making a quick batch of overnight oats that will sit happily in the fridge for up to 3 days, ready to be transformed with all kinds of different flavours, is a really helpful, nutritious, delicious thing to have in your life. This is the mothership recipe, which is perfectly tasty in its own right, but when you turn the page, you'll see there's a whole lot more to love about this breakfast . . .

MAKES 6 PORTIONS
10 MINUTES
PLUS OVERNIGHT SOAKING

2 ripe bananas (320g)

700ml semi-skimmed milk or your favourite unsweetened, fortified plant milk

2 teaspoons vanilla bean paste

300g porridge oats

2 eating apples

1 In a blender, blitz the peeled bananas with the milk and vanilla until smooth, then pour over the oats in a bowl. Coarsely grate in the apples, mix well, then cover and pop into the fridge overnight to do its thing.

2 The next day, stir well, correct the consistency with a little extra milk, if needed, then either tuck in as it is, adding a handful of your favourite seasonal fruit, unsalted nuts or seeds, or choose one of the epic flavour combos over the page – each makes one tasty portion when paired with 220g of Mothership overnight oats. Fill. Your. Boots.

HELPFUL HINT

Prepping for one? It's easy to halve the recipe here, giving you 3 portions (220g each) for the days ahead.

TURN THE PAGE FOR INSPO!

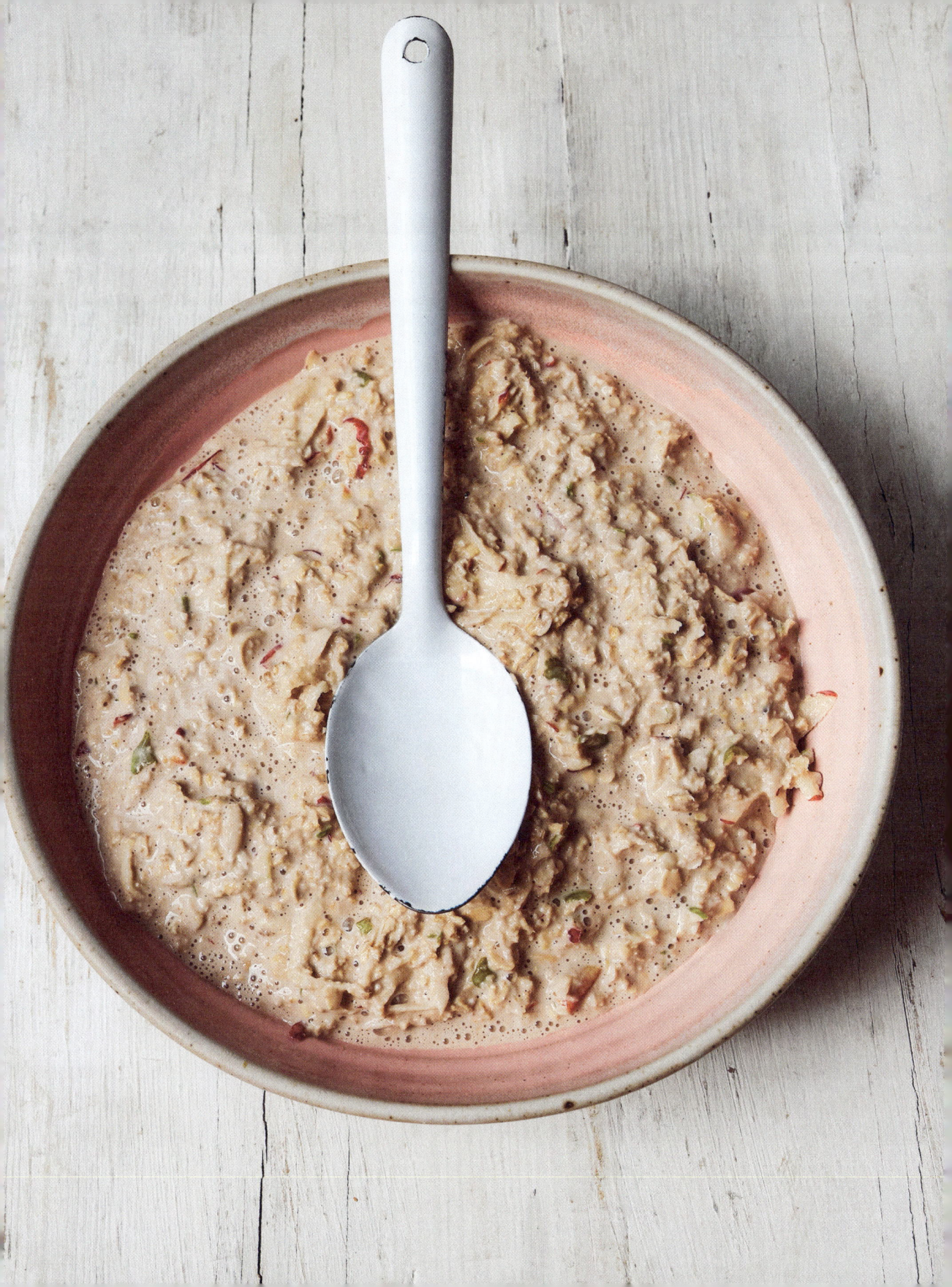

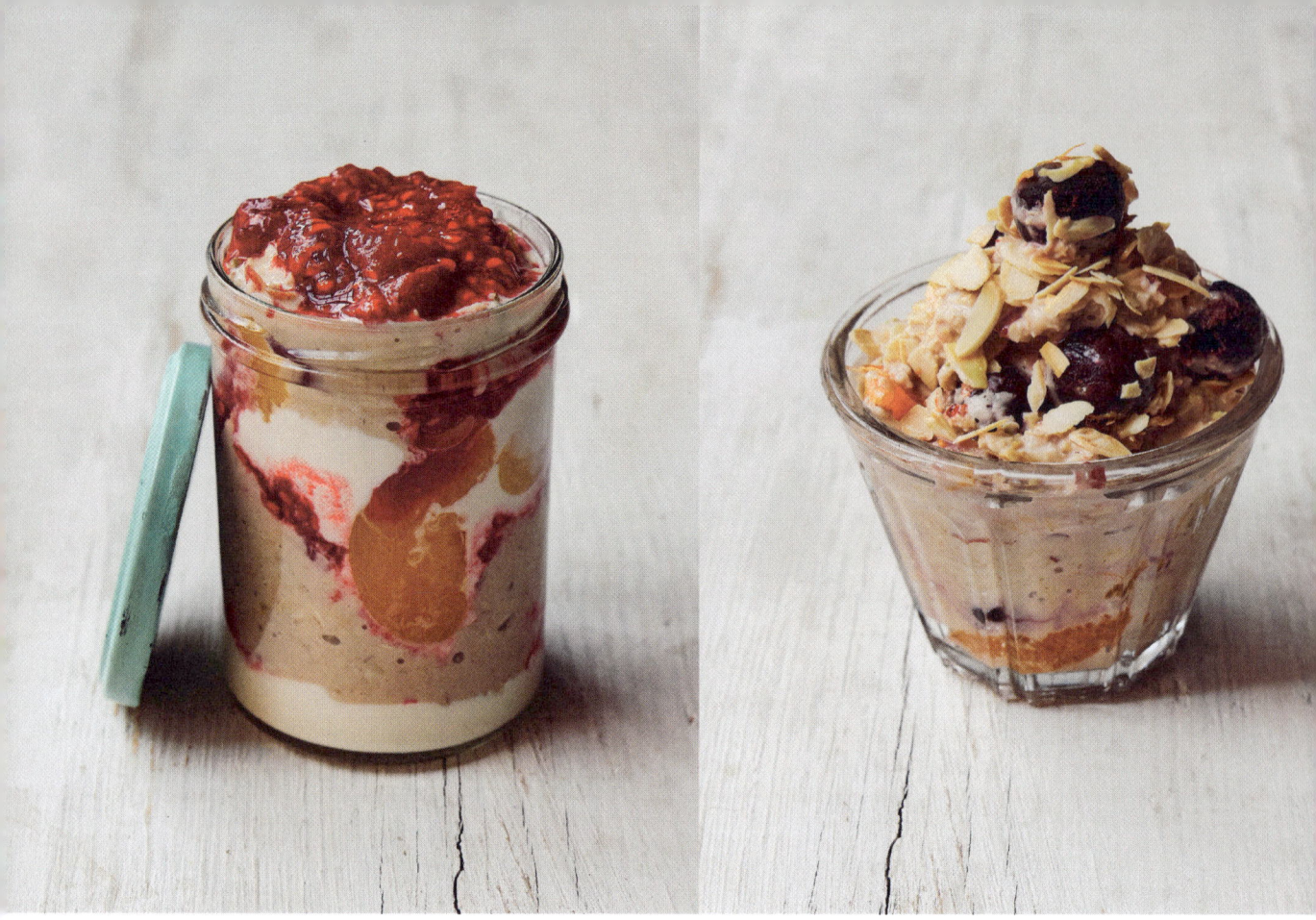

Peach melba

Crush **80g of raspberries** with a fork and layer up in a jar or pot with **220g of Mothership overnight oats**, **80g of drained tinned peaches** and **2 tablespoons of Greek yoghurt**.

Cherry Bakewell

Finely grate the zest of **1 orange**, segment the fruit, and layer up with **220g of Mothership overnight oats**, **80g of frozen cherries** and **1 heaped tablespoon of toasted flaked almonds**.

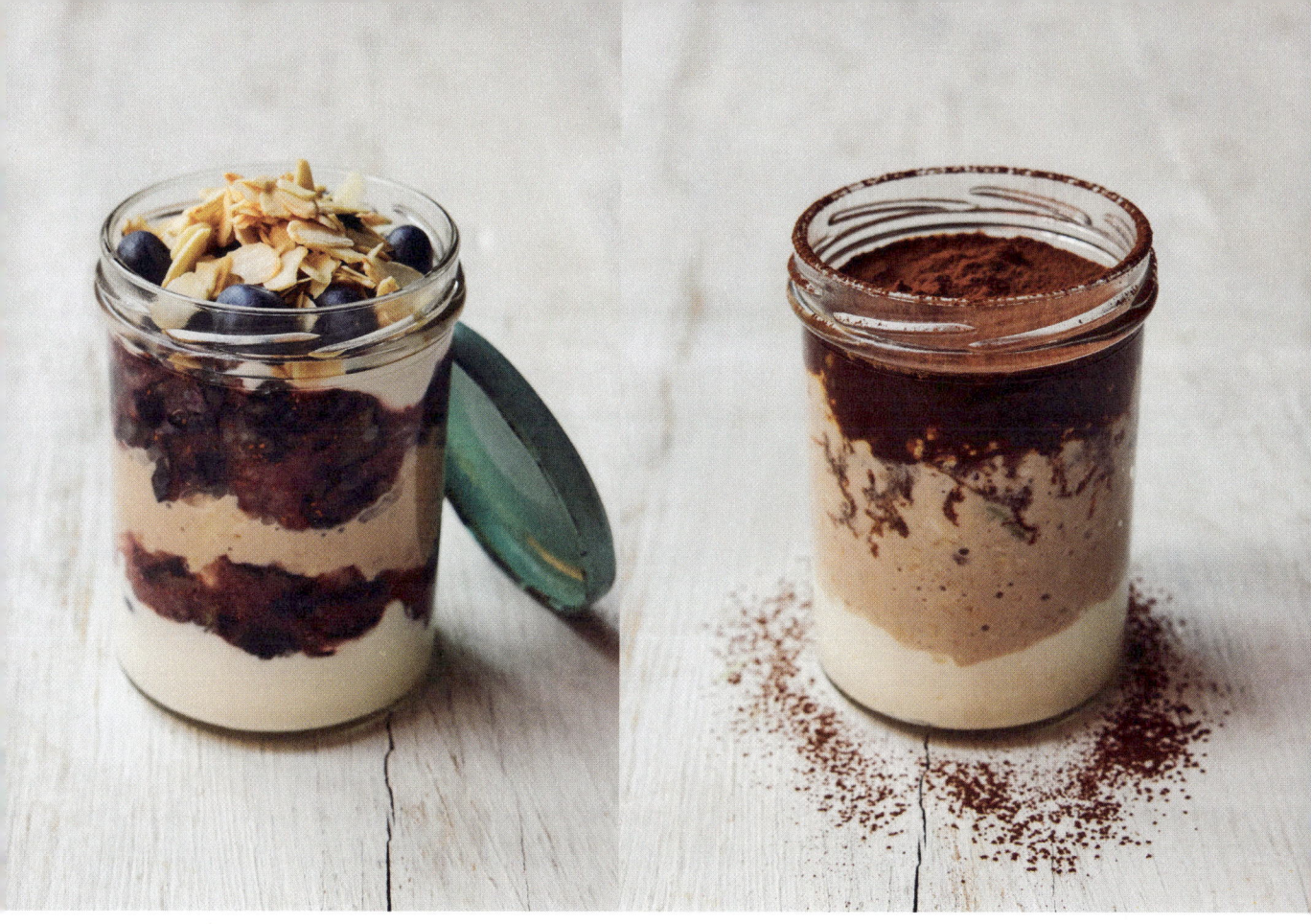

Berry cheesecake

Layer up **80g of blueberries** (crushing half with a fork) with **220g of Mothership overnight oats**, **2 tablespoons of soured cream** and **1 heaped tablespoon of toasted flaked almonds**.

Tiramisù

Add **1 shot of espresso** (as strong as you like it!) to **220g of Mothership overnight oats** and layer up with **2 tablespoons of Greek yoghurt** and a nice dusting of **cocoa powder**.

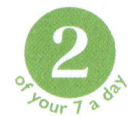

Spicy tofu & sweet pepper eggs

Invest in a good crunchy peanut and sesame chilli oil to add big flavour to lots of dishes

SERVES 1
10 MINUTES

100g oyster mushrooms

100g firm tofu

1 large jarred roasted pepper (80g)

1 tablespoon crunchy peanut & sesame chilli oil

1 teaspoon low-salt soy sauce

½ a lemon

2 medium eggs

2 sprigs of coriander

1 Trim the mushrooms and place in a large non-stick frying pan on a high heat. Chunk up and add the tofu, then dry fry and char it all for 4 minutes. Tear in the pepper and char for 1 more minute.

2 Off the heat, add ½ a tablespoon of chilli oil, the soy and a squeeze of lemon juice. Toss for 1 minute, then tip on to your plate.

3 Working swiftly, wipe out the pan, return it to the heat, spritz it with oil, then season, beat and pour in the eggs. Stir gently until you've got beautiful silky strips of just-cooked egg, surrounded by softer, custardy egg, then slide the eggs on to your plate as one. Pick over the coriander, drizzle with the remaining chilli oil, and serve. Nice with steamed rice, if you like.

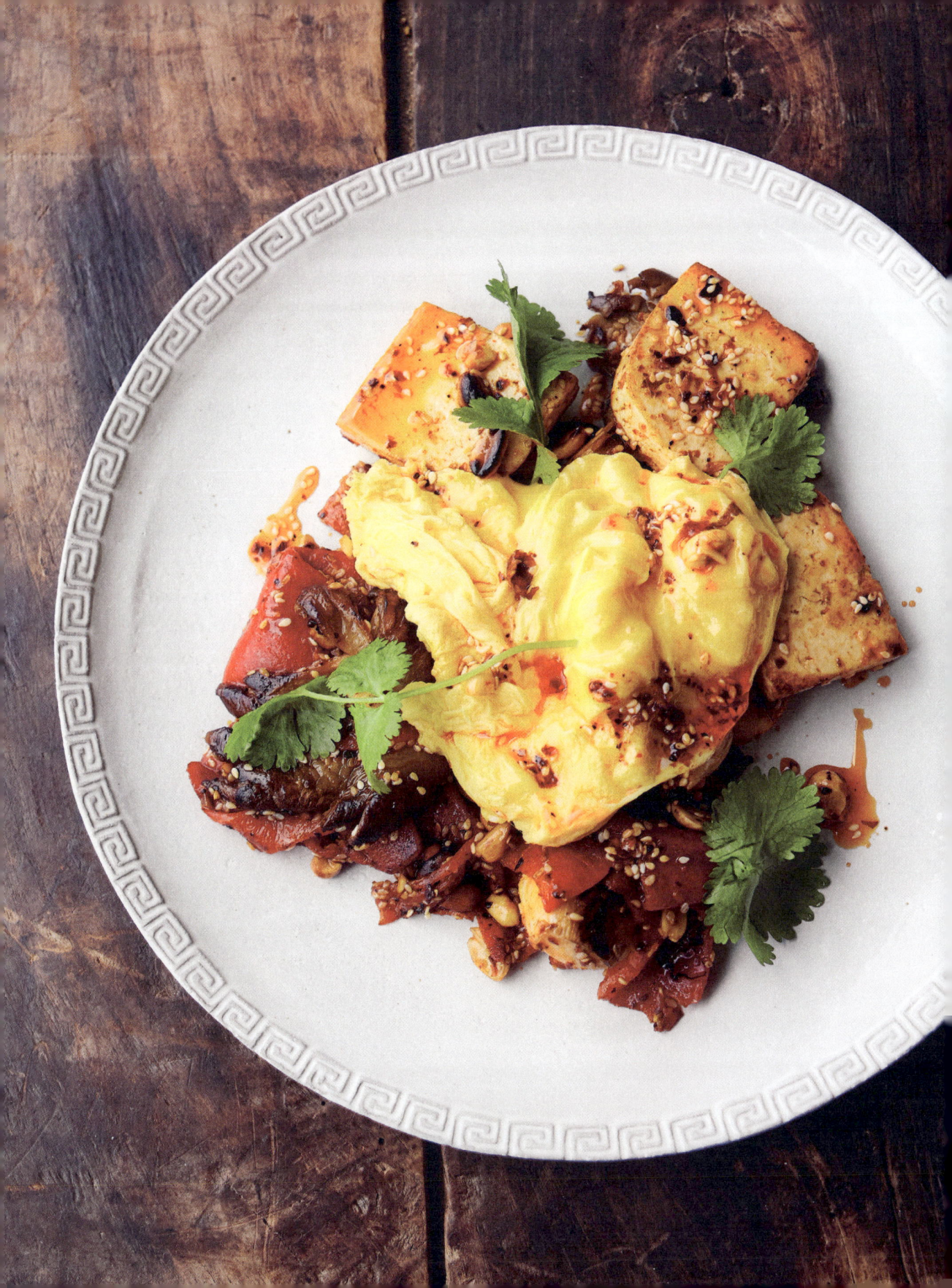

Golden cheese & jammy berries

In the Mediterranean, fried cheese is often served with fresh or jammy fruits – a magical combo

SERVES 2
12 MINUTES

80g halloumi or paneer cheese

320g mixed berries, such as strawberries, raspberries, blueberries

1 teaspoon balsamic vinegar

2 sprigs of basil

2 slices of wholemeal sourdough bread

1 teaspoon runny honey

1 Put a non-stick frying pan on a medium heat with 1 tablespoon of olive oil. Slice and add the cheese, cook until golden on both sides, then remove.

2 Hull and halve any strawberries, then put all the berries into the pan. Cook for 3 minutes, or until soft, gently stirring occasionally. Drizzle over the balsamic, pick in most of the basil leaves, and stir gently until just wilted.

3 Toast the bread and divide between your plates, then spoon the jammy fruit on top. Pick over the remaining basil leaves, add the golden cheese, drizzle over the honey, and tuck right in.

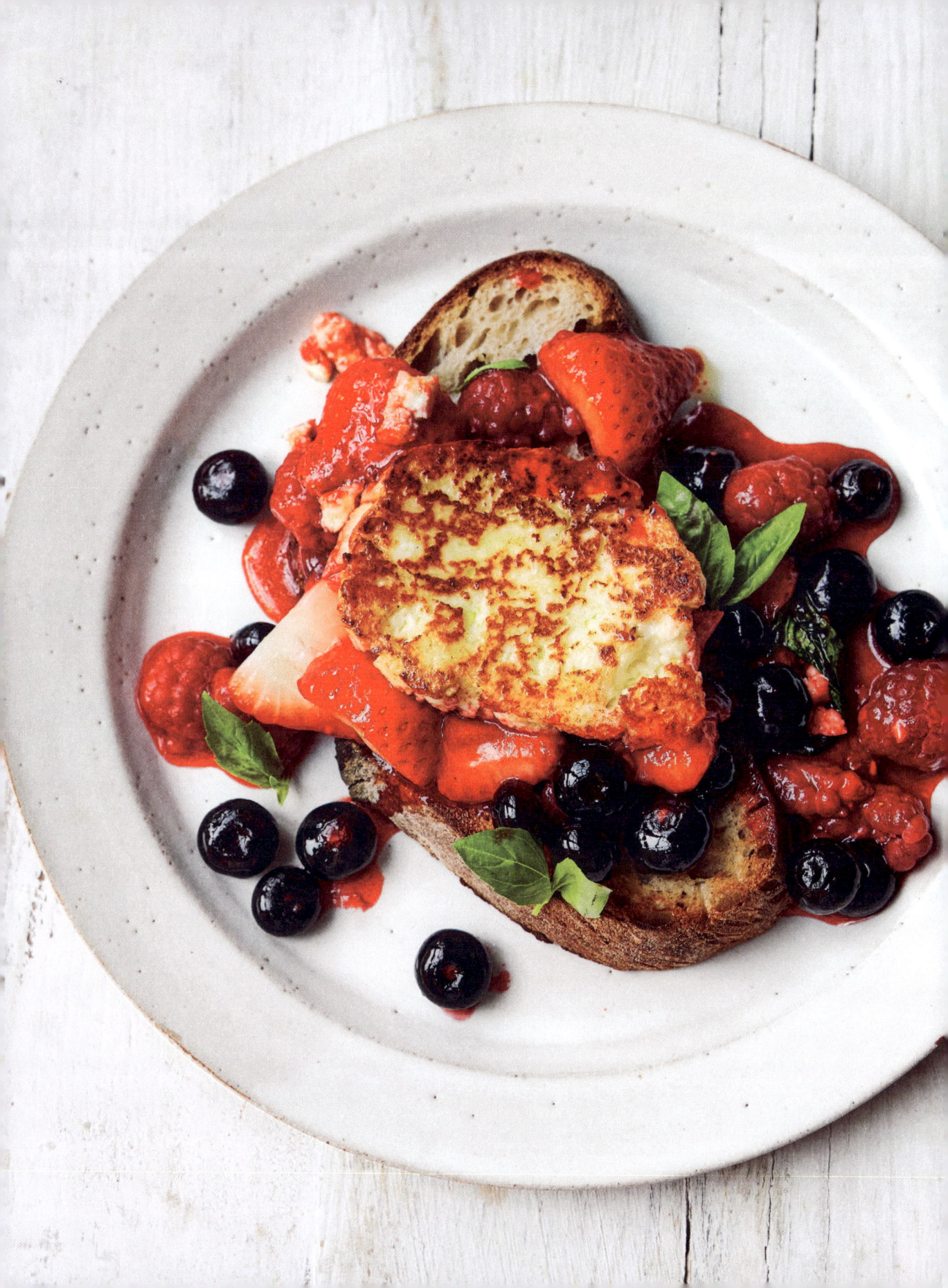

Dukkah poached eggs

Exciting, sumptuous and delicious, this dish is perfect for brekkie, brunch, lunch or a light meal

SERVES 1
14 MINUTES

1 small sweet potato (160g)

80g ripe mixed-colour cherry tomatoes

1 fresh red chilli

½ a bunch of flat-leaf parsley (15g)

½ a lemon

2 eggs

1 tablespoon dukkah

optional: 1 flatbread

1 Prick the sweet potato and microwave for 6 minutes at 800W, or until soft.

2 Chop the tomatoes, chilli and parsley, stalks and all, reserving a few leaves. Dress with the lemon juice and a little pinch of sea salt and black pepper.

3 Half fill a pan with water, add a pinch of salt and bring to a light simmer. Crack one of the eggs into a mug, gently pour it into the water, then repeat. Poach for 2 to 4 minutes, depending on how you like your eggs.

4 Meanwhile, mash the sweet potato with 2 teaspoons of extra virgin olive oil, discarding the skin, season to perfection, and spread across your plate. Pile the dressed tomatoes on top. Use a slotted spoon to add the poached eggs, sprinkle over the dukkah and reserved parsley leaves, and add a drizzle of extra virgin olive oil, to finish, if you like. Nice with a flatbread.

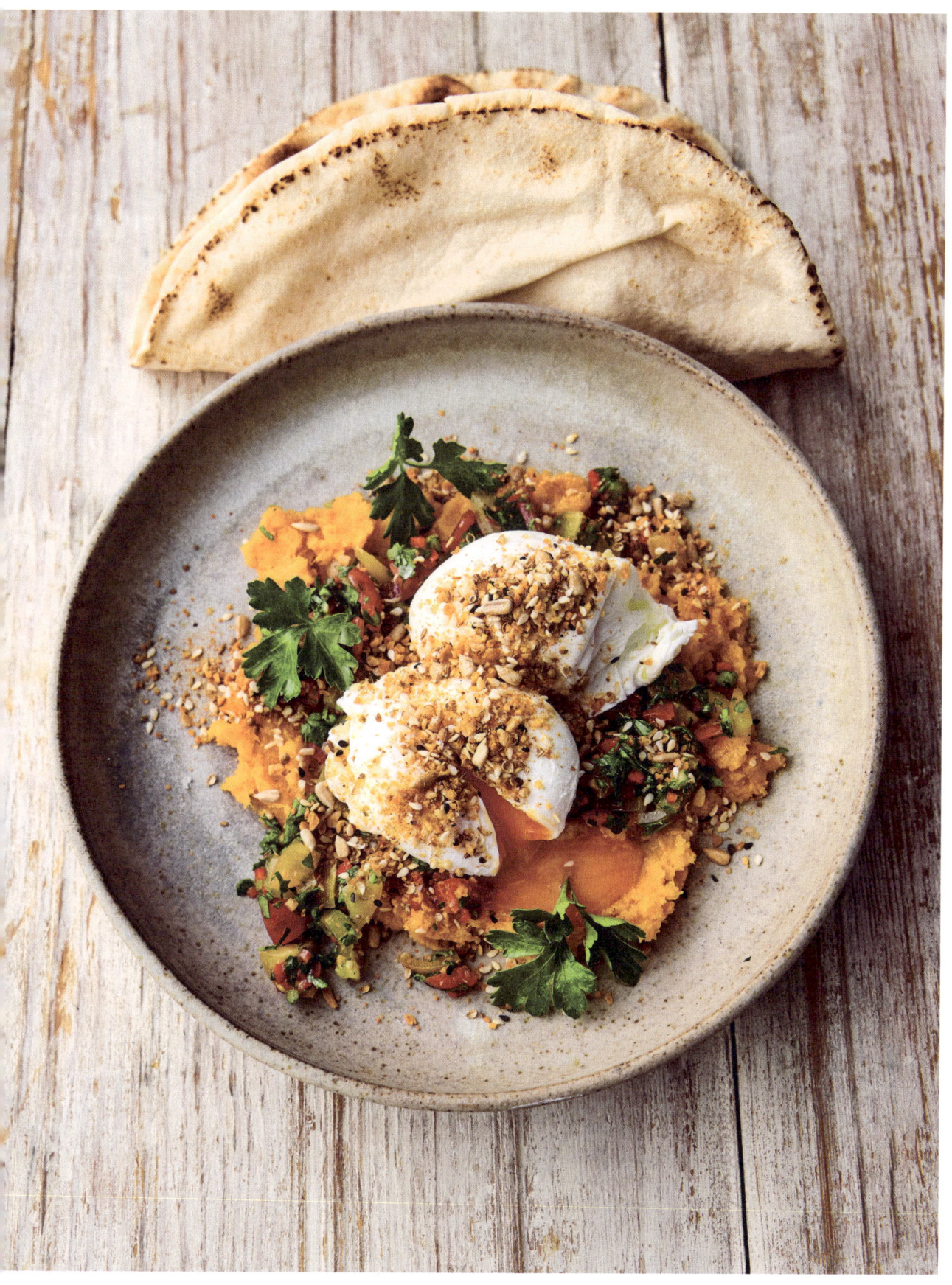

Extraordinary brekkie smush-in

Deliciously satisfying, quick caramelized banana makes all the difference on the flavour front

SERVES 1
14 MINUTES

1 thick slice of wholemeal sourdough bread

1 small ripe banana (80g)

30g pitted Medjool dates

1 teaspoon mixed seeds

1 tablespoon crunchy peanut butter

1 teaspoon cocoa powder, plus extra for dusting

1 heaped tablespoon Greek yoghurt

40g raspberries

1 Toast the bread in a dry non-stick frying pan on a medium heat. Peel the banana and flatten it in alongside, add the dates and seeds, and cook it all until golden. Put the toast on a serving plate and everything else in a bowl.

2 Use a fork to mash up the caramelized banana with the dates, seeds, peanut butter and cocoa, mixing as you go until you have a fine mush, then slather it on to the toast. Spoon over the yoghurt, dust with a little extra cocoa, press in the raspberries and tuck on in.

EASY SWAPS

Feel free to swap in any seasonal berries here – blackberries, blueberries or sliced strawberries would all work a treat.

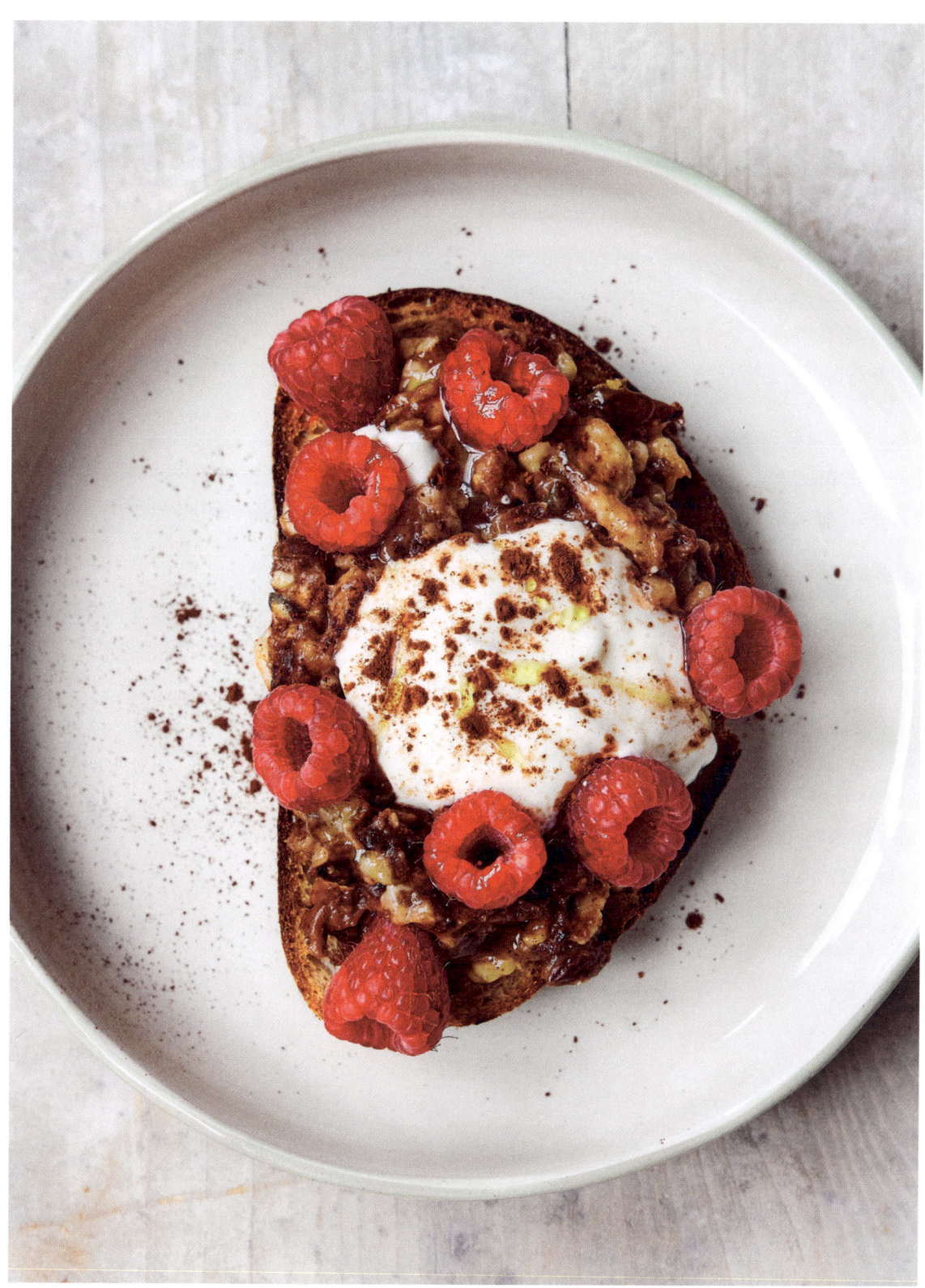

One-cup pancakes

Pancakes allow you to have a bit of fun – they're a wonderful vehicle for additional flavour, and a great way to try a whole rainbow of fruits and veggies, for both kids and adults alike. Plus, by introducing a savoury option, you can enjoy pancakes for brekkie, brunch, lunch or dinner! Just grab a mug, use it to measure both the flour and the milk, add an egg, mix and go!

SERVES 4
18 MINUTES

1 mug of wholemeal self-raising flour

1 mug of semi-skimmed milk or your favourite unsweetened, fortified plant milk

1 large egg

Sweet pancakes
1 teaspoon vanilla bean paste

Savoury pancakes
50g crumbled feta cheese

1 Put all the ingredients into a large bowl with a small pinch of sea salt (for fatter, fluffier pancakes use a heaped mug of flour) and whisk well, adding the extra sweet or savoury ingredient, if you wish.

2 Put a large non-stick frying pan on a medium heat. Spritz with olive oil, then go in with a few separate tablespoons of batter. Add your chosen fruit or veg to each (turn the page for inspo), then, once golden on the base, gently flip over, until lightly golden on the fruit or veg side, too. Serve, and repeat!

KEEPING IT SWEET?

A dollop of yoghurt, a sprinkling of your favourite unsalted nuts and seeds, and a little runny honey, to taste, will always work a treat on the side.

GOING SAVOURY?

A spoonful of cottage cheese or soured cream over the top and a handful of lemony-dressed rocket will complete your plate nicely.

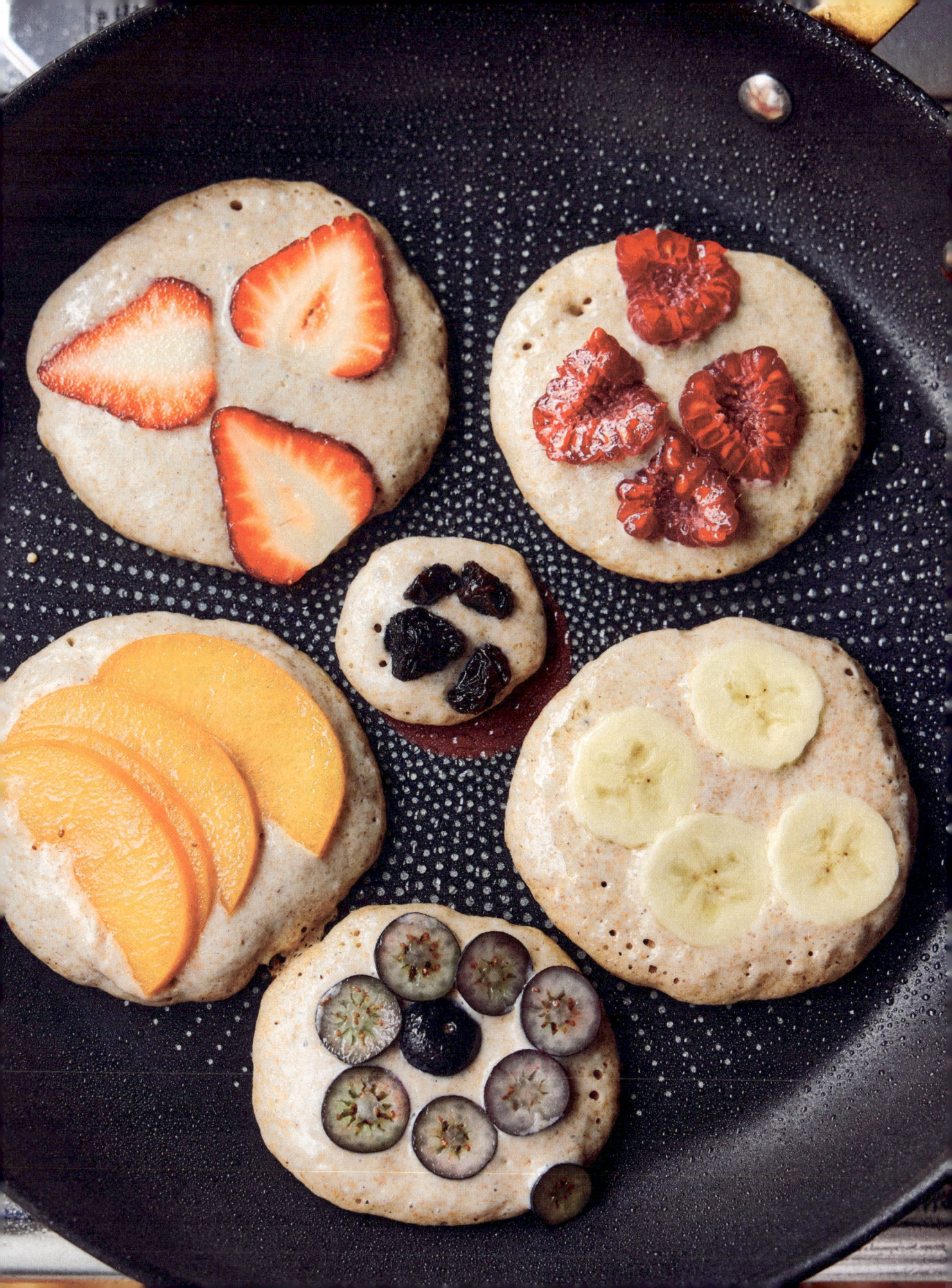

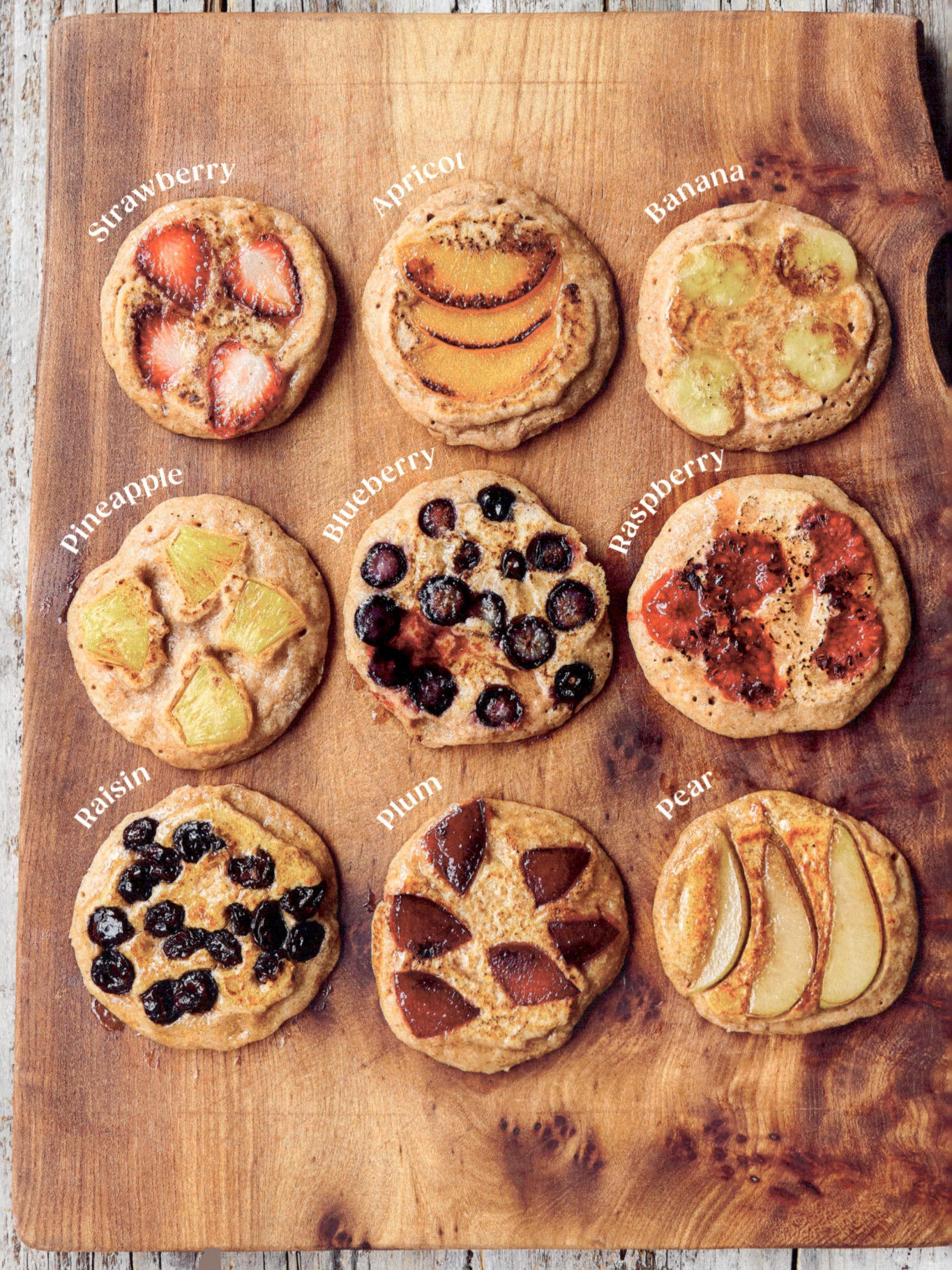

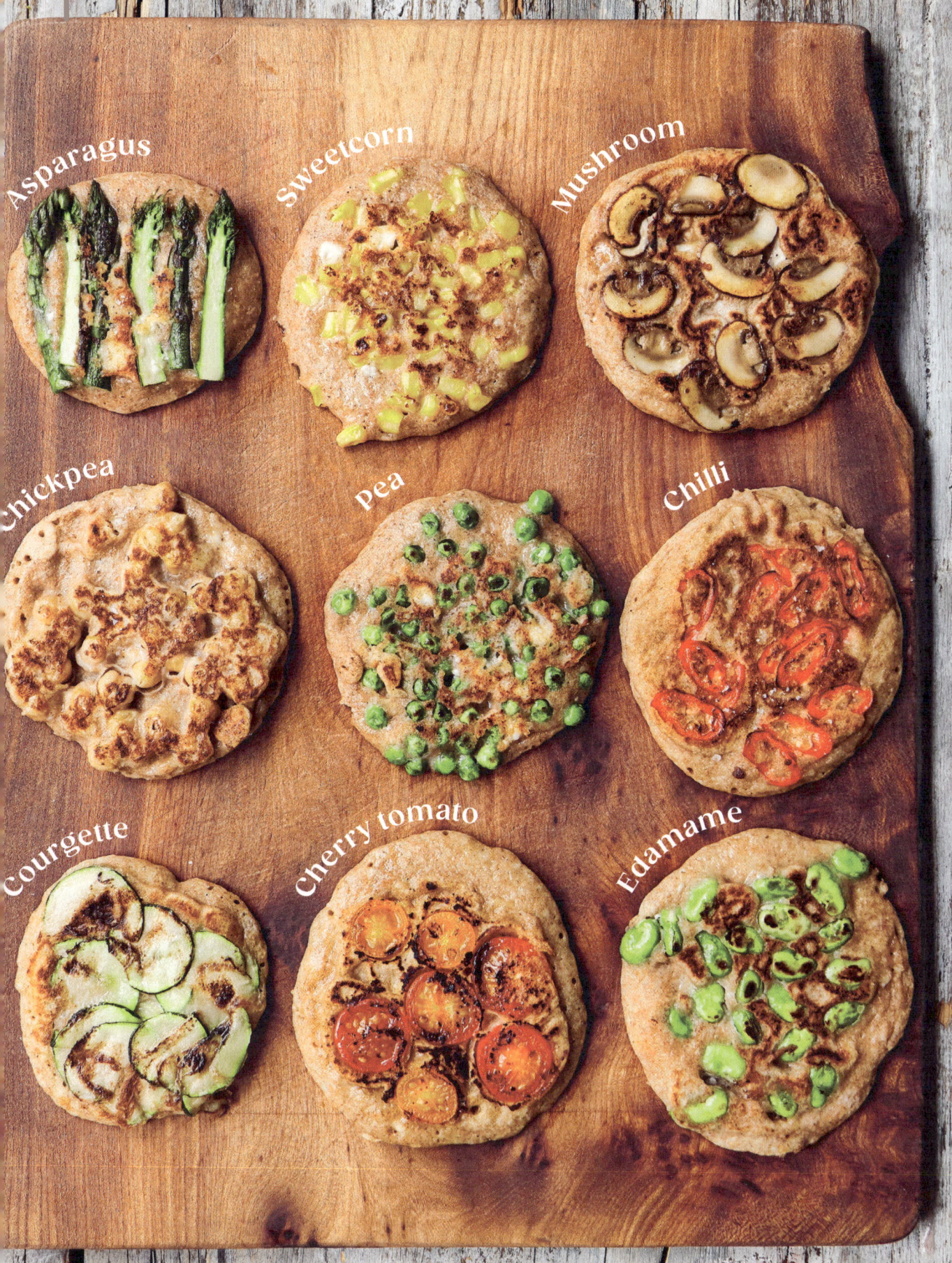

Cheesy beans on toast

Quick to rustle up and full of the good stuff, this is a delicious breakfast, brunch, lunch or dinner

SERVES 2
18 MINUTES

1 clove of garlic

½ a fresh red chilli

2 sprigs of sage

200g ripe mixed-colour cherry tomatoes

1 x 400g tin of butter beans

2 teaspoons thick balsamic vinegar

2 slices of wholemeal sourdough bread

80g halloumi or paneer cheese

1. Peel the garlic and finely slice with the chilli. Pick the sage leaves. Halve the tomatoes. Put a non-stick frying pan on a high heat with ½ a tablespoon of olive oil, the garlic, chilli and sage. Fry until it all starts to sizzle and get lightly golden, removing the sage leaves to kitchen paper once crispy, then go in with the tomatoes, beans, juice and all, and the balsamic. Simmer for 5 minutes, or until starting to thicken nicely, stirring occasionally.

2. Toast the bread, then put on your serving plates. Season the beans to perfection and divide over the top, then quickly wipe out the pan and return to a high heat with ½ a tablespoon of oil. Slice and add the cheese. Fry until lightly golden on both sides, then break over the beans, scatter over the crispy sage, add an extra drizzle of balsamic, if you like, and serve.

EASY SWAPS

Try your favourite beans here – cannellini or borlotti would be delicious.

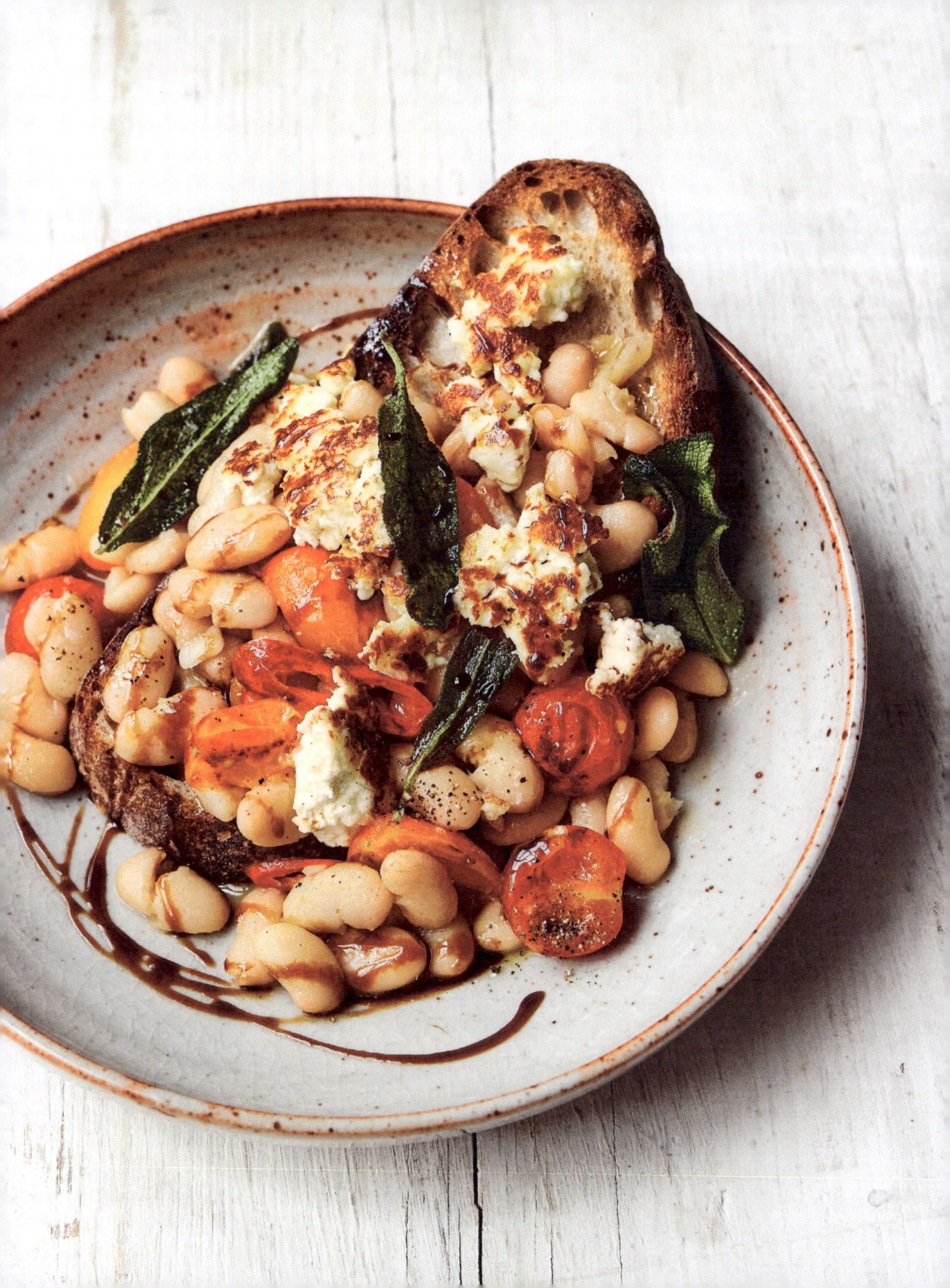

Easy egg & bean filo twists

Filo is such a versatile pastry. No matter how you put this together, the results are always fun

SERVES 4
22 MINUTES

8 sheets of filo pastry

2 x 400g tins of haricot beans

2 heaped tablespoons tomato purée

1 heaped tablespoon harissa paste

4 large eggs

40g Cheddar cheese

2 teaspoons sesame seeds

2 mixed-colour peppers (320g)

2 spring onions

1 bunch of dill (20g)

1. Preheat the oven to 200°C. Spritz 2 sheets of filo with olive oil, line up the two short sides so they slightly overlap, then scrunch up lengthways and twist into a nest about 15cm wide, making sure it has a base. Place on an oil-spritzed baking tray, and repeat.

2. Drain the beans, toss with the harissa, tomato purée and ½ a tablespoon of red wine vinegar, then divide evenly between the filo nests. Crack an egg on to each one, season with sea salt and black pepper, grate over the cheese, then divide and sprinkle over the sesame seeds. Bake for 15 minutes, or until golden and crisp.

3. Meanwhile, deseed and very finely chop the peppers. Trim and finely chop the spring onions. Finely chop the dill, mix together, then dress with 2 tablespoons of red wine vinegar, 1 tablespoon of extra virgin olive oil, and a good pinch of salt.

4. Serve the egg filo twists with the pepper salsa on the side.

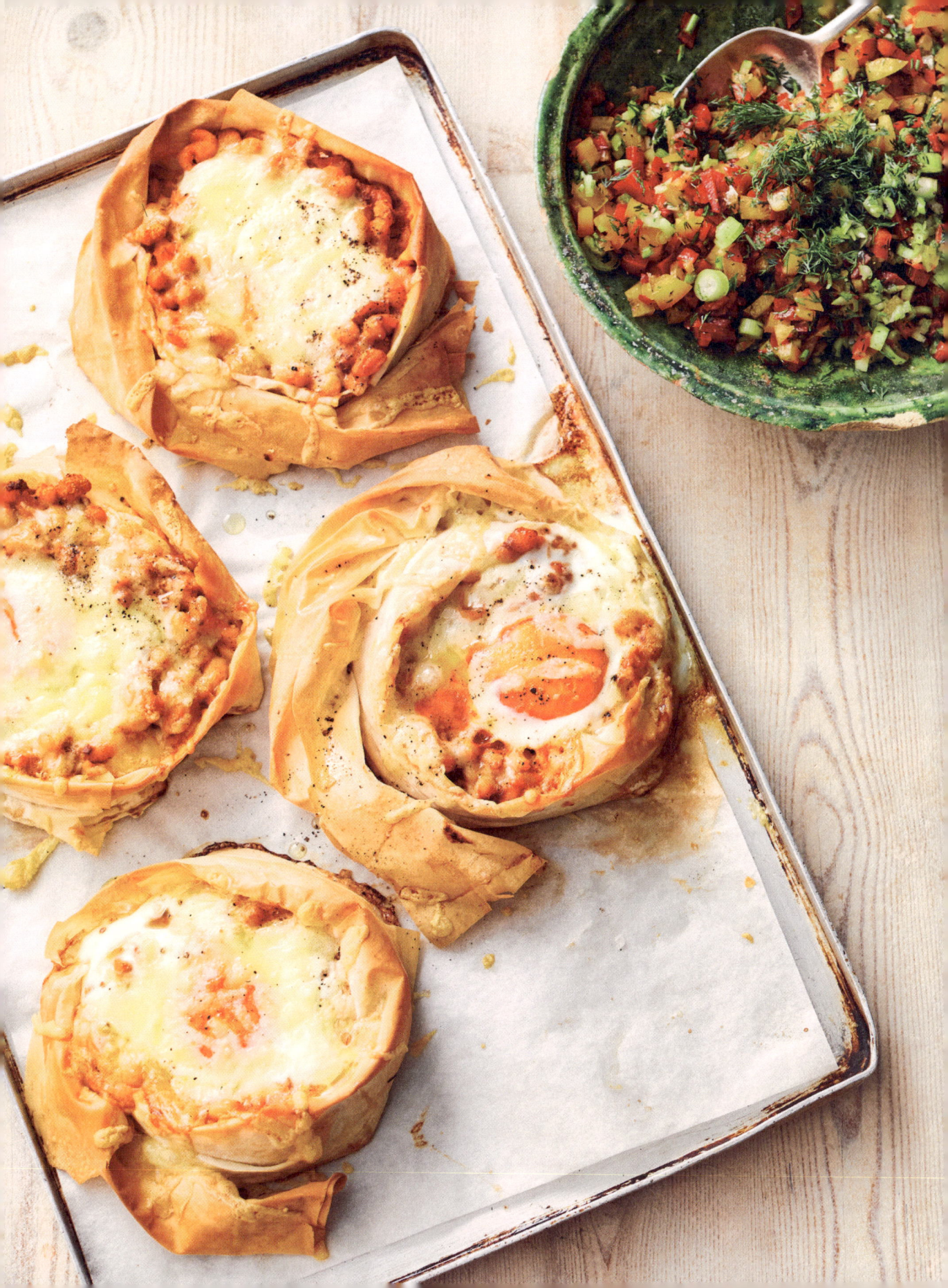

1 of your 7 a day

Granola fruit cups

Sweet roasted stone fruit, an easy-to-make granola and yoghurt is a perfect portable brekkie

MAKES 6 PORTIONS
26 MINUTES

800g ripe peaches, plums or apricots

1 teaspoon vanilla bean paste or 1 vanilla pod

1 orange

100g porridge oats

30g mixed seeds, such as pumpkin, sunflower, linseed

1 teaspoon ground ginger

50g maple syrup

2 tablespoons of your favourite nut butter

30g unsalted nuts, such as pecans, hazelnuts, walnut halves

Greek or plant-based yoghurt, to serve

1. Preheat the oven to 180°C. Halve and destone your chosen stone fruit, and place in a large roasting tray with the vanilla paste (or halve the vanilla pod lengthways and scrape out the seeds, then add both to the tray). Finely grate over the orange zest, squeeze over the juice, toss together, then arrange the fruit in a single layer. Roast for 20 minutes, or until soft and sweet.

2. For the granola, put the oats, seeds, ginger, maple syrup and nut butter into a large bowl with a pinch of sea salt. Roughly chop and add the nuts. Mix well, using your thumbs and fingertips to create both little clumps and loose crumbs. Spread across a large roasting tray and cook beneath the fruit for the last 10 minutes, or until beautifully golden.

3. Serve the fruit warm, or cool and stash in the fridge until needed, when you can portion up to order. Let the granola cool, then store in an airtight jar until needed. I like to layer up fruit and granola in little cups, pots or glasses to order, finishing with a dollop of cool, creamy yoghurt.

BATCH IT UP

It's super-easy and convenient to double up on the granola and make a bigger batch to stash in an airtight jar, ready for brekkie, puds, or even snacking!

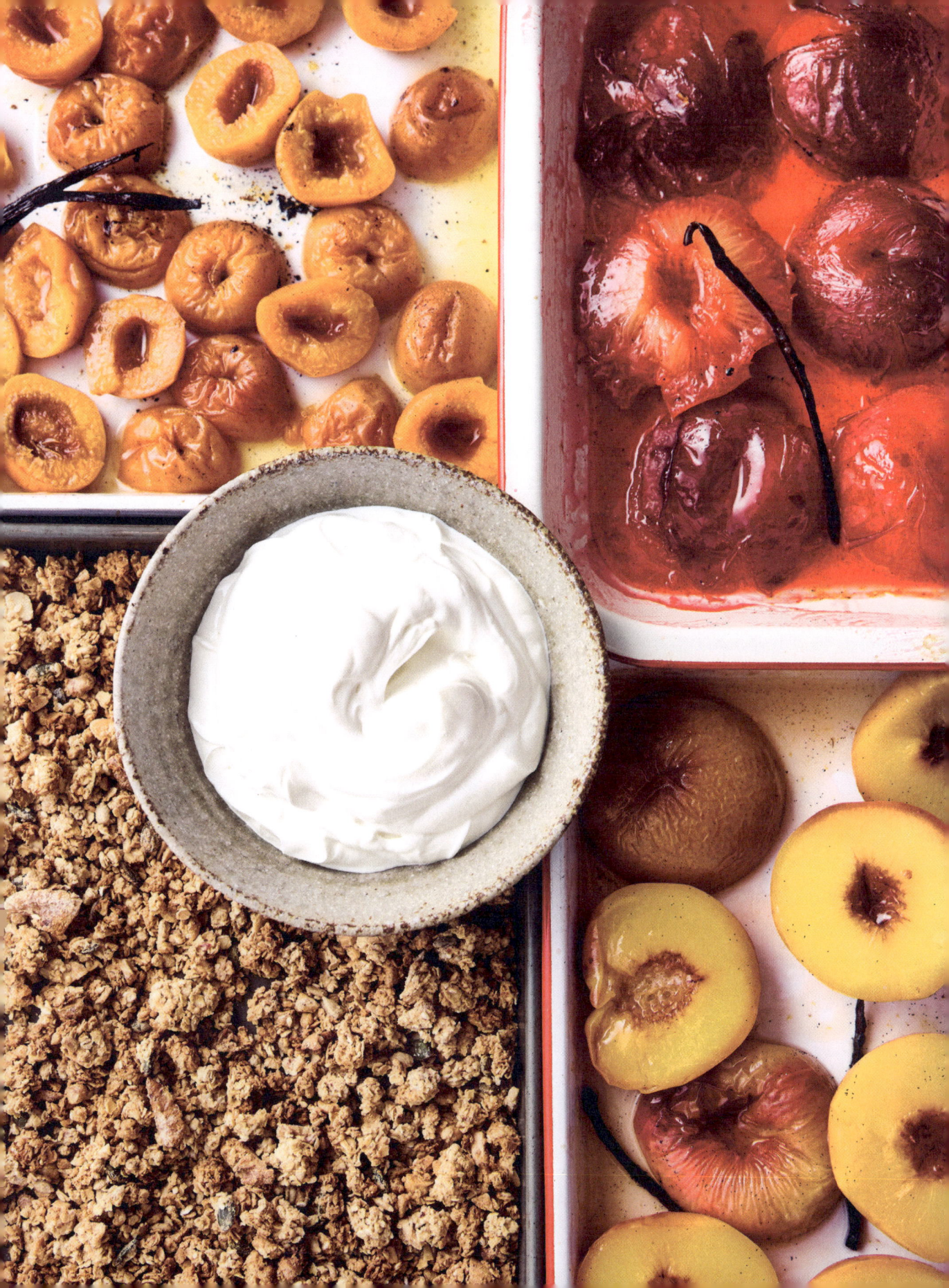

Batch-it-up protein rolls

Bump up your protein fix while filling your house with the nicest baking aromas. It's a win–win

MAKES 12
35 MINUTES
PLUS PROVING

1 x 7g sachet of yeast

150g mixed unsalted nuts, such as almonds, cashews, walnut halves

2 tablespoons sunflower seeds

2 tablespoons pumpkin seeds

3 large eggs

850g wholemeal self-raising flour

300g cottage cheese

1 teaspoon Marmite

1 In a jug, stir the yeast into 300ml of tepid water and leave for 5 minutes.

2 Place the nuts and seeds in a food processor and pulse to roughly chop. Crack in 2 eggs, then add 1 teaspoon of sea salt, the flour, cottage cheese and Marmite. Pour in the yeast mixture and blitz until just combined.

3 Tip on to a clean work surface and knead for 5 minutes, then cover and leave to prove somewhere warm for 1 hour, or until doubled in size.

4 Divide the dough equally into 12, roll each piece into a long roll-shape and line them up on a large greaseproof-paper-lined tray (you may need to work in batches). Score lengthways down each one, then beat the remaining egg and eggwash each roll. Prove for 1 more hour, or until doubled in size.

5 Preheat the oven to 190°C. Bake the rolls for 20 minutes, or until golden and hollow-sounding when tapped on the bottom. Cool on a wire rack.

FREEZER STASH

You can cover and freeze excess rolls after the second prove (end of step 4). Simply cook straight from frozen for 25 minutes at 190°C.

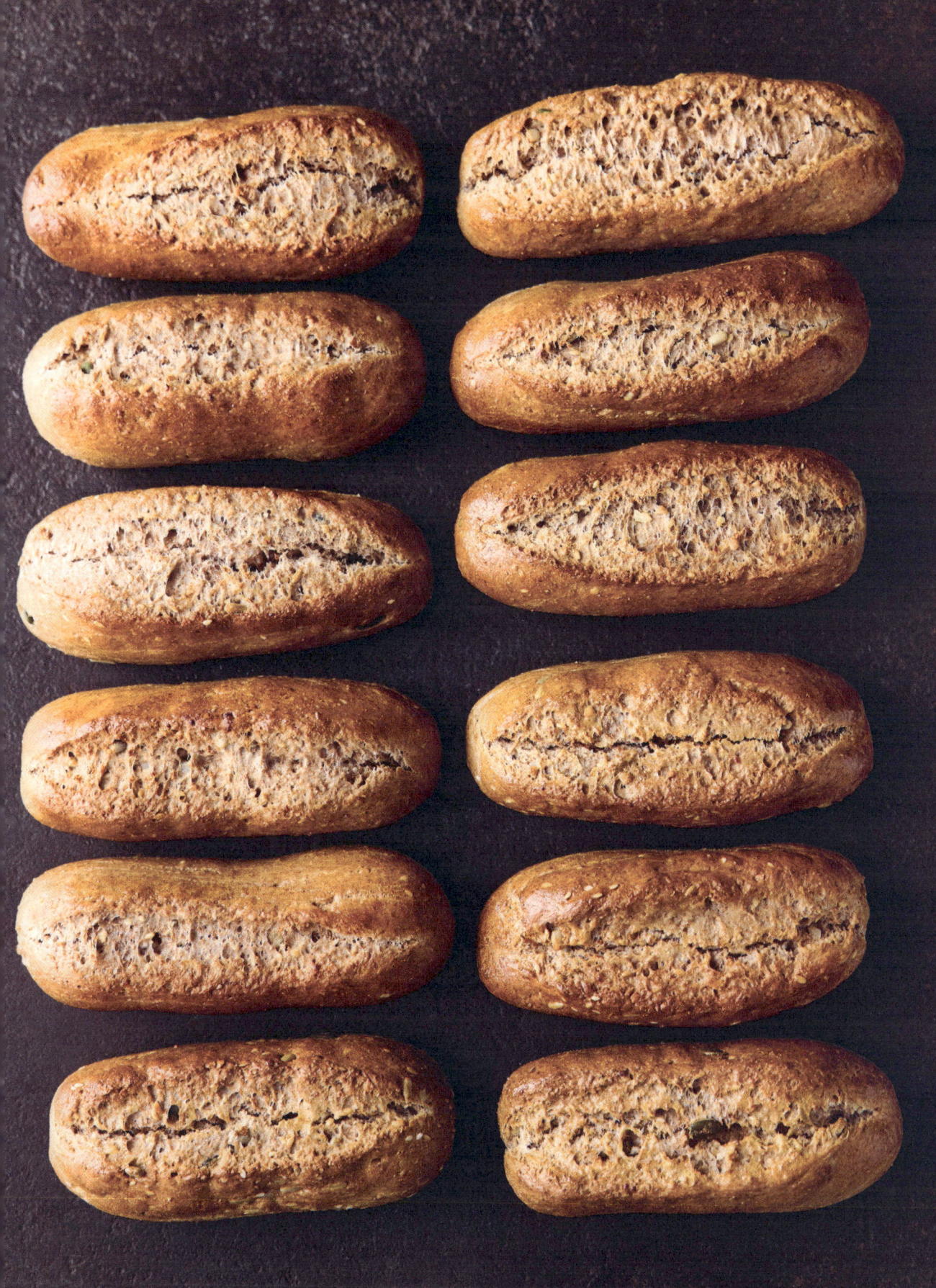

Lunch

Prawn cocktail for one

Prawn cocktail is one of my favourite things, and this re-imagination is truly delicious

SERVES 1
6 MINUTES

2 heaped tablespoons Greek yoghurt

1 heaped tablespoon tomato ketchup

1 teaspoon Worcestershire sauce

1 lemon

150g cooked peeled prawns

1 small perfectly ripe mango

80g iceberg lettuce

80g tinned sweetcorn

80g cucumber

1 tablespoon jarred sliced jalapeños

1 To make the cocktail sauce, in a serving bowl mix the yoghurt, ketchup and Worcestershire sauce with half the lemon juice. Stir in the prawns.

2 Peel, slice, dice and add the mango, also squeezing in any juice from around the stone. Very finely shred the lettuce and stir into the prawns with the sweetcorn, then season to perfection with sea salt and black pepper.

3 Use a speed-peeler to add the cucumber in ribbons. Scatter over the jalapeños and a pinch of black pepper, and serve with lemon wedges. Nice with a slice of wholemeal bread, a handful of croutons or crackers.

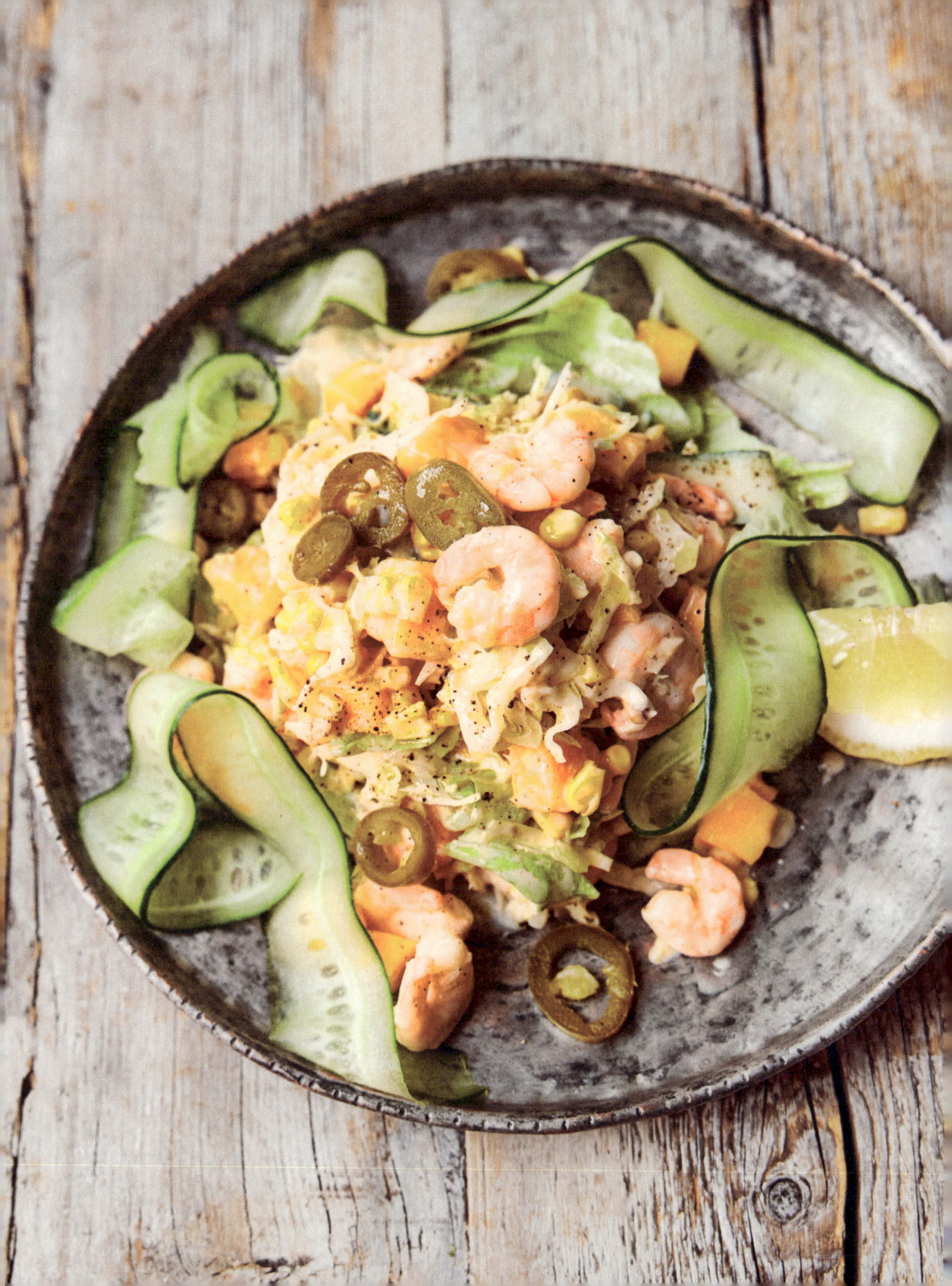

Speedy kedgeree

Great for lunch or brunch, kedgeree is nourishing, comforting and a really good go-to fast meal

SERVES 1
9 MINUTES

1 x 90g hot-smoked trout or salmon fillet, skin on

½ an onion (80g)

1 heaped teaspoon of your favourite curry paste

½ x 250g packet of cooked wholegrain basmati rice

80g baby spinach

80g frozen peas

1 lemon

1 egg

1 heaped teaspoon toasted flaked almonds

1 heaped tablespoon natural yoghurt

1. Place a large non-stick frying pan on a medium-high heat. Pull the skin off the fish fillet and place the skin only in the pan to crisp up, then remove.

2. Reduce the heat to medium. Peel, very finely chop and add the onion with a spritz of olive oil and a good splash of water and cook for 3 minutes, stirring regularly. Stir in the curry paste, followed by the rice, spinach, peas and half the lemon juice. Flake in the fish and cook for 2 minutes, then push everything to one side. Spritz the gap with oil, crack in the egg, fry for 1 minute per side, then mix it through the rice and season to perfection.

3. Flake in the crispy fish skin, add the almonds, and toss well. Plate up and serve with dollops of yoghurt, and a lemon wedge.

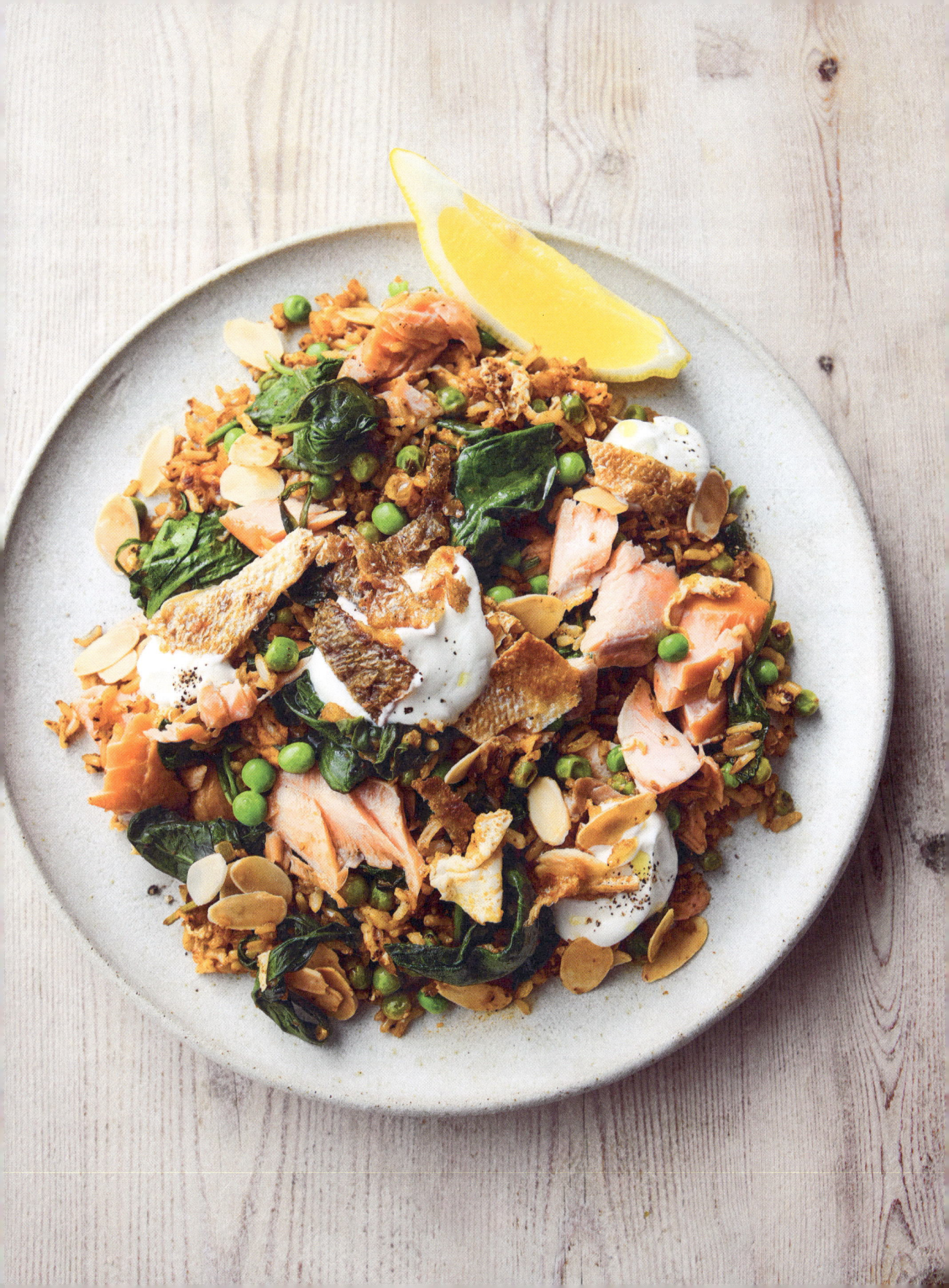

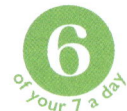

Creamy walnut coleslaw

SERVES 1 | 9 MINUTES

80g each
carrot, celeriac, red onion, pear, Savoy cabbage

30g dried apple

10g walnut halves

2 sprigs of flat-leaf parsley

2 tablespoons Greek yoghurt

2 teaspoons wholegrain mustard

Trim and peel the fresh veg and fruit, as needed, then coarsely grate it on a box grater, or finely shred using good knife skills or a mandolin (use the guard!). Finely chop the dried apple, walnuts and the parsley, stalks and all. Scrunch everything with the yoghurt, mustard and 1 tablespoon each of red wine vinegar and extra virgin olive oil, then season to perfection. Great with a jacket potato, fried eggs, roast chicken or simply as it is.

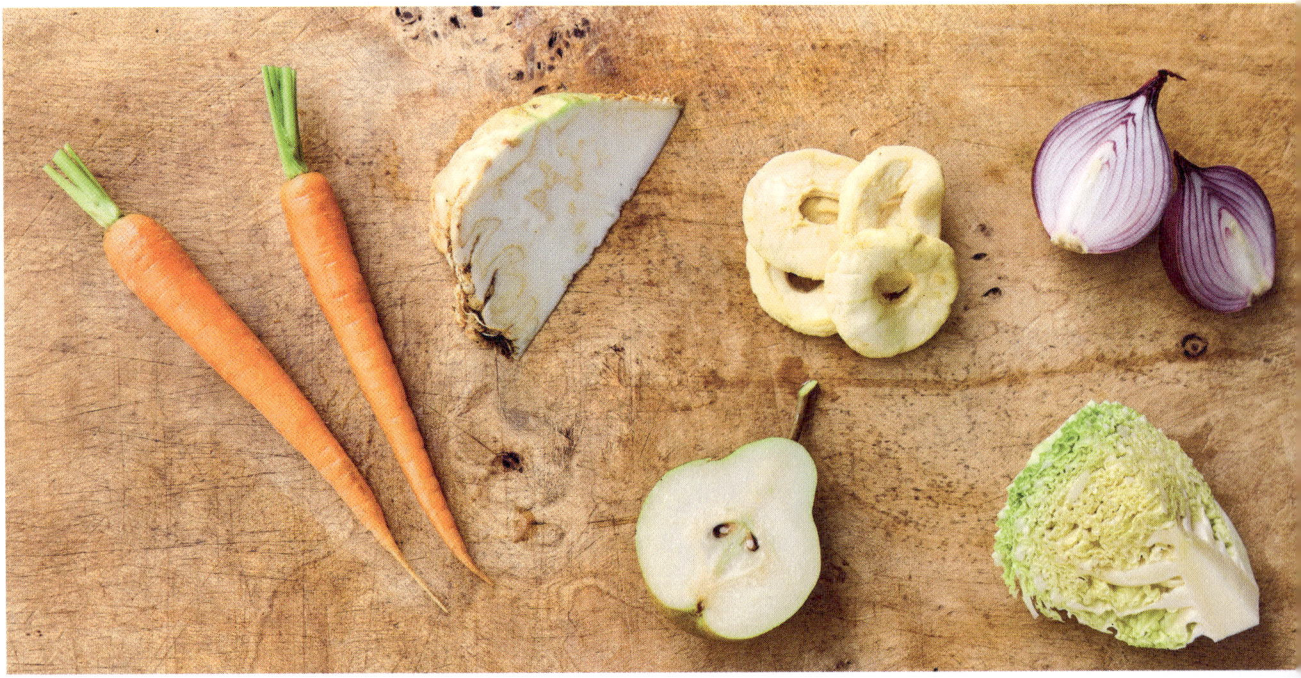

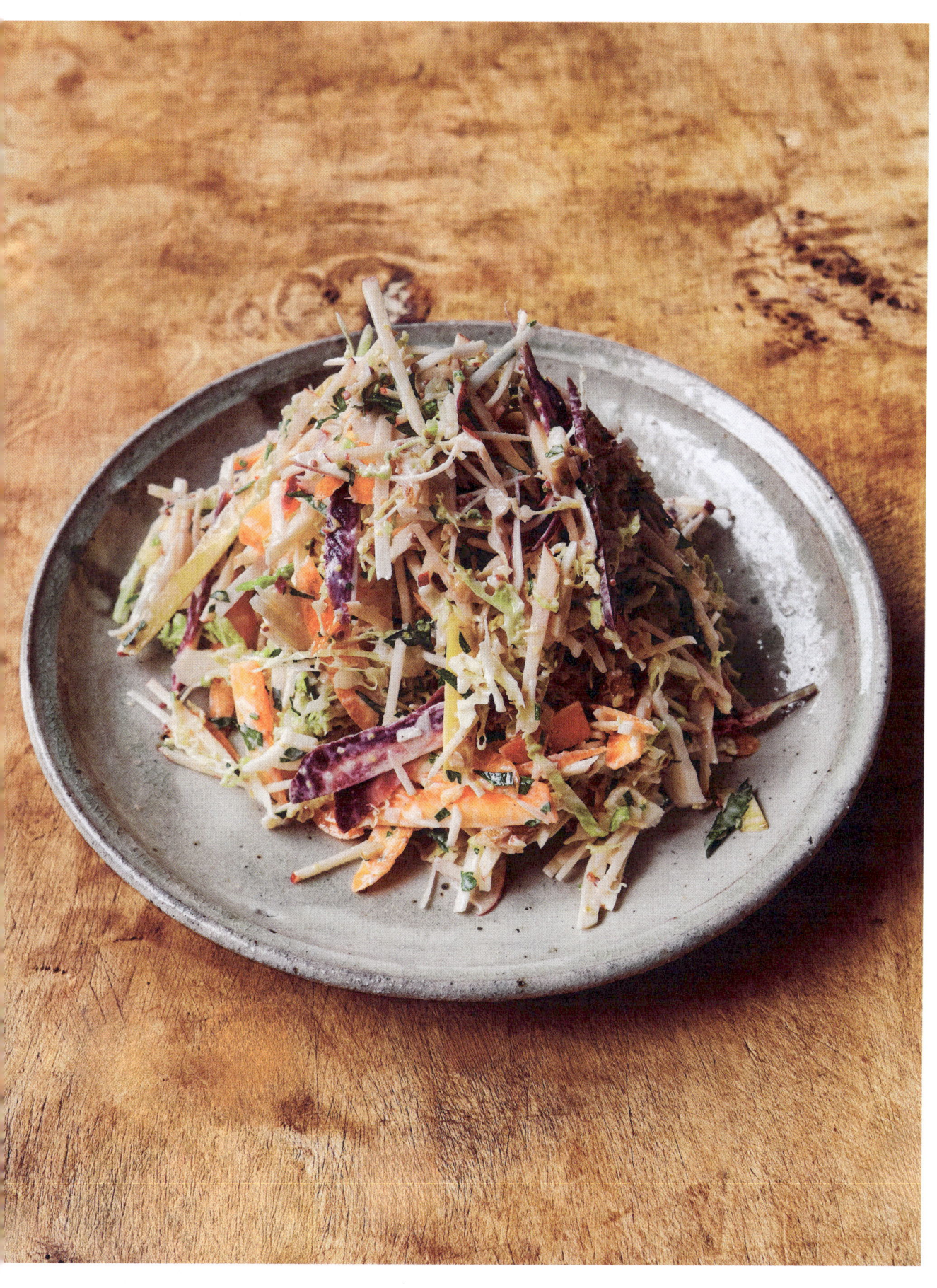

Warm lentil salad

Tasty, warm lentils, the cold crunch of salad and a creamy mustard dressing is a classy combo

SERVES 2
9 MINUTES

1 red onion (160g)

1 clove of garlic

160g ripe mixed-colour tomatoes

½ a bunch of basil (15g)

2 teaspoons Dijon mustard

½ a lemon

2 tablespoons balsamic vinegar

1 x 400g tin of lentils

½ a soft round lettuce

4 baby mozzarella balls

1. Put a large non-stick frying pan on a high heat with a spritz of olive oil. Peel, very finely slice and add the onion and garlic, stirring regularly for 5 minutes.

2. Meanwhile, slice, halve or quarter the tomatoes and place in serving bowls. Pick and reserve the baby basil leaves, then finely slice the rest, stalks and all. In a bowl, whisk the mustard with the lemon juice and 2 tablespoons of extra virgin olive oil, then season to perfection to make a dressing.

3. Stir the balsamic and lentils, juice and all, into the pan. As soon as the lentils are bubbling, mash half of them to achieve a creamier texture. Toss in the sliced basil, season to perfection and spoon over the tomatoes.

4. Click apart the washed lettuce, divide between the bowls, tear over the mozzarella, drizzle over the dressing and sprinkle over the reserved basil leaves. Use the lettuce leaves as a receptacle to scoop a bit of everything up. Nice with a bit of crusty wholemeal bread on the side.

VEGAN LOVE

Simply ditch the mozzarella or swap in a bit of vegan yoghurt or vegan feta.

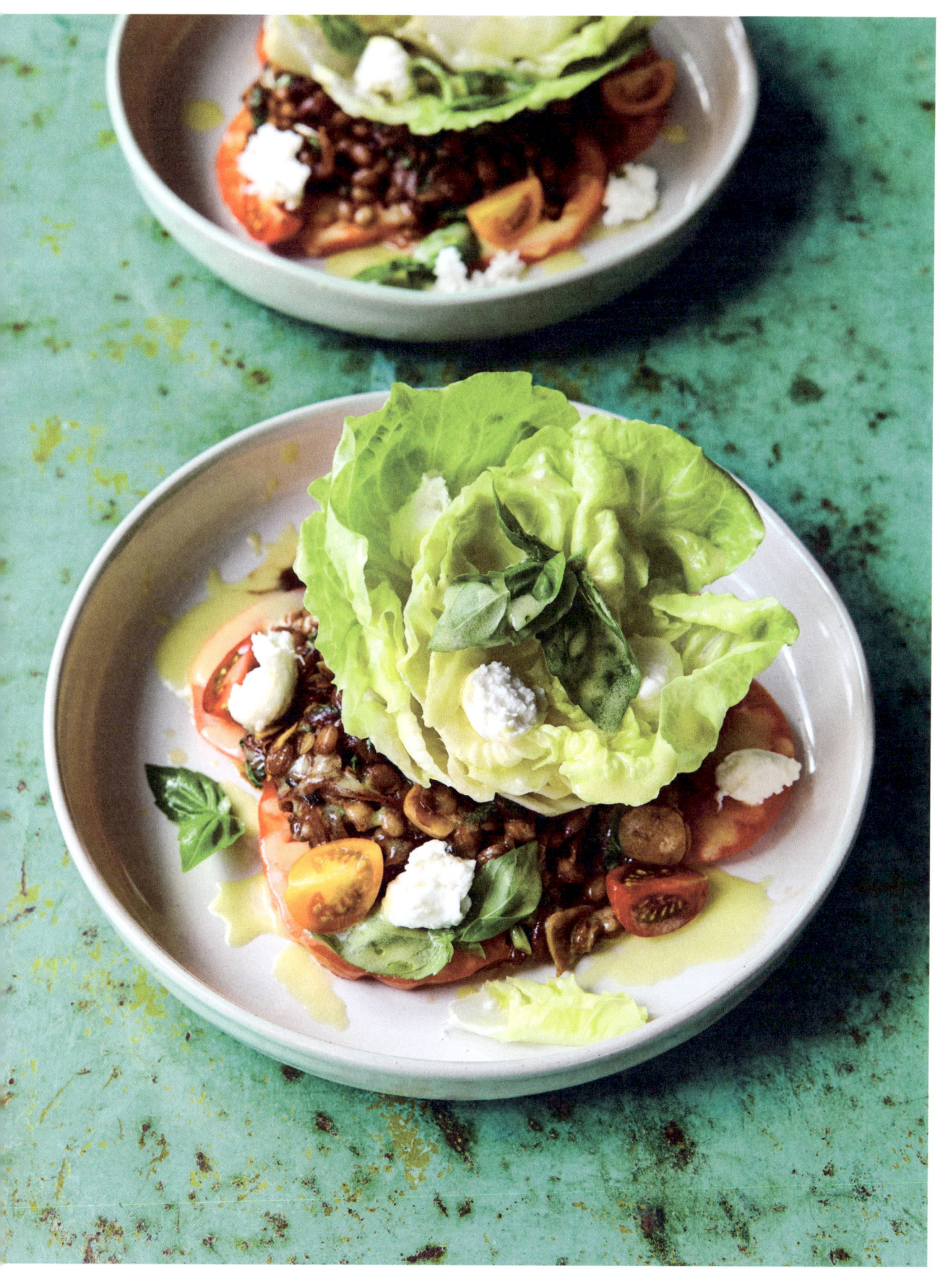

Harissa tuna platter

This pretty no-cook assembly salad is full of vibrancy, joy, big taste and texture

SERVES 2
9 MINUTES

2 spring onions

1 small bulb of fennel (160g)

2 carrots (160g)

1 lemon

1 clementine

2 tablespoons crispy fried onions

1 x 220g jar of tuna in olive oil or 1 x 145g tin of tuna in spring water

4 tablespoons Greek yoghurt

4 teaspoons harissa paste

8 oatcakes

1 Trim and very finely slice the spring onions, fennel, reserving any leafy tops, and carrot (I like to use a speed-peeler to peel the carrot into ribbons), then toss it all with half the lemon juice. Peel the clementine and slice into rounds. Arrange it all on your serving plates and scatter over the crispy onions.

2 Drain and flake over the tuna. Dollop over the yoghurt and ripple with the harissa. Sprinkle over any reserved fennel tops and drizzle with a little extra virgin olive oil. Serve with oatcakes and lemon wedges, for squeezing over.

EASY SWAPS

Tuna is the perfect companion in this salad, but you can swap in other tinned fish, such as salmon or mackerel, if you prefer.

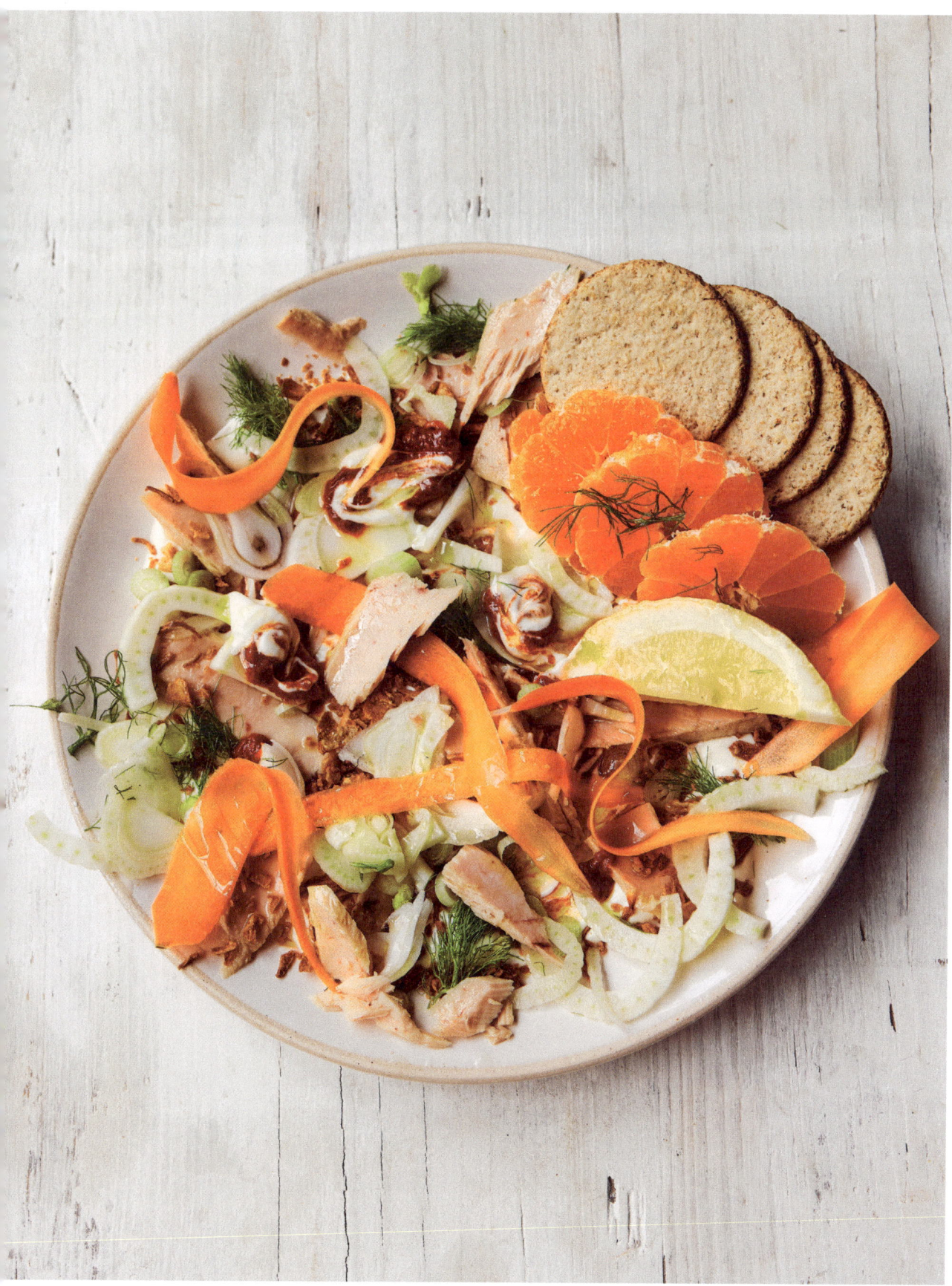

Curried fried eggs & grain salad

I love adding extra value to cooked grain packets for a tasty, quick, working-from-home lunch

SERVES 2
10 MINUTES

1 x 250g packet of cooked mixed grains

2 carrots (160g)

2 little gem lettuces

½ a bunch of mint (15g)

1 lemon

½–1 fresh red chilli

1 teaspoon curry powder, plus extra for sprinkling

4 eggs

2 heaped tablespoons mango chutney

2 heaped tablespoons natural yoghurt

1 Heat the grains according to the packet instructions. Wash the carrot, then coarsely grate on a box grater. Trim and shred the lettuce. Pick the mint, slicing the larger leaves, then put it all into a large bowl.

2 Tip in the hot grains, toss together, then dress it all with the lemon juice, season to perfection and divide between two serving bowls.

3 Put a frying pan on a medium heat with 1 tablespoon of olive oil. Finely chop and sprinkle in the chilli, along with the curry powder. When it starts to sizzle, crack in the eggs, season with sea salt, black pepper, and an extra pinch of curry powder, then cover the pan. Leave to fry and coddle to your liking, while you ripple the mango chutney through the yoghurt. Plate up the eggs, and serve with the jazzed-up yoghurt.

VEG BOOST

Feel free to mix up the veg, swapping in mangetout, cucumber or spring onions in place of some of the lettuce, or even adding extra for a boost!

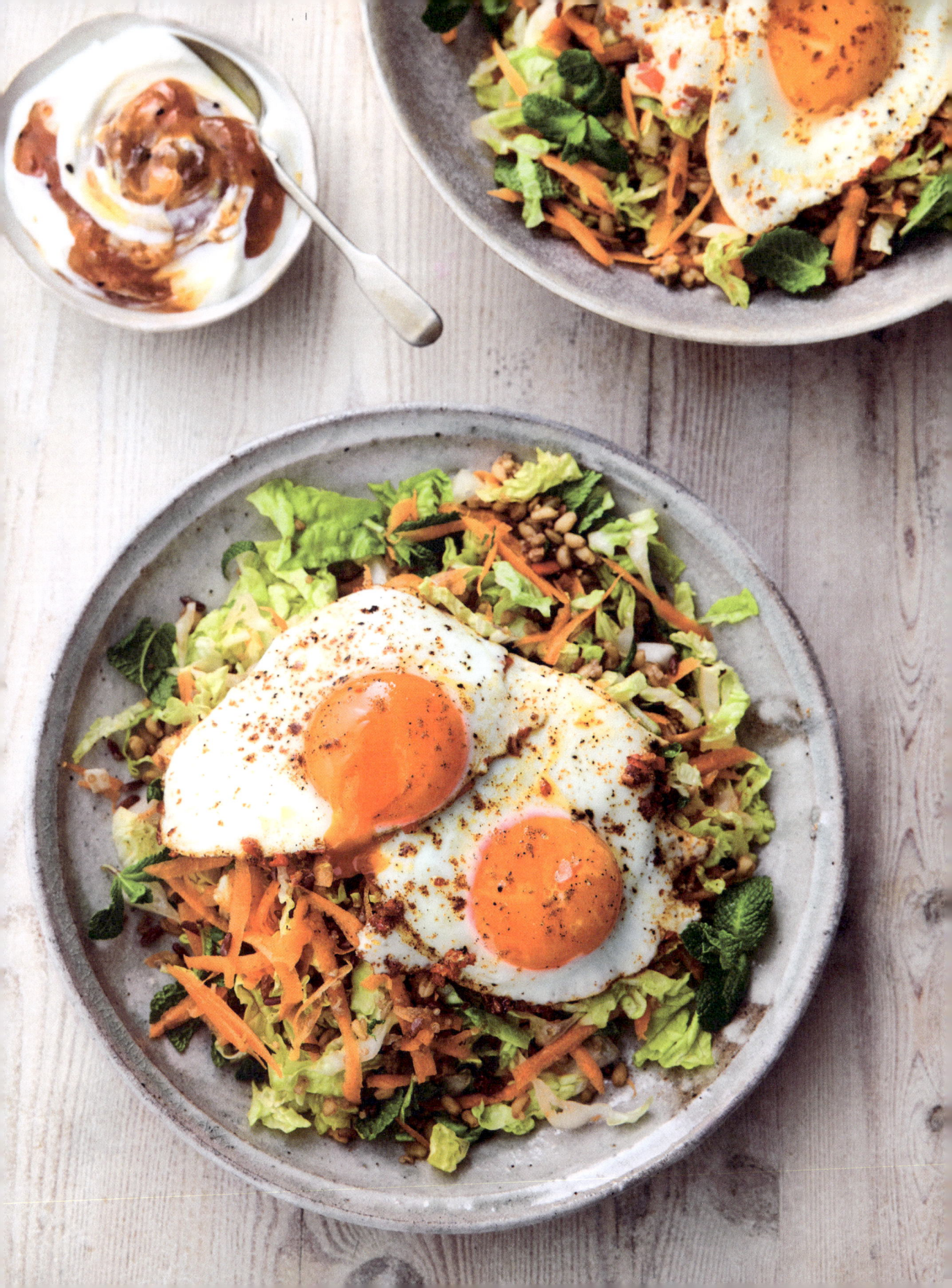

Speedy silky omelette

A great lunch, or perfect anytime of the day, this simple one-pan wonder is sure to hit the spot

SERVES 1
10 MINUTES

80g asparagus

80g ripe cherry tomatoes

1 x 400g tin of cannellini beans

2 black olives, stone in

2 sprigs of basil

2 medium eggs

15g Parmesan cheese

1 Trim the woody ends off the asparagus and place the spears in a dry non-stick frying pan on a high heat with the tomatoes. Cook for 4 minutes, or until starting to char, tossing occasionally, then remove the asparagus.

2 Pour in the beans, juice and all, add 1 teaspoon of red wine vinegar, and boil down until creamy. Squash, destone and tear in the olives, tear in most of the basil, saving the nice baby leaves for garnish, toss together with the asparagus, season to perfection and pour on to your plate.

3 Working swiftly, wipe out the pan, then spritz with olive oil. Beat and pour in the eggs, swirling them around the pan. Finely grate over most of the Parmesan, by which point the eggs will be almost cooked, so turn the heat off. Angle the pan and use a rubber spatula to gently ease the omelette away from the edges, folding it up a few times, then slide on to your plate.

4 Finely grate over the remaining Parmesan and scatter over the reserved basil leaves. I like to add a dash of chilli sauce, and a slice of wholemeal toast.

EASY SWAPS

Borlotti or butter beans would also be delicious here.

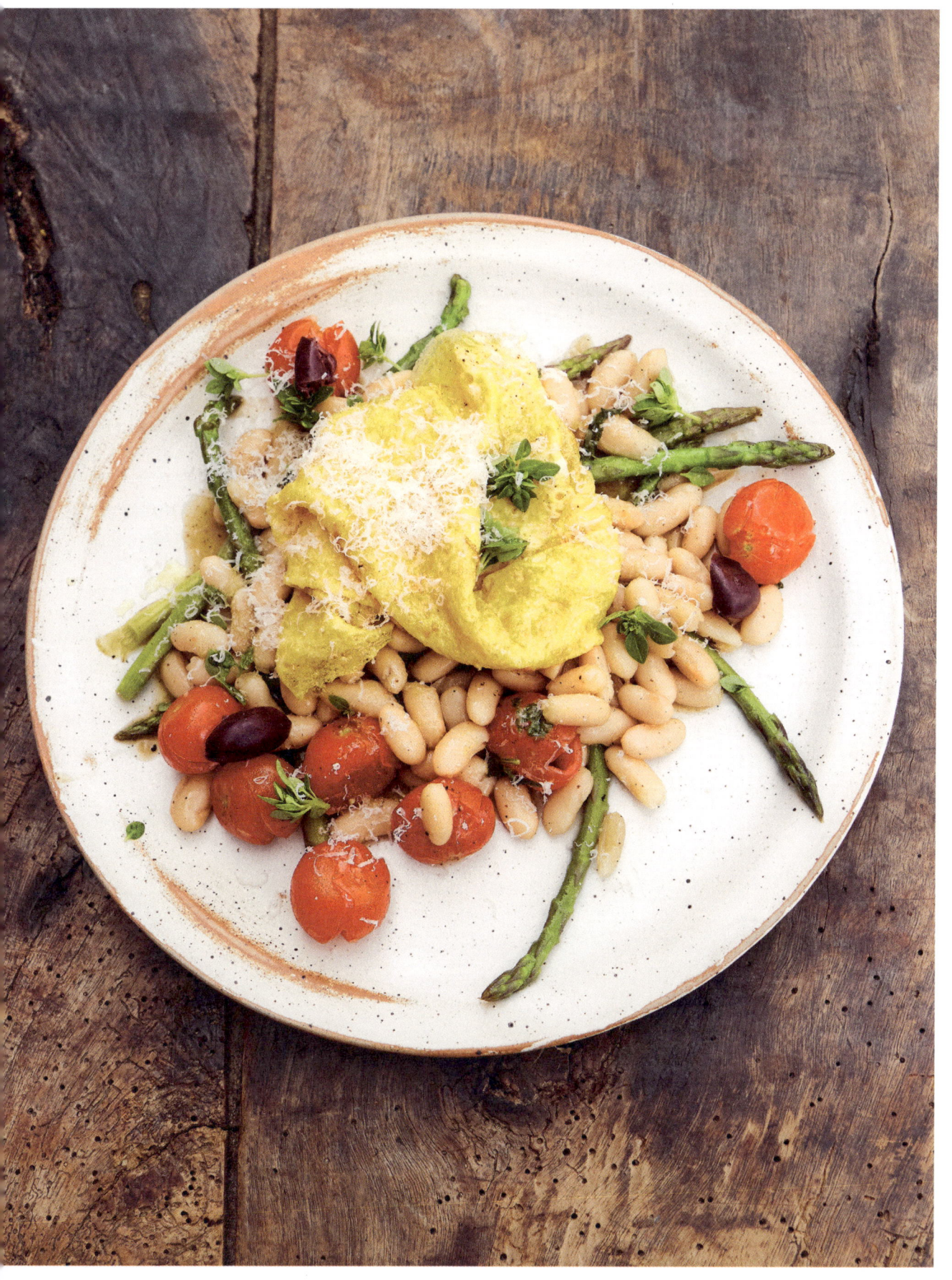

Prawn & noodle salad

Vibrant and joyful, this is all about contrast – think sweet, salty, charred, crunchy, soft

SERVES 2
10 MINUTES

250g ripe mixed-colour cherry tomatoes

1 x 410g tin of peach slices in juice

1 lime

½ a bunch of mint (15g)

2 nests of instant vermicelli rice noodles (90g total)

160g mangetout

165g raw peeled king prawns

1 tablespoon low-salt soy sauce

1 teaspoon crunchy peanut & sesame chilli oil, plus extra to serve

1. Boil the kettle. Halve the tomatoes, drain and chop the peaches. Place three-quarters of it all in a large bowl and finely grate over the lime zest. Reserving the baby mint leaves, finely chop the rest and add to the bowl.

2. In another bowl, just cover the noodles with boiling kettle water and leave to rehydrate for a few minutes, then drain and add to the large bowl.

3. Char the mangetout and prawns in a dry non-stick frying pan on a high heat for 4 minutes, or until cooked through, tossing regularly. Add to the salad.

4. Place the reserved tomato and peach chunks in a blender with the soy, lime juice and chilli oil. Blitz until smooth, season to perfection and pour over the salad, then gently toss together. Serve scattered with the baby mint leaves and a little extra drizzle of chilli oil, if you like.

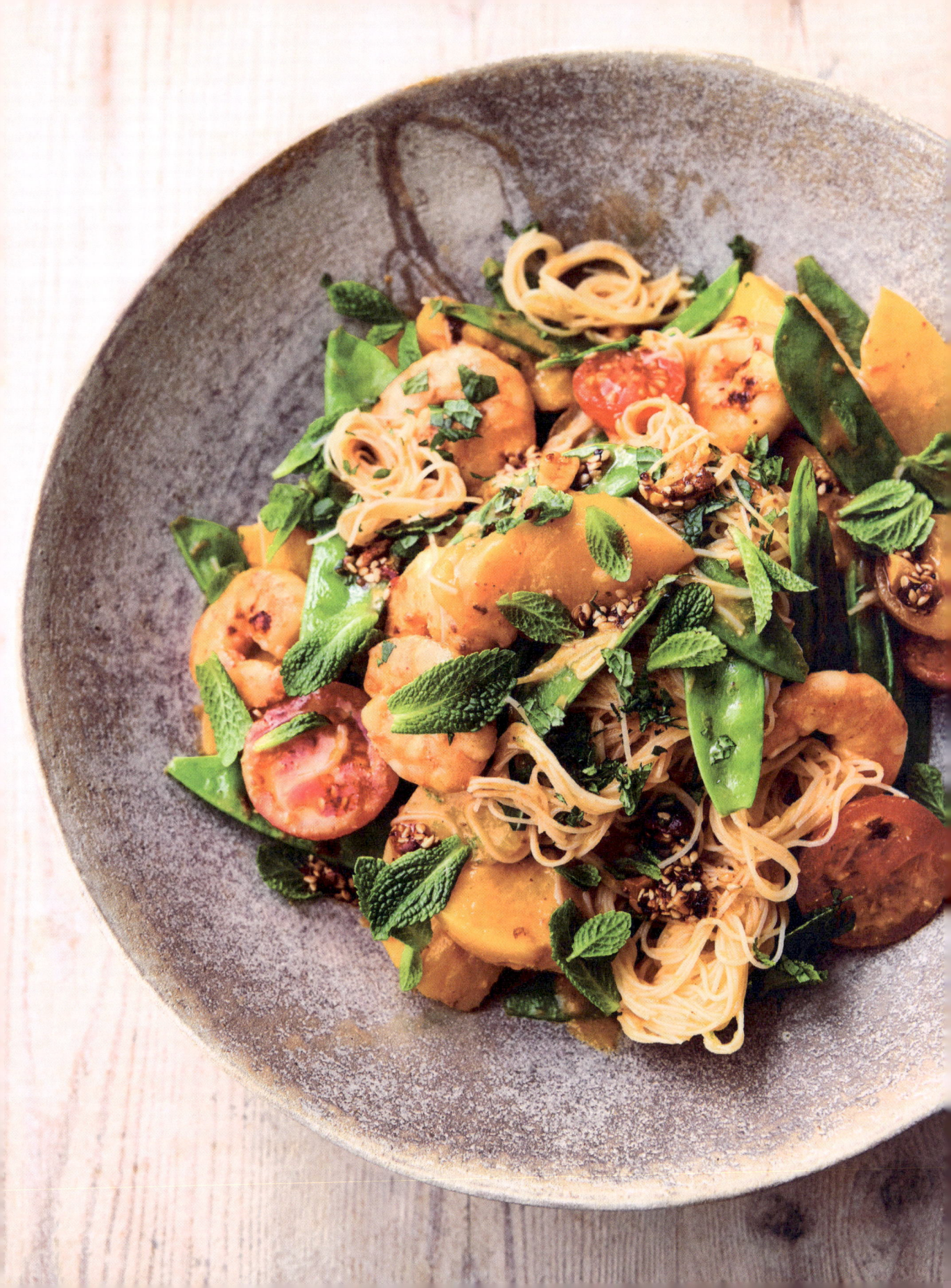

Crispy sardine & avo wrap

A fun mix of flavour and texture – hot, cold, smooth, crunchy, fragrant, zingy and chilli heat

SERVES 1
10 MINUTES

1 x 105g tin of sardines in spring water

1 pinch of fennel seeds

½–1 fresh red chilli

1 large wholemeal tortilla

1 ripe tomato (80g)

1 lime

80g white cabbage

½ a small ripe avocado (80g)

1 tablespoon cottage cheese

2 sprigs of coriander

1. Drain the sardines, place in a large non-stick frying pan, spritz with olive oil, sprinkle over the fennel seeds, then finely slice and add half the chilli. Cook on a high heat for 5 minutes, or until golden and crisp, shaking occasionally and warming the tortilla on top for just the last minute.

2. Meanwhile, halve the tomato and finely grate cut side down into a bowl with the remaining chilli, discarding the tomato skin. Squeeze in half the lime juice, then season to perfection. Coarsely grate the cabbage, dress with the remaining lime juice and season. Halve, destone, peel and slice the avocado.

3. Place the warm tortilla on your plate, dollop over the cottage cheese, scatter over the cabbage and avo, sit the crispy sardines and chilli on top, then spoon over the tomato salsa and pick over the coriander. Enjoy!

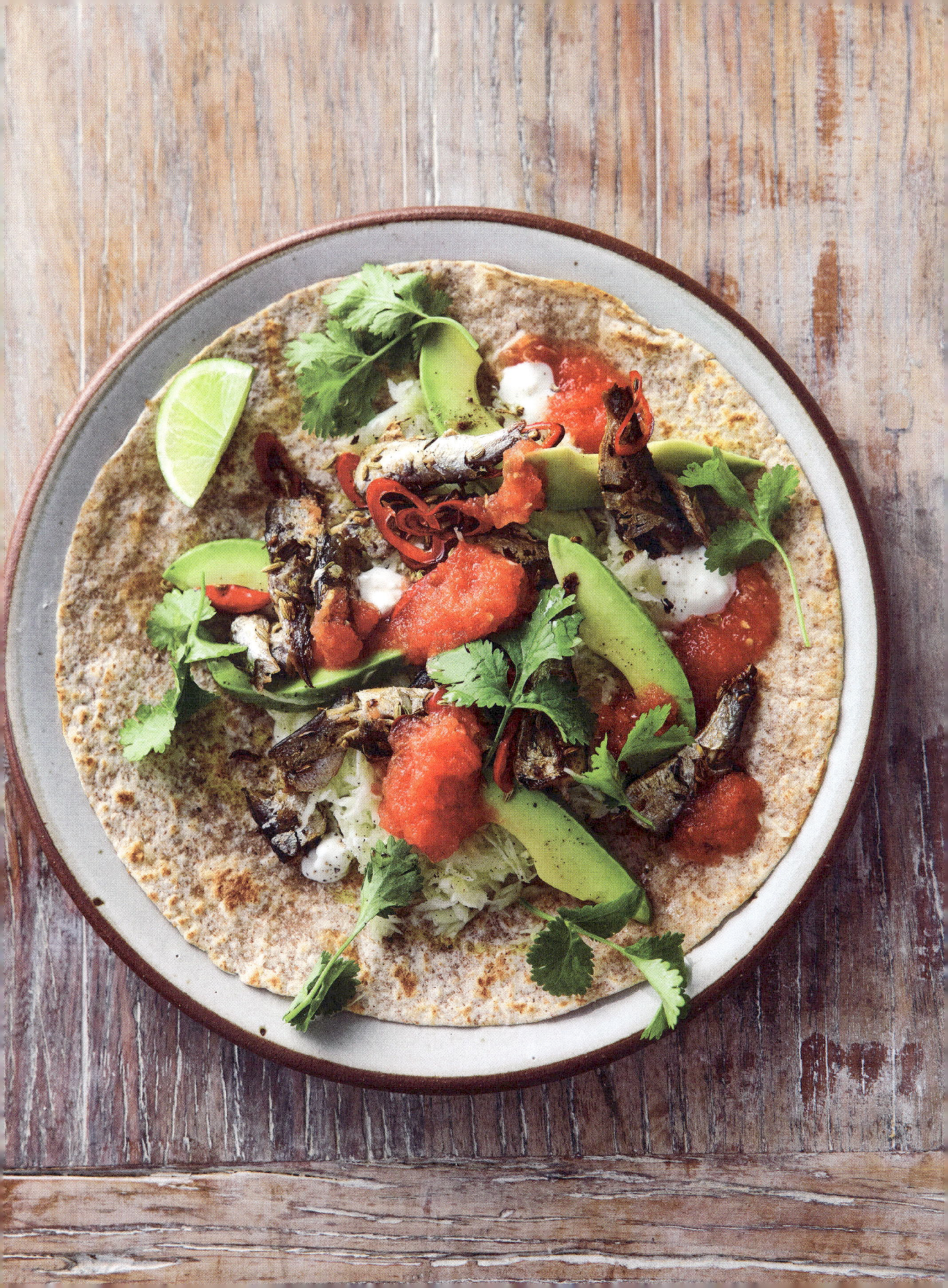

Chopped rainbow salad

SERVES 1 | 11 MINUTES

80g each
pomegranate seeds, yellow pepper, ripe tomatoes, red onion, cucumber, tinned chickpeas, radishes, ripe avocado, little gem lettuce

30g dried mango

½ a bunch of mint (15g)

1 lime

Leaving the chickpeas and pomegranate seeds whole, trim, peel or deseed and finely chop all the veg and fruit, along with the dried mango and the mint leaves, then dress with the lime juice and 1 tablespoon of extra virgin olive oil. Season to perfection with sea salt and black pepper, and serve. Delicious just as it is, or paired with couscous or a steaming jacket potato.

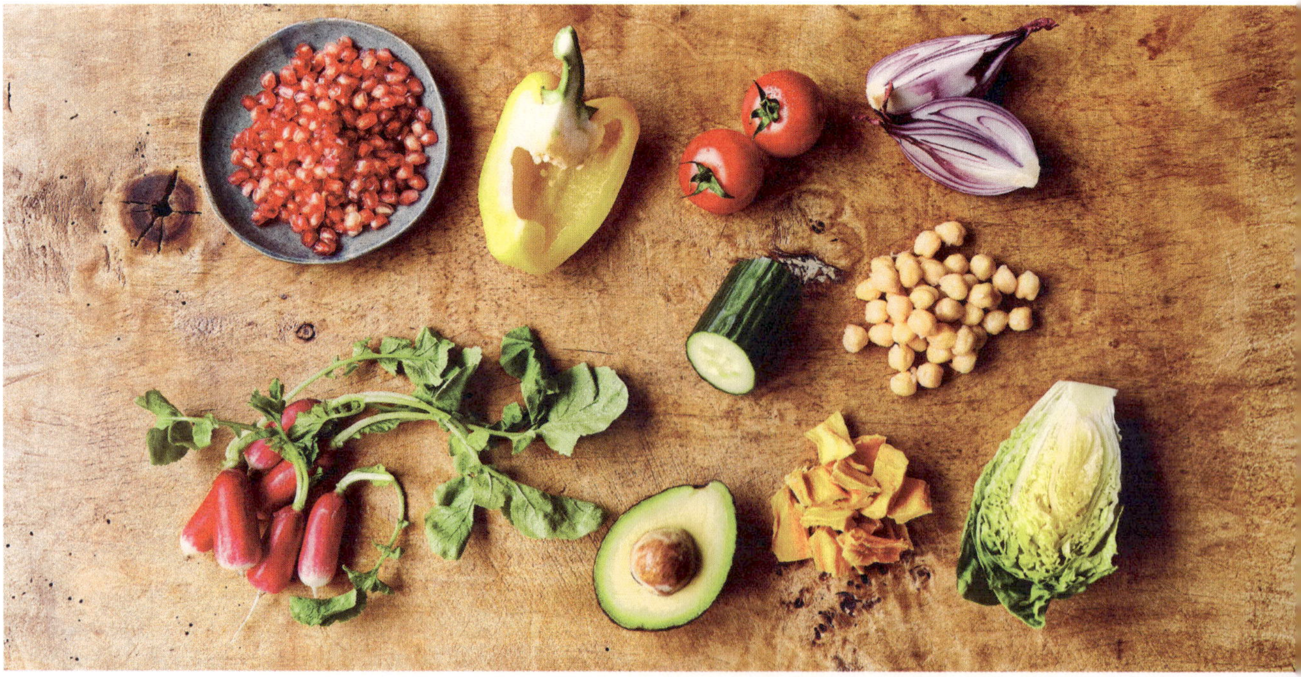

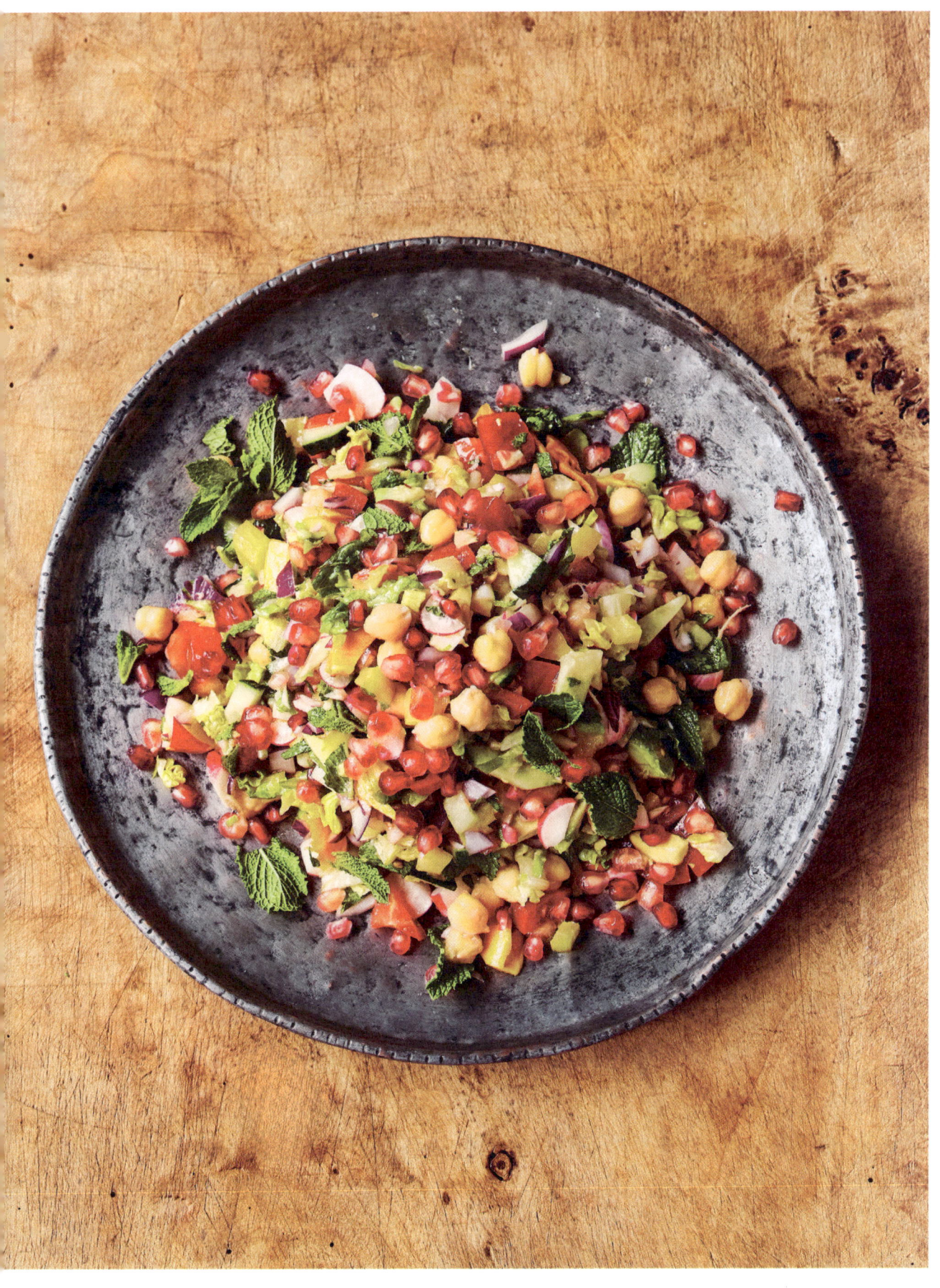

Salmon, beet & potato salad

Packet, tinned and smoked items unite in this simple but vibrant, fun and tasty meal

SERVES 2
11 MINUTES

280g vac-packed beetroot

1 x 567g tin of peeled new potatoes

2 tablespoons Greek yoghurt

1 tablespoon wholegrain mustard or jarred grated horseradish

1 lemon

1 bunch of dill (20g)

4 spring onions

½ cucumber (160g)

2 x 90g fillets of hot-smoked salmon or trout

4 multigrain Ryvita or other crispbread

1 Still in their packet, squash the beets, then empty into a large bowl, draining away any excess juice. Drain, roughly chop and add the potatoes, along with the yoghurt and mustard or horseradish. Finely grate in the lemon zest and squeeze in half the juice. Finely chop the dill, add most to the bowl, mix well, season to perfection, then divide between your plates.

2 Trim and finely slice the spring onions. Squash along the length of the cucumber with the heel of your hand, then roughly chop it and toss with the spring onions and 1 tablespoon each of red wine vinegar and extra virgin olive oil. Season to perfection, and add to your plates.

3 Flake over the salmon, sprinkle over the remaining dill, and crack over the Ryvita. Tuck in as is, or toss it all together before digging in, giving a range of soggy and crispy bits of Ryvita, which is really rather delicious.

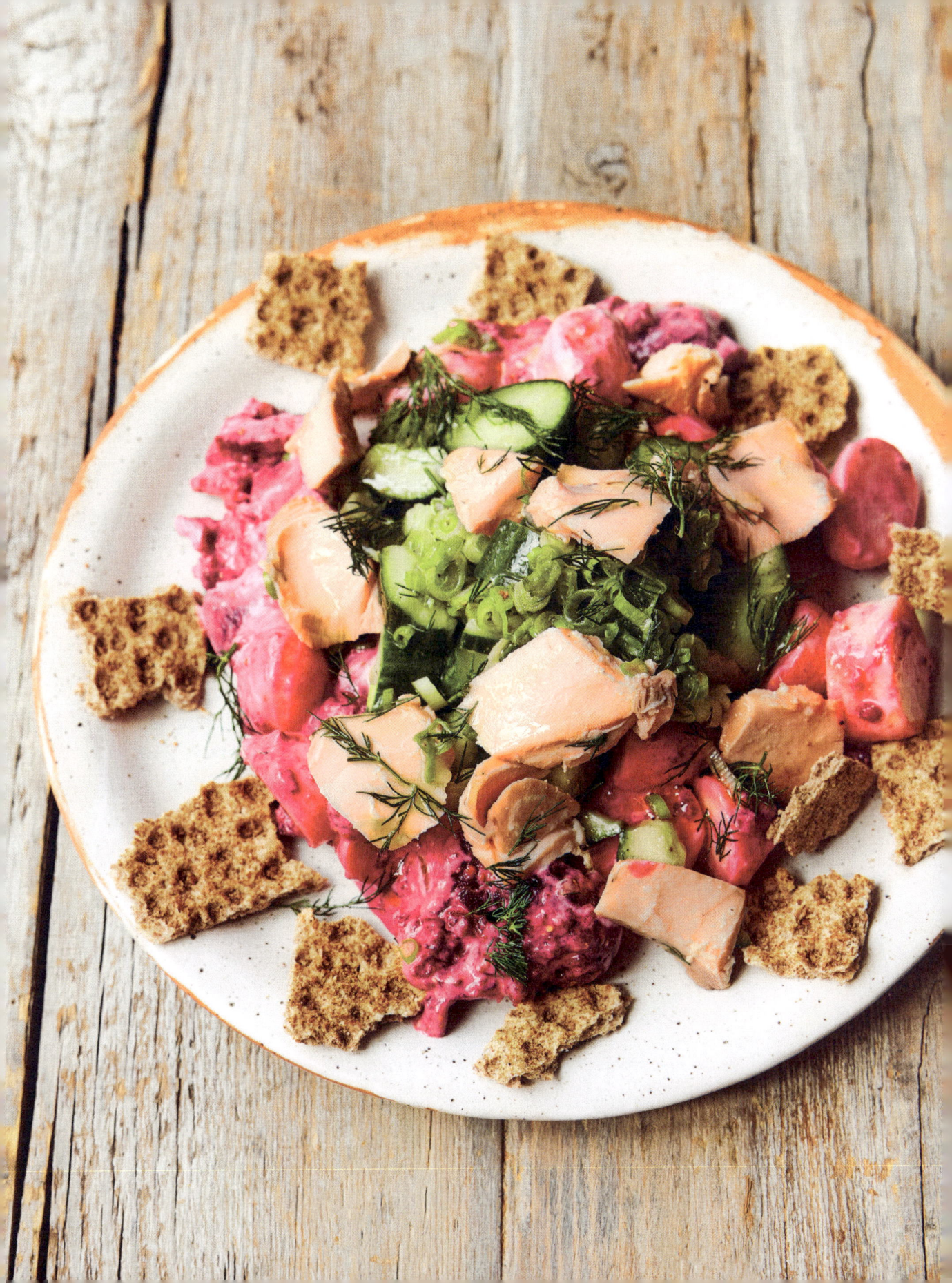

Sardines on toast & tomato salad

I love making simple working lunches like this that are colourful, tasty and big up tinned oily fish

SERVES 2
11 MINUTES

1 red onion (160g)

1 fresh red chilli

1 small bulb of fennel (160g)

1 x 400g tin of cannellini beans

160g jarred roasted red peppers

300g ripe mixed-colour cherry tomatoes

8 black olives, stone in

2 slices of wholemeal sourdough bread

1 x 105g tin of sardines in spring water

1 Peel the onion, deseed the chilli and trim the fennel, reserving any leafy tops. Very finely slice or speed-peel it all, place in a large bowl with 2 tablespoons each of red wine vinegar and extra virgin olive oil, and massage well.

2 Drain and add the beans, slice and add the peppers. Chop and add the tomatoes. Destone and tear in the olives, then mix really well and season to perfection with sea salt and black pepper.

3 Toast the bread. Drain the sardines (I like to toss the liquor into the salad), arrange on the toasts, sprinkle with any reserved fennel tops and divide between your plates. Finish with a drizzle of extra virgin olive oil, to serve.

EASY SWAPS

Swap out the tinned sardines for tuna or mackerel, or go veggie and use baby mozzarella balls or goat's cheese in place of the fish.

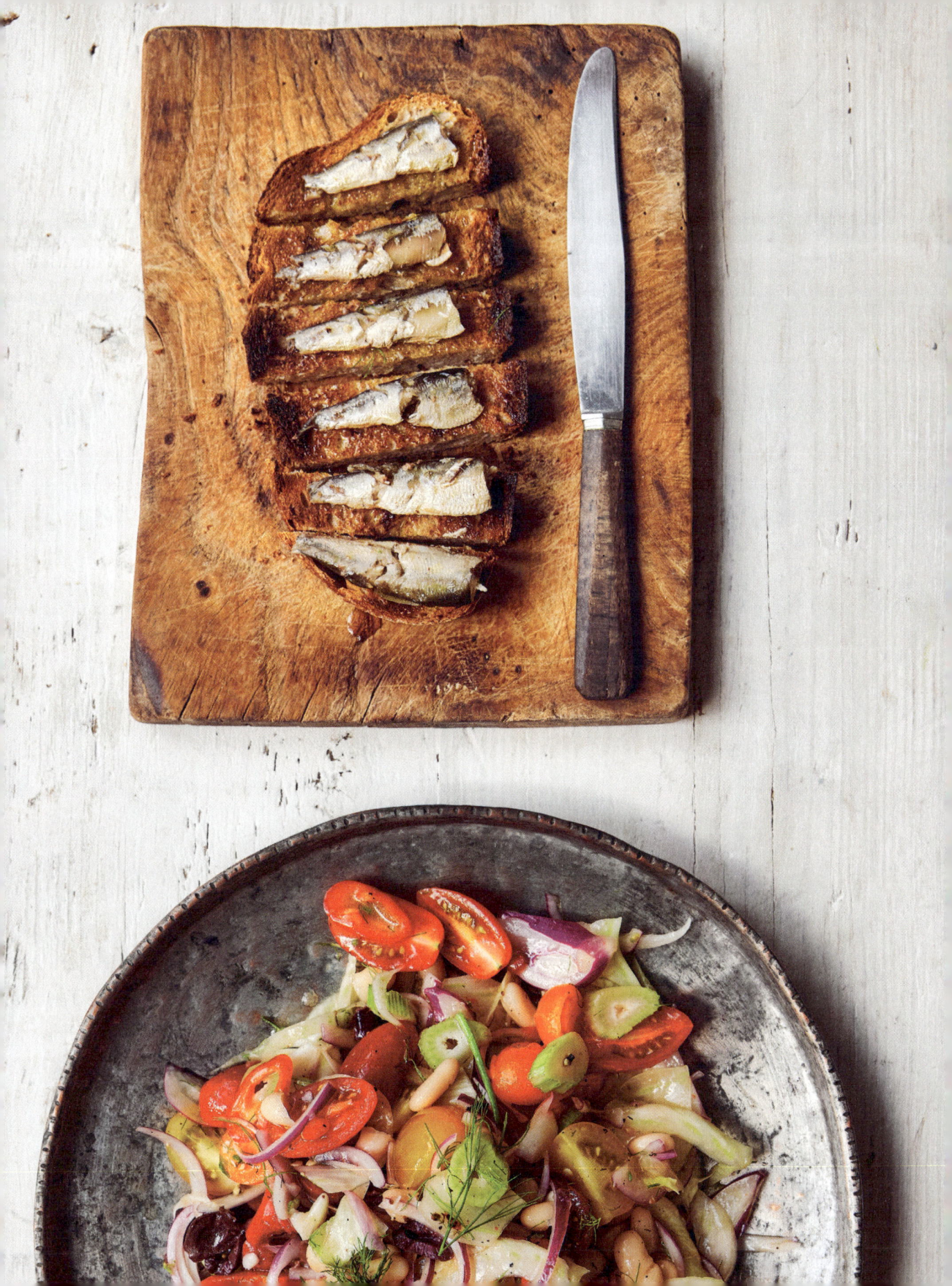

Sesame miso shred salad

SERVES 1 | 12 MINUTES

80g each
sugar snap peas, white cabbage, yellow pepper, carrot, asparagus

1 fresh red chilli

1 lime

1 heaped teaspoon tahini

1 heaped teaspoon white miso

1 heaped teaspoon toasted sesame seeds

2 sprigs of coriander

Trim or deseed the veg, as needed, then finely shred it all with a speed-peeler, or by hand with good knife skills. Finely chop the chilli (deseed if you like), then gently scrunch it all in the lime juice, tahini, miso and 1 tablespoon of extra virgin olive oil. Season to perfection, then scatter over the sesame seeds and pick over the coriander. Great with wholegrain rice or noodles, if you like.

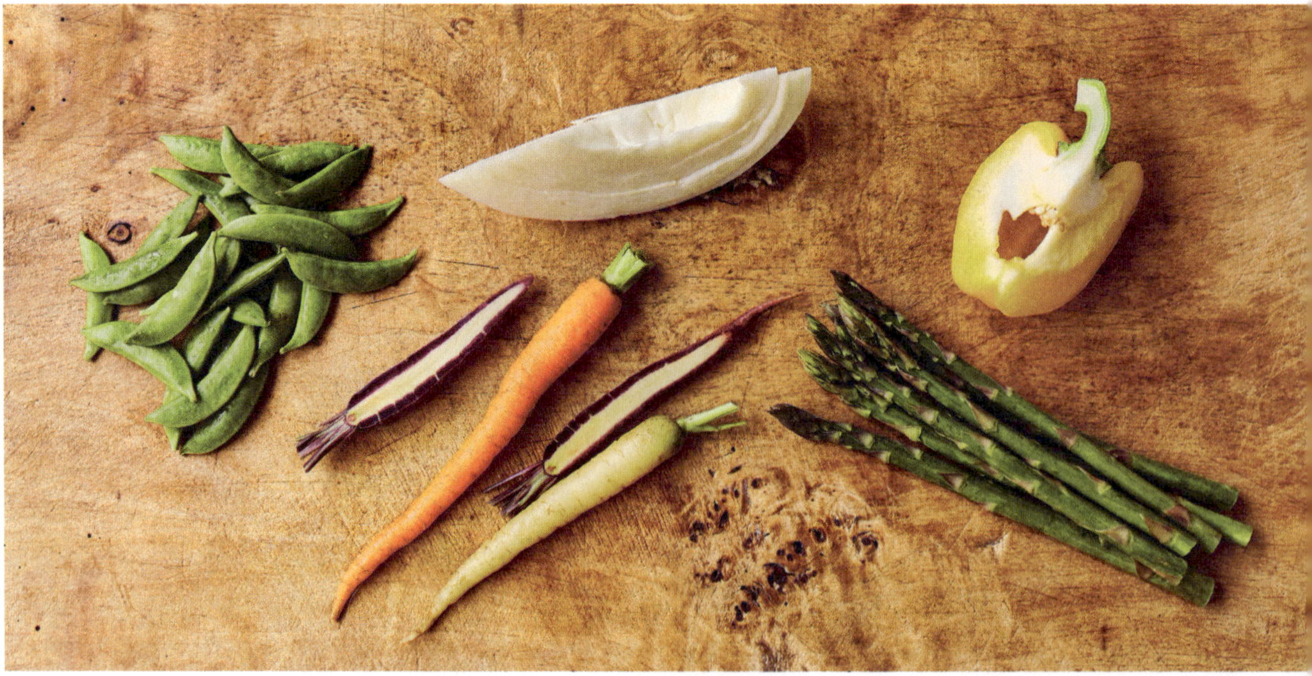

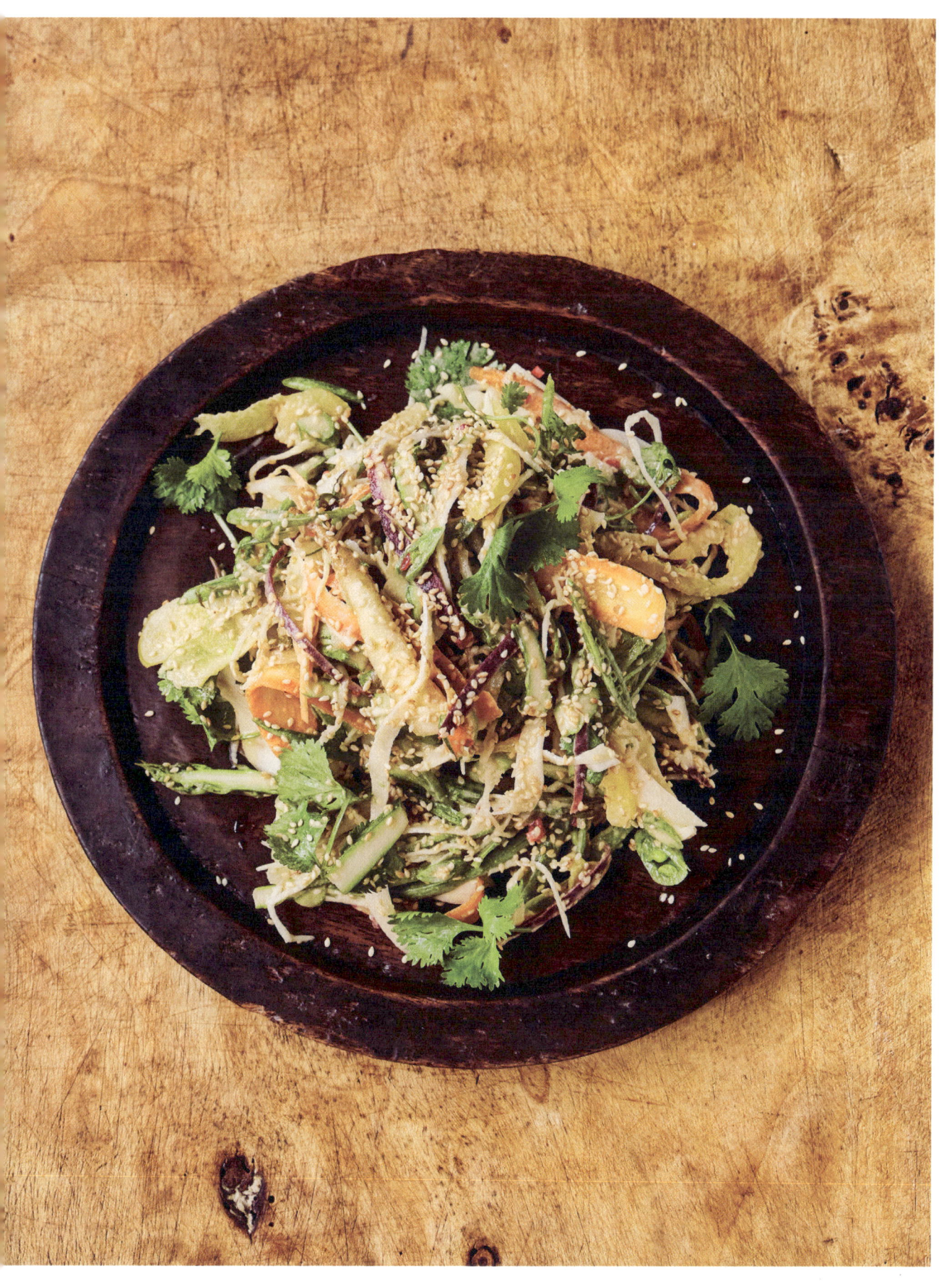

Black bean houmous salad wrap

Making a kinda houmous from different nutritious beans is a great flavour and health hack

SERVES 2
12 MINUTES

1 x 400g tin of black beans

1 tablespoon tahini

1 lime

½ a clove of garlic

160g radishes

1 small ripe avocado (160g)

1 ripe beef tomato (160g)

2 large seeded wholewheat tortillas

1 teaspoon dukkah

30g feta cheese

1 Put the beans into a blender, reserving the juice. Add the tahini, finely grate and reserve the lime zest, then squeeze in the juice. Peel and add the garlic, then blitz until smooth, loosening to your desired consistency with splashes of bean juice, if needed. Season to perfection.

2 Lightly crush the radishes. Halve, destone, peel and slice the avocado. Gently toss with 1 tablespoon of red wine vinegar and ½ a tablespoon of extra virgin olive oil, and season to perfection. Slice the tomato.

3 Warm the tortillas, slather on the houmous, then pile on all the veg, sprinkle over the lime zest and dukkah, and crumble over the feta. Finish with a little drizzle of extra virgin olive oil, if you like, and get stuck in.

EASY SWAPS

Swap out the radishes for baby carrots, courgettes or beets, or a mixture!

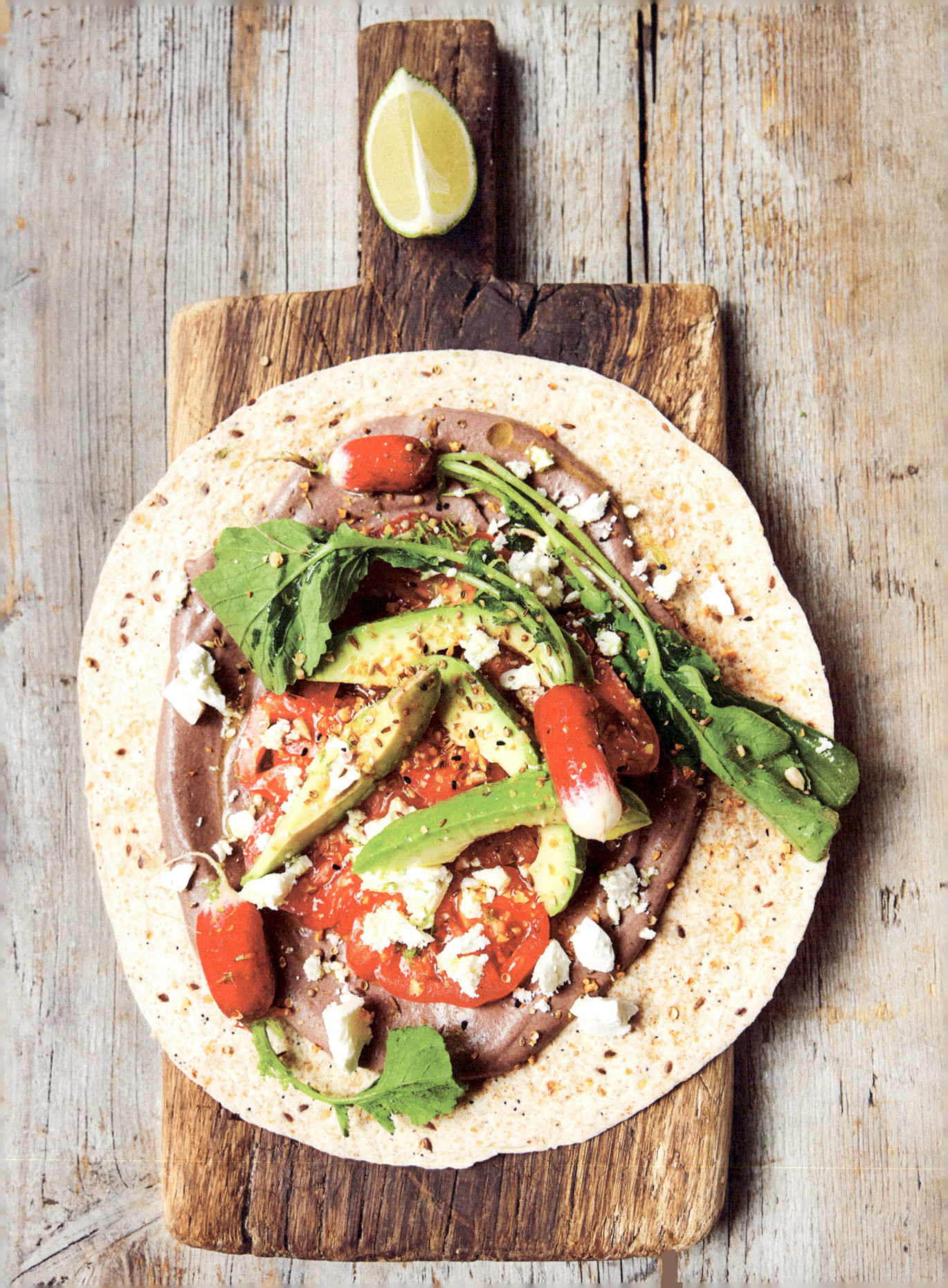

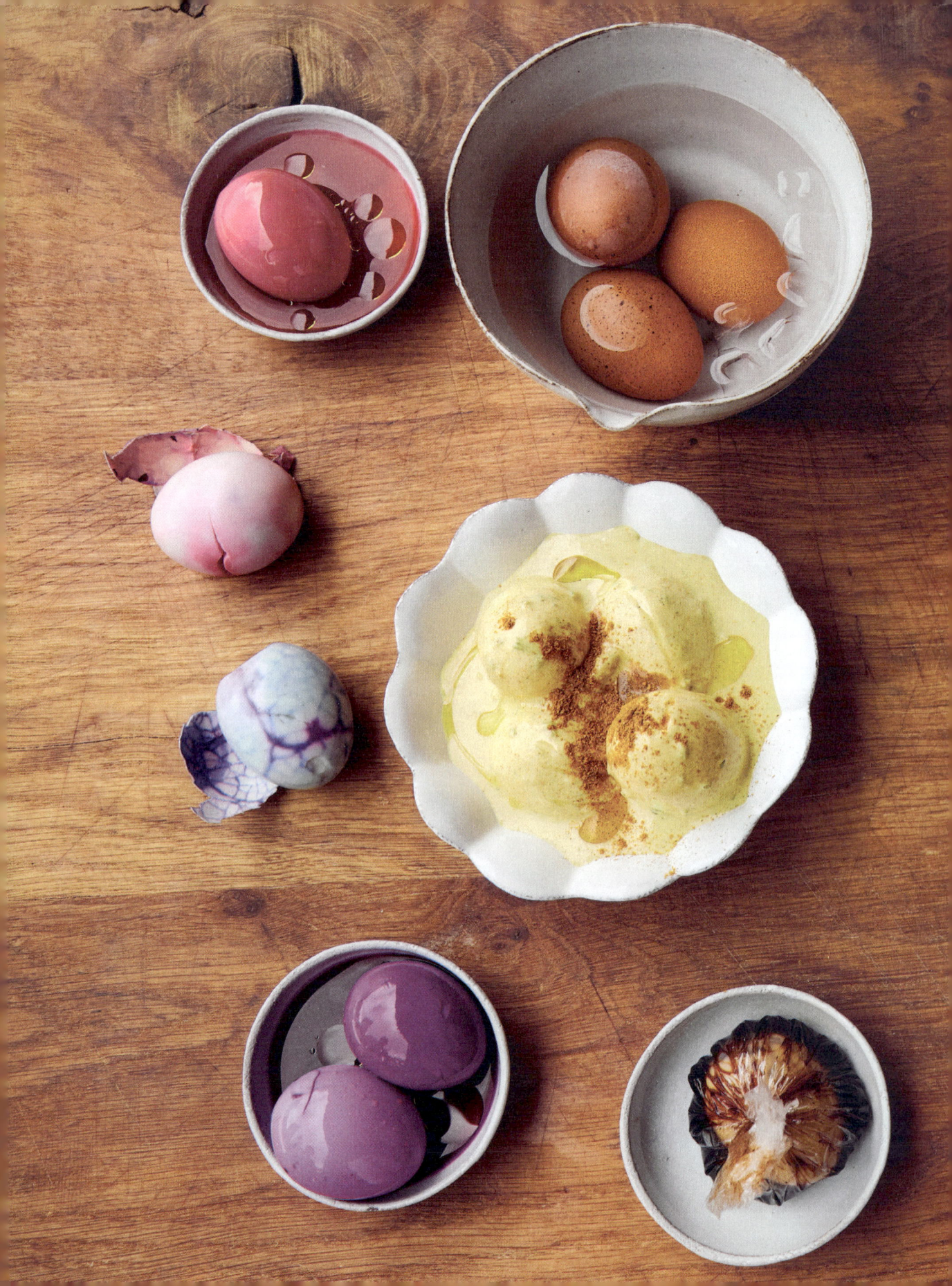

BONUS HACK

Boiled egg fridge stash

Having boiled eggs in the fridge ready to go is really handy for putting quick meals together; from salads and sandwiches to ramens and noodle dishes, there's so much you can use them for. If I put 6 boiled eggs in the fridge at home, they're always gone within a day.

You can have a bit of fun by marinating them in a 50/50 water and soy sauce mix, or in the leftover pickling liquor from jarred beetroot or red cabbage. It gives a very subtle, delicious flavour, and they look incredible, too, depending on how long you marinate them for (just 30 minutes for a light pickle, or up to 2 days in the fridge). Before submerging, either peel them, or simply crack the shell multiple times, which will create a marbled effect. You can also try marinating them in a curried yoghurt mixture (see recipe, page 118). Once removed from the marinade, they'll keep in the fridge for up to 3 days.

Fluffy spring veg omelette

Tasty omelettes are a great vehicle for getting more veg into your life. Get creative!

SERVES 1
12 MINUTES

2 spring onions

80g baby spinach

80g asparagus

2 sprigs of mint

2 eggs

2 teaspoons harissa paste

2 tablespoons cottage cheese

2 small slices of seeded sourdough bread

½ a lemon

1. Put a medium non-stick frying pan on a high heat with a good spritz of olive oil. Trim, finely slice and add the spring onions, then the spinach, tossing regularly. Trim the woody ends off the asparagus, then roughly chop the spears, leaving the tips whole, and add both to the pan. Pick in most of the mint and cook for 3 minutes, or until starting to soften, stirring regularly.

2. Meanwhile, crack the eggs into a large bowl and whisk with a pinch of sea salt and black pepper until frothy and doubled in size.

3. Tip the veg into the frothy eggs, fold through with half the harissa, then spritz the empty pan with oil and pour the mixture back in. Spread it out and cook gently on a very low heat for 5 minutes, or until almost set.

4. Spoon over the cottage cheese and remaining harissa, then use a fish slice to fold the omelette in half. Cook to your liking while you toast the bread, then slide the omelette on to a plate. Sprinkle over the remaining mint leaves, finely grate over the lemon zest, and serve with the toast.

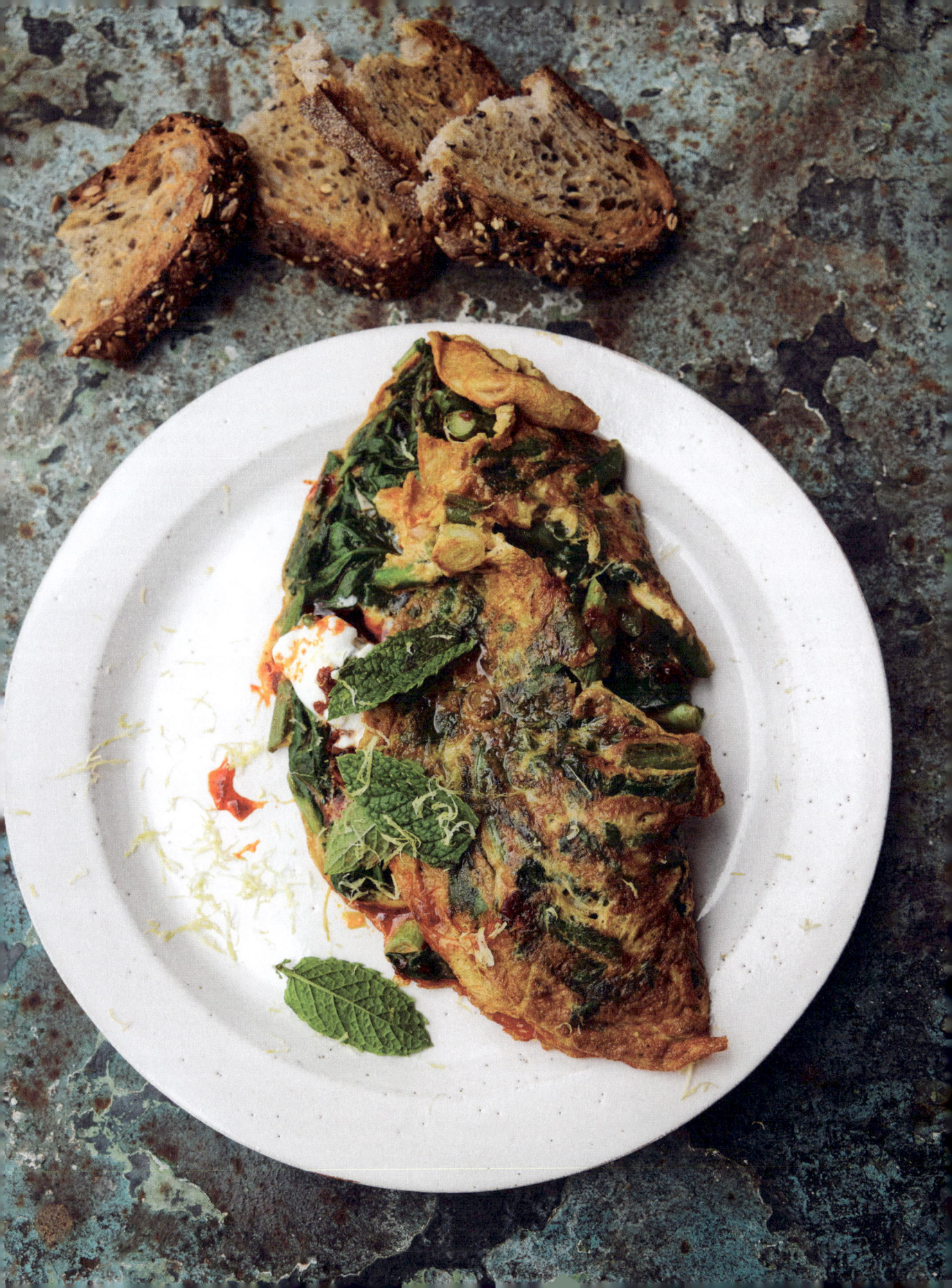

Carrot gazpacho

Refreshing, surprising and vivacious, you must try this beautiful cool soup

SERVES 1
12 MINUTES

2 carrots (160g)

80g cucumber

20g blanched almonds

160g ice cubes

1 slice of wholemeal sourdough bread (50g)

80g celery

80g ripe mixed-colour cherry tomatoes

80g mixed-colour grapes

1 sprig of mint or basil

20g feta cheese

1 Peel the carrot and cucumber, roughly chop, then place in a blender with the almonds, ice cubes and 2 tablespoons of red wine vinegar. Tear in the bread and blitz until beautifully smooth, loosening with splashes of water to achieve a soupy consistency – you may need to work in batches. Season to absolute perfection with sea salt and black pepper.

2 Trim and peel the celery, then finely dice and scrape into a serving bowl. Chop the tomatoes, slice the grapes, and scatter on top. Pick and tear over the herb leaves, crumble over the feta, then pour over the soup. Nice with an extra slice of bread on the side for dunking, if you like.

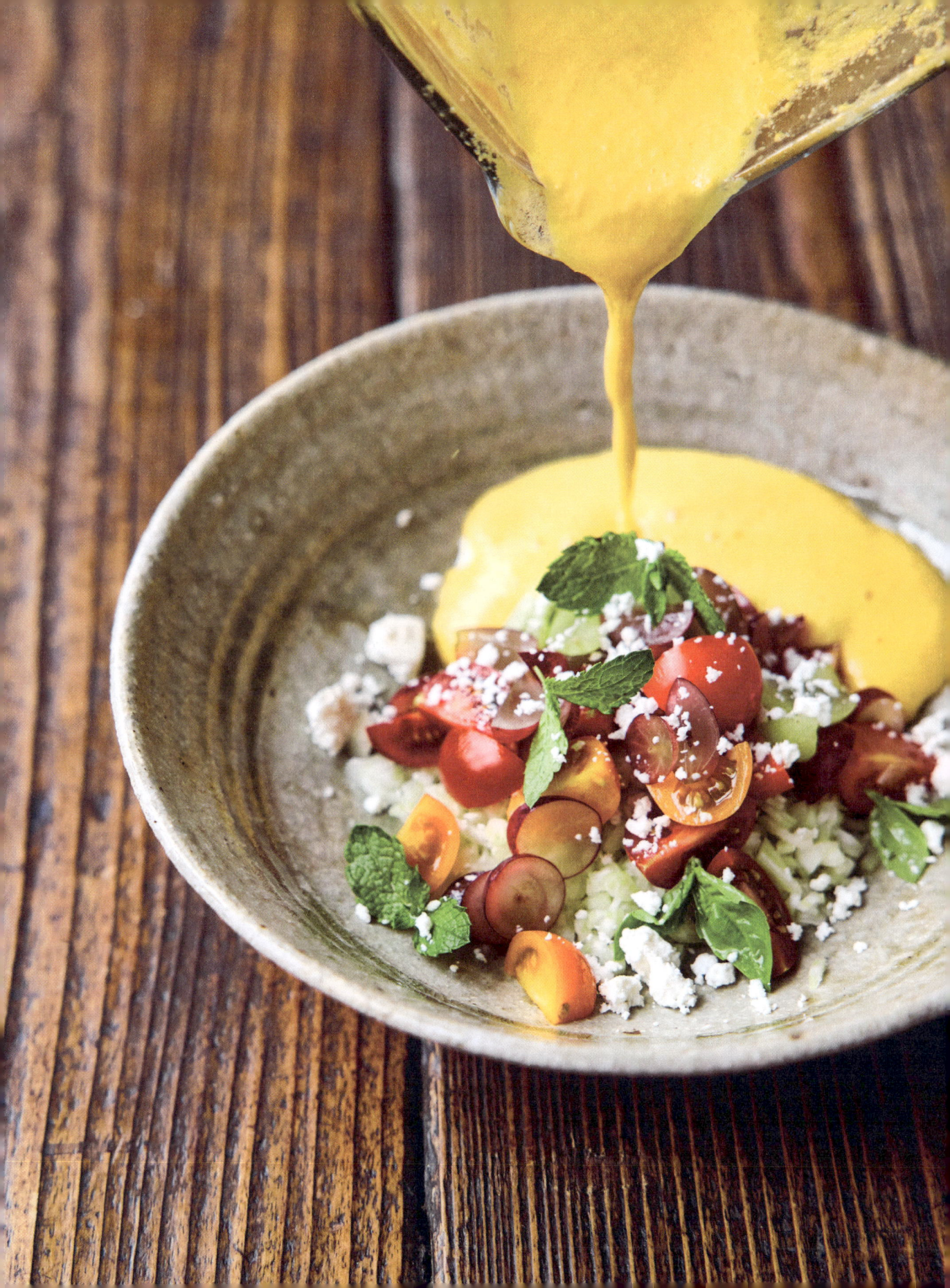

Pea & feta egg warm salad

Using freezer and store-cupboard favourites makes this tasty salad super-quick to put together

SERVES 2
12 MINUTES

160g jarred roasted red peppers

1 tablespoon balsamic vinegar

4 sprigs of mint

4 eggs

160g frozen peas

30g feta cheese

80g baby spinach

1 x 250g packet of cooked mixed grains

1 Put the jarred peppers into a blender, add the balsamic, pick in most of the mint leaves, reserving a few nice ones, then blitz until smooth, season to perfection and pour most of the sauce into a large bowl.

2 Put a large non-stick frying pan on a medium-high heat. Spritz with olive oil, crack in the eggs, sprinkle the frozen peas over the whites, crumble over the feta, and season with black pepper and a little sea salt. Add a small splash of water to the pan to create steam, cover, and cook the eggs to your liking.

3 Scatter the spinach around your plates. Microwave the grains according to the packet instructions, then toss into the bowl of pepper sauce and pile on top of the spinach, making a little well in the middle of each portion.

4 Pour the remaining pepper sauce into the wells, then sit the pea and feta eggs proudly on top, scatter over the reserved mint leaves, drizzle with a little extra balsamic, if you like, and tuck on in.

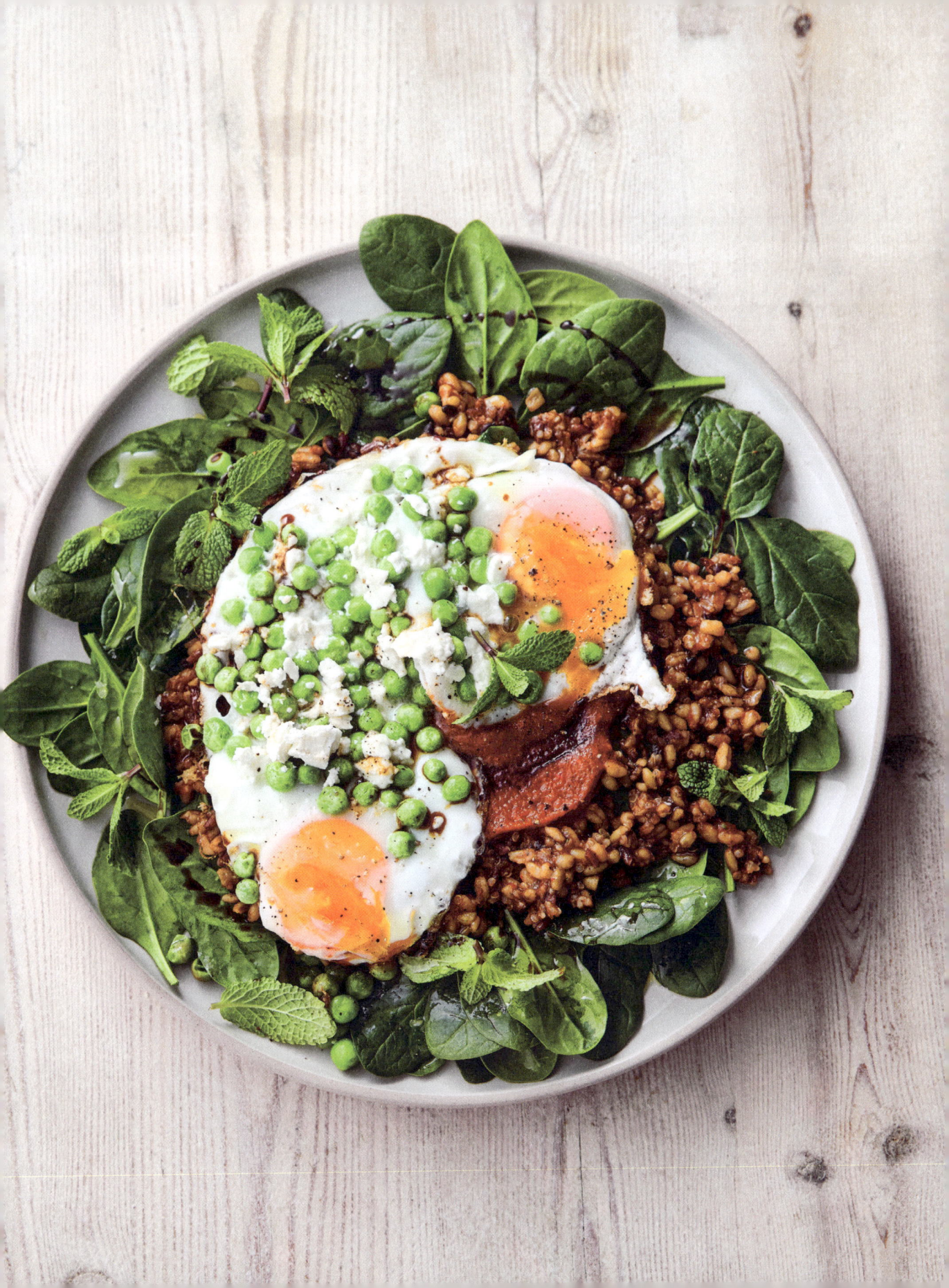

Soy eggs & crispy mackerel rice

Quick, hot cooking with fragrant ingredients consistently gives an exhilaratingly delicious result

SERVES 2
12 MINUTES

6cm piece of ginger

1 clove of garlic

½–1 fresh red chilli

2 spring onions

160g tenderstem broccoli

1 x 125g tin of mackerel in spring water

160g frozen edamame beans, peas or broad beans

1 x 250g packet of cooked wholegrain rice

2 tablespoons low-salt soy sauce

4 medium eggs

1 Peel and finely chop the ginger and garlic. Finely slice the chilli. Trim and finely slice the spring onions and tenderstem stalks, leaving the tips whole.

2 Put a large non-stick frying pan on a medium-high heat, spritz with olive oil, drain and flake in the mackerel, then fry until crispy. Add the broccoli and frozen edamame, the ginger, garlic and most of the spring onions and chilli. Cook for 2 minutes, tossing regularly, then stir in the rice and soy, and cook for a final 2 minutes, or until the rice is hot through. Season to perfection and tip on to a platter or divide between two plates.

3 Working swiftly, wipe out the pan, get it back on the heat, and spritz it with oil, then beat and pour in the eggs, stirring gently until you've got beautiful silky strips of just-cooked egg, surrounded by softer, custardy egg. Slide them on to the rice, scatter over the remaining spring onions and chilli, drizzle with a little extra soy, if you like, and serve.

EASY SWAPS

I've used tinned mackerel here, but you can get the same oily fish benefits from tinned sardines, salmon or trout, too.

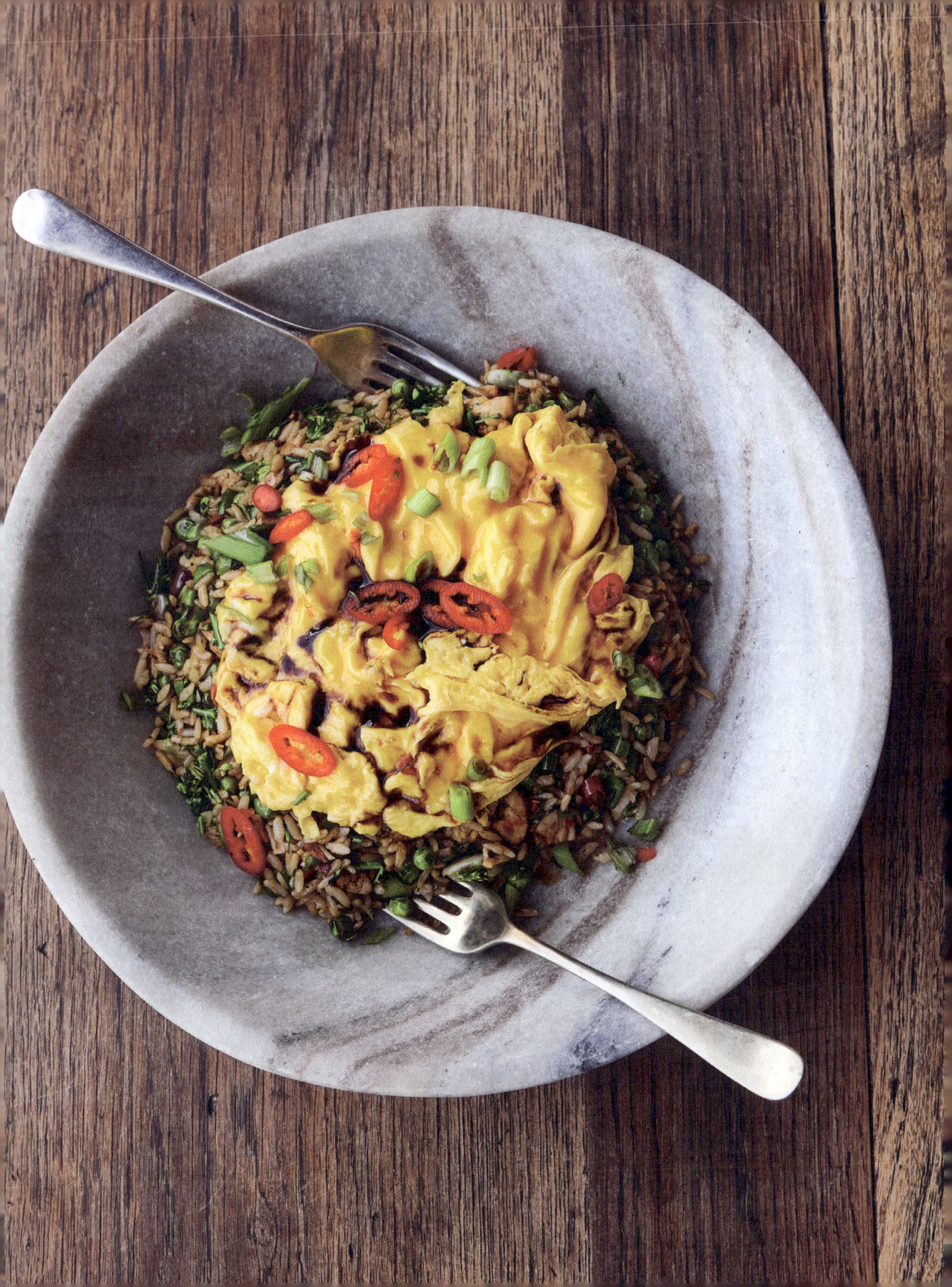

Chickpea arrabbiata

Fast, spicy and delicious, this is the perfect midweek meal to put a smile on your face

SERVES 1
13 MINUTES

1 clove of garlic

1 fresh red chilli

200g passata

½ × 400g tin of chickpeas

125g fresh lasagne sheets

30g rocket

20g Parmesan cheese

1 Boil the kettle. Put a 28cm frying pan on a medium-high heat with ½ a tablespoon of olive oil. Peel the garlic and finely slice with the chilli, reserving a little chilli for garnish, then add to the pan and fry until lightly golden.

2 Tip in the passata, add the chickpeas and half the juice from the tin, and let it bubble for 2 minutes, stirring occasionally, while you slice the lasagne sheets into 2cm strips. Roughly chop most of the rocket, reserving a few leaves.

3 Scatter the chopped rocket and the pasta into the pan, then pour in enough boiling water to just cover the pasta – about 300ml. Let it bubble away for 4 minutes, or until the pasta has absorbed most of the water and you've got a nice sauce, stirring regularly. Turn the heat off and season to perfection.

4 Scatter over the reserved rocket and chilli, finely grate over the Parmesan and finish with a kiss of extra virgin olive oil, if you like.

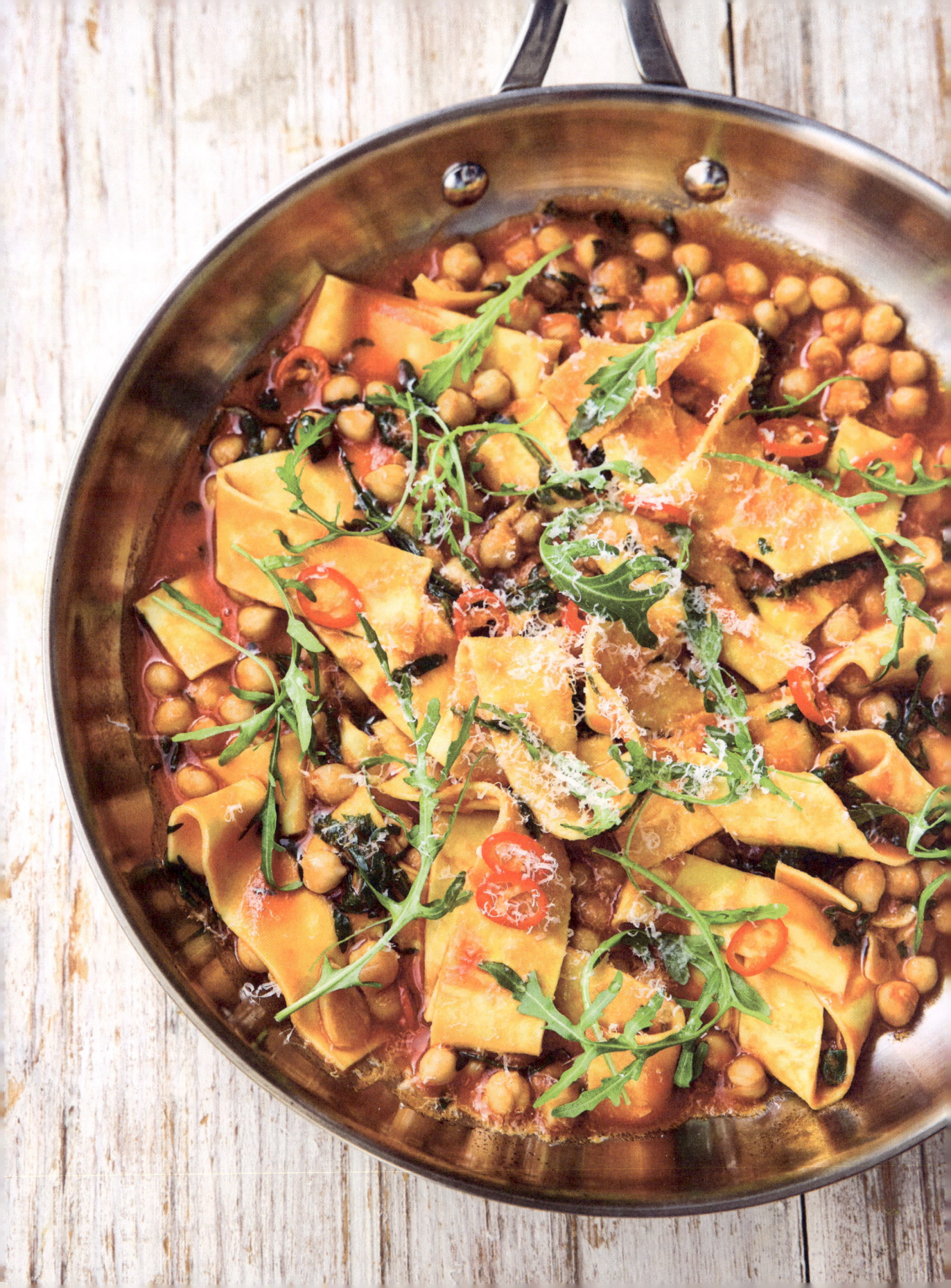

Crispy bean & anchovy eggs

Trust me, when used with elegance and restraint, anchovies are genius

SERVES 2
14 MINUTES

1 x 400g tin of butter beans

½ a red onion (80g)

1 lemon

½ a bunch of oregano (10g)

½ a cucumber (160g)

160g ripe mixed-colour tomatoes

4 eggs

2 anchovy fillets in oil

smoked paprika

20g feta cheese

1 Put a large non-stick frying pan on a medium-high heat and spritz with olive oil, then drain and add the beans. Cook for 7 minutes, or until starting to char and pop, tossing occasionally while you make the salad.

2 Peel and very finely chop the red onion, place in a bowl with 1 tablespoon of extra virgin olive oil, finely grate in the lemon zest, squeeze in the juice, then tear in the oregano leaves. Use the heel of your hand to squash along the length of the cucumber, then roughly chop it and add to the bowl. Chop and add the tomatoes, mix well, and season to perfection.

3 Make four little wells in the beans and crack in the eggs. Reduce to a low heat, then halve the anchovies lengthways and lay one piece around each egg yolk. Season it all with sea salt, black pepper and a pinch of paprika, then cover the pan and leave until the eggs are cooked to your liking.

4 Divide the salad, eggs and beans between your plates, crumble the feta over everything, dust with another pinch of paprika, and serve. Nice with bread.

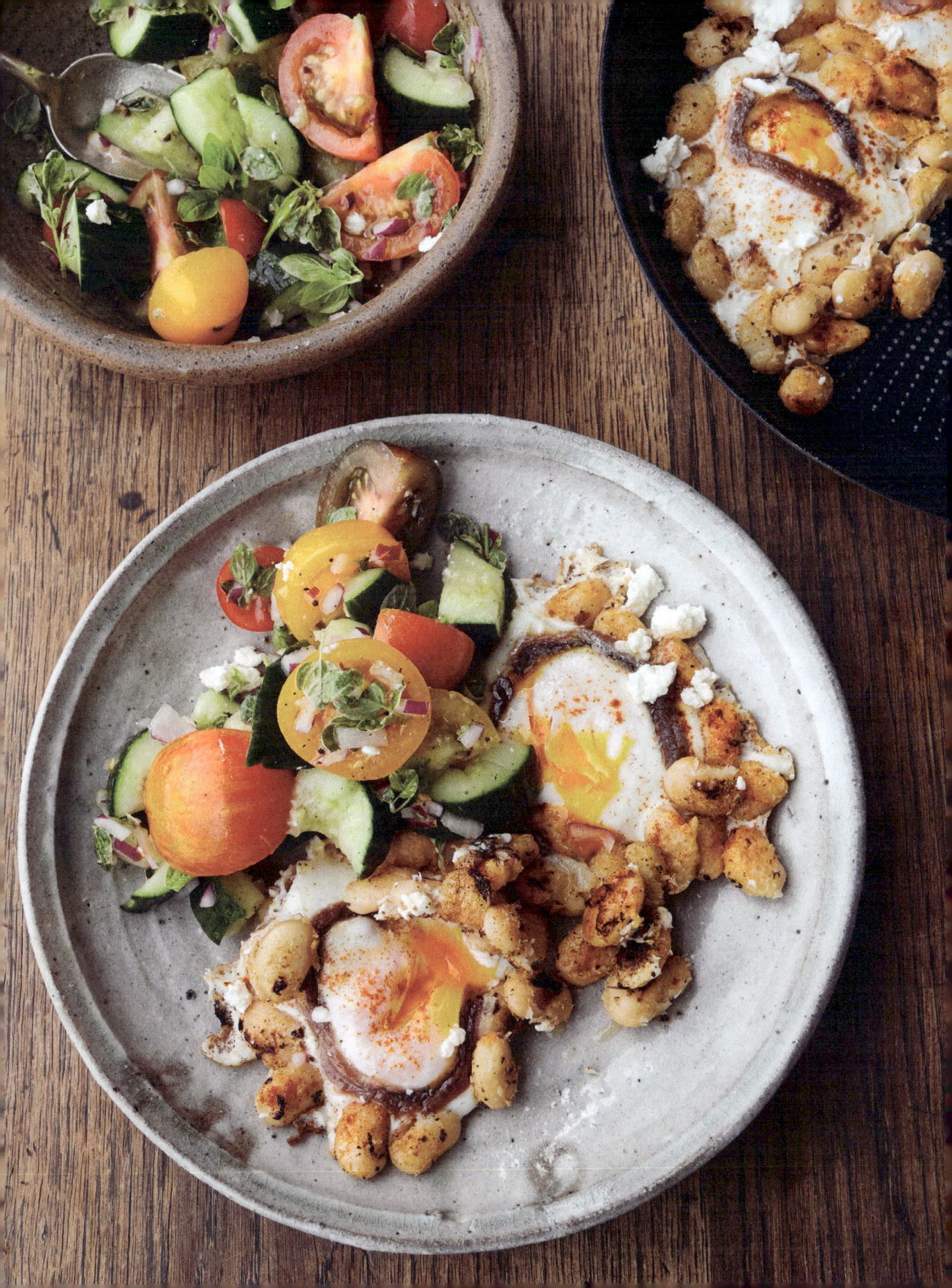

Smashed salad

SERVES 1 | 14 MINUTES

80g each
cucumber, eating apple, carrots, raw baby beets, red pepper, radishes

½ a clove of garlic

1 tablespoon mixed seeds

1 bunch of mixed soft herbs (30g), such as dill, mint, parsley, basil, tarragon

15g feta cheese

In a pestle and mortar, pound the peeled garlic with the seeds and a pinch of sea salt, then muddle in 1 tablespoon each of red wine vinegar and extra virgin olive oil, and season to perfection. Trim and roughly chop the veg and fruit, then either smash it up in the pestle and mortar, or wrap it in a clean tea towel and give it a good bashing with a rolling pin. Toss with the dressing and herb leaves, then crumble over the feta. Delicious with crusty wholemeal bread.

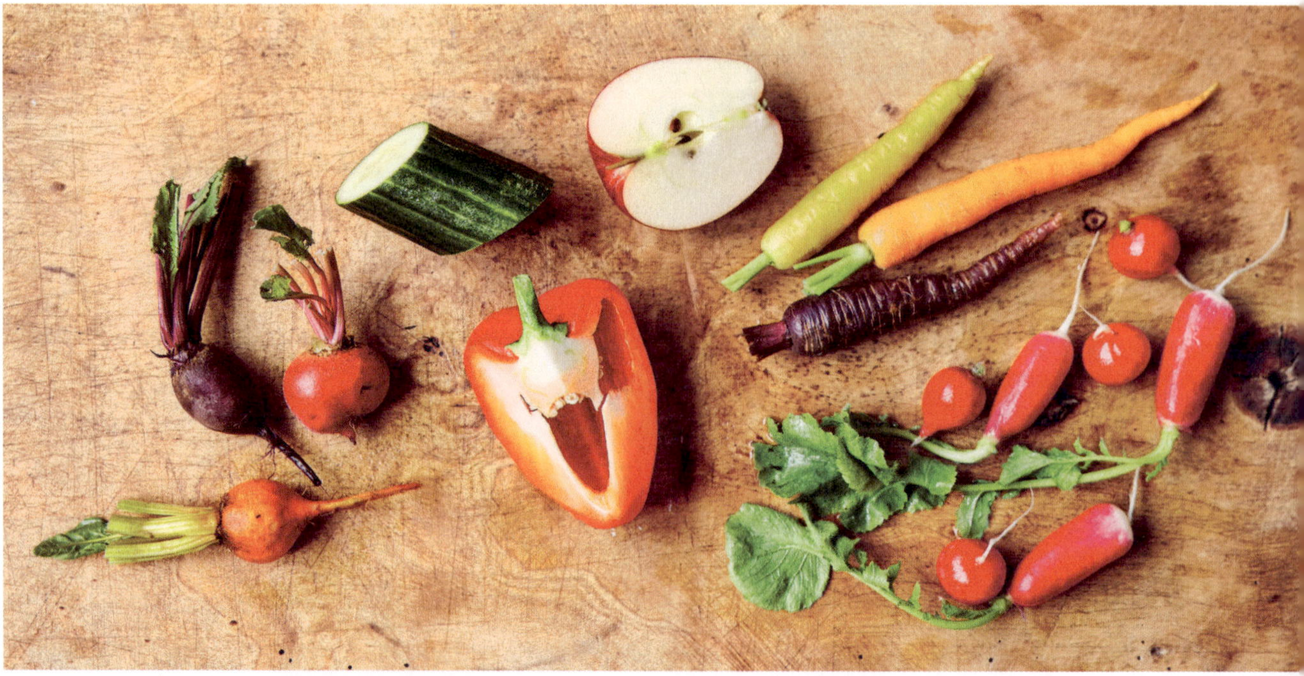

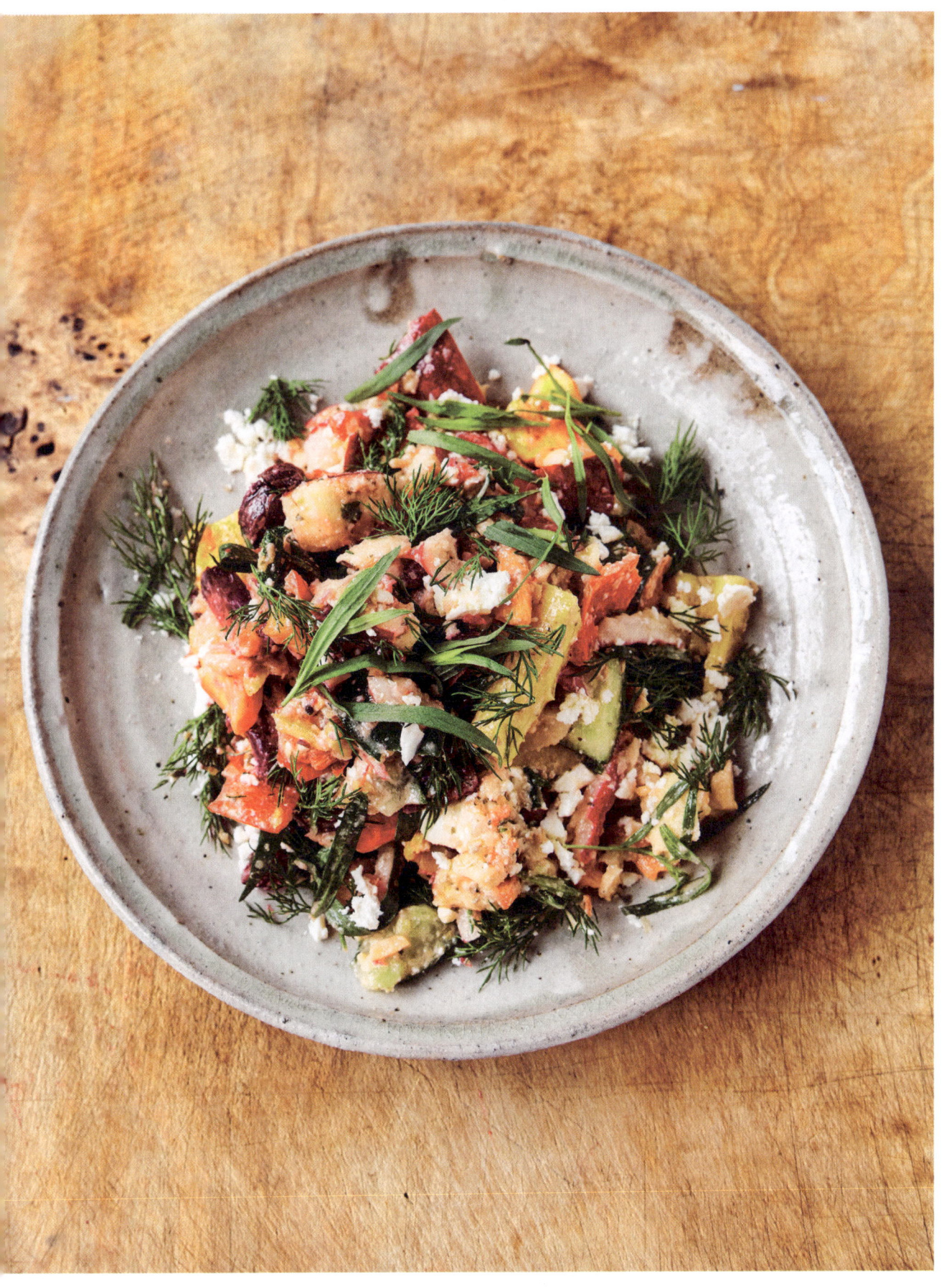

Herby chickpea & feta salad

This lovely salad is lifted by an incredible tomato dressing that goes big on flavour

SERVES 2
16 MINUTES

150g wholewheat couscous

1 lemon

300g ripe tomatoes

1 clove of garlic

½–1 fresh red chilli

1 x 400g tin of chickpeas

2 teaspoons dried oregano

2 carrots (160g)

1 courgette

40g feta cheese

1 Boil the kettle. Put the couscous into a bowl, just cover with boiling kettle water, cover and put aside. Finely grate the lemon zest into another bowl, squeeze in half the juice, then halve the tomatoes and finely grate in cut side down, discarding the skins. Peel and finely grate in the garlic. Add 1 tablespoon of extra virgin olive oil and season to perfection to make your dressing. Finely slice the chilli.

2 Drain the chickpeas, then toss with the oregano and season to perfection. Fluff up the couscous with a fork, peel the carrots, then coarsely grate over with the courgette (or leave the carrots whole, for added crunch), mix well and season to perfection. Plate up the couscous and the chickpeas, spoon over the tomato dressing, crumble over the feta, sprinkle over the chilli, and serve with lemon wedges.

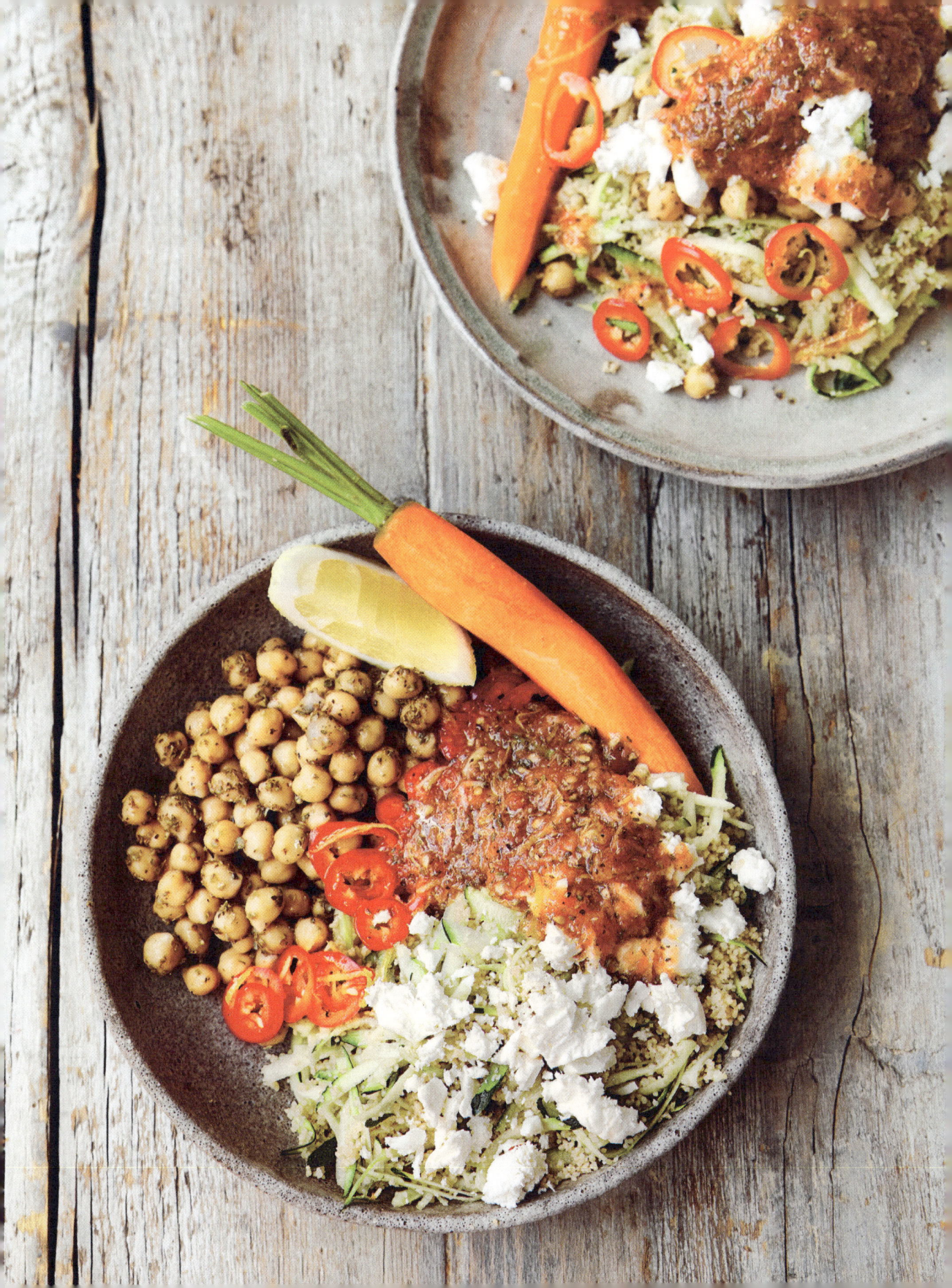

Curried egg & rice pots

A great solution for lunches on the go, have fun playing with different pulses and grains here

SERVES 2
16 MINUTES

4 medium eggs

250g baby spinach

½ a bunch of coriander (15g)

100g natural yoghurt

1 tablespoon mango chutney

2 teaspoons curry powder

1 lemon

1 x 400g tin of chickpeas

1 x 250g packet of cooked wholegrain basmati rice

30g Bombay mix

1. Cook the eggs in a pan of boiling salted water for 6½ minutes for soft-boiled, or until cooked to your liking. Wilt the spinach in a colander on top, then remove, leave to cool, squeeze out excess moisture and season to perfection. Refresh and cool the eggs under cold running water, then peel.

2. Very finely chop the coriander stalks, reserving the leaves, and mix with the yoghurt, mango chutney, curry powder and half the lemon juice, then season to perfection. Coat the eggs in the yoghurt mixture, and they're good to go, or you can marinate them in the fridge for up to 3 days.

3. To make your egg pots, drain the chickpeas, divide between two lidded pots, squeeze over the remaining lemon juice, add a drizzle of extra virgin olive oil and season to perfection. Divide up the spinach and the rice.

4. Halve and add the eggs, along with the curried yoghurt mixture, which will act as your dressing. To tuck in, bash up and scatter over the Bombay mix, and pick over the coriander leaves. If you're on the go, keep the Bombay mix and coriander in a separate pot until ready to eat, for maximum crunch.

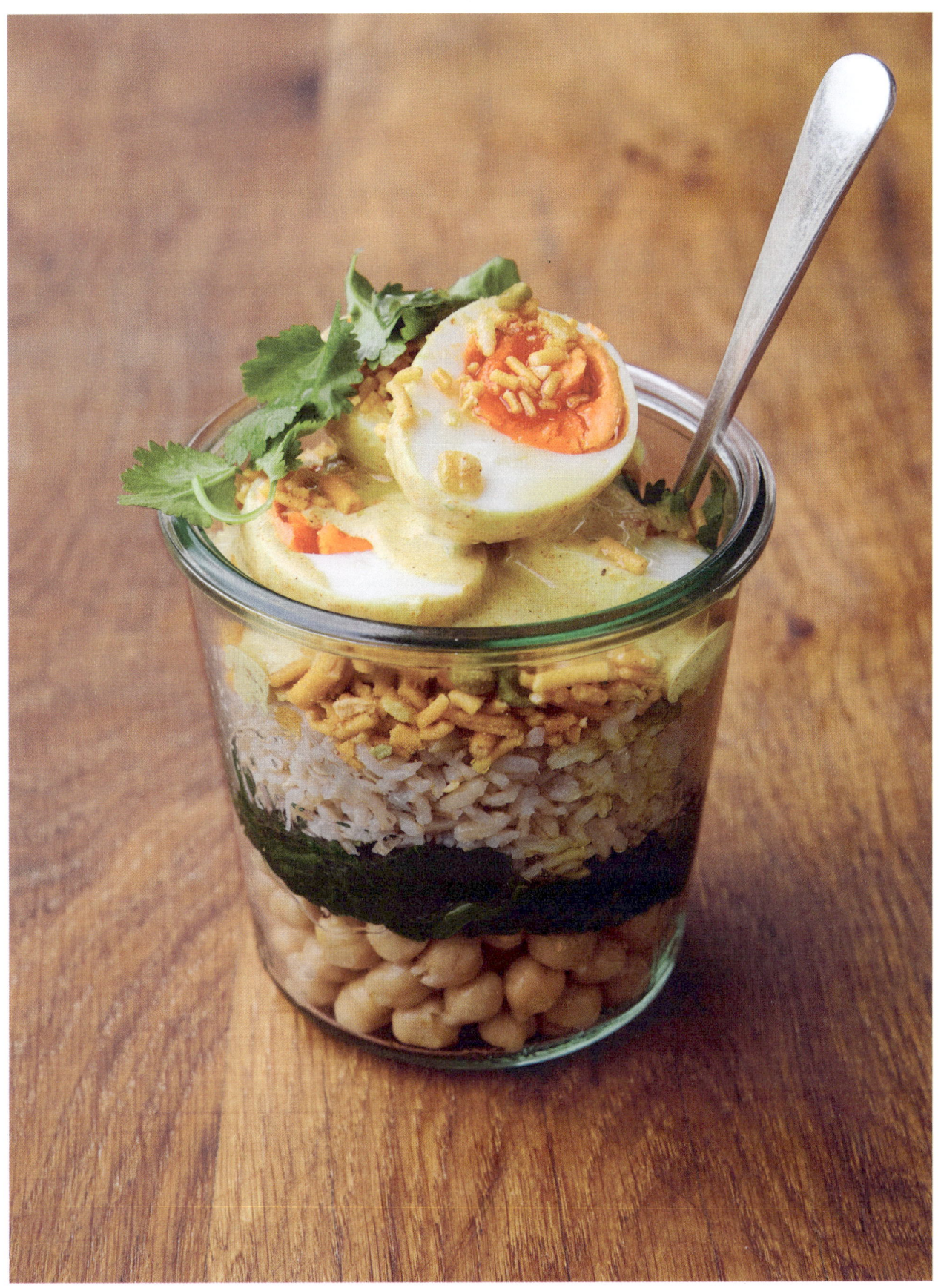

Tuna & broccoli pasta

It might look super-simple, but this recipe gives you very satisfying layers of delicious flavour

SERVES 1
18 MINUTES

125g fresh lasagne sheets

1 clove of garlic

½ a fresh red chilli

2 sprigs of rosemary

80g purple sprouting broccoli

80g ripe cherry tomatoes

½ a lemon

40g jarred or tinned tuna in oil

1 level tablespoon baby capers in brine

1 level tablespoon black olive tapenade

1. Boil the kettle. Cut the lasagne sheets into random 5cm shapes to make stracci (rags). Peel the garlic, then finely slice with the chilli. Strip and finely chop the rosemary leaves. Trim the broccoli and finely slice the stalks, leaving the tips whole. Halve the tomatoes. Finely grate the lemon zest.

2. Put a 28cm frying pan on a high heat. Go in with a little drizzle of oil from the tuna jar (or use olive oil), then add the garlic, chilli, rosemary, broccoli and capers, then the tomatoes and lemon zest, finally flaking in the tuna.

3. Scatter the pasta into the pan, then pour in enough boiling water to just cover the pasta – about 300ml. Let it bubble away for 4 minutes, or until the pasta has absorbed most of the water and you've got a nice sauce, stirring regularly and loosening with an extra splash of water, if needed.

4. Turn the heat off, crush the tomatoes with the back of your spoon, squeeze over the lemon juice, season to perfection, then bomb over the tapenade. Finish with a kiss of extra virgin olive oil, if you like.

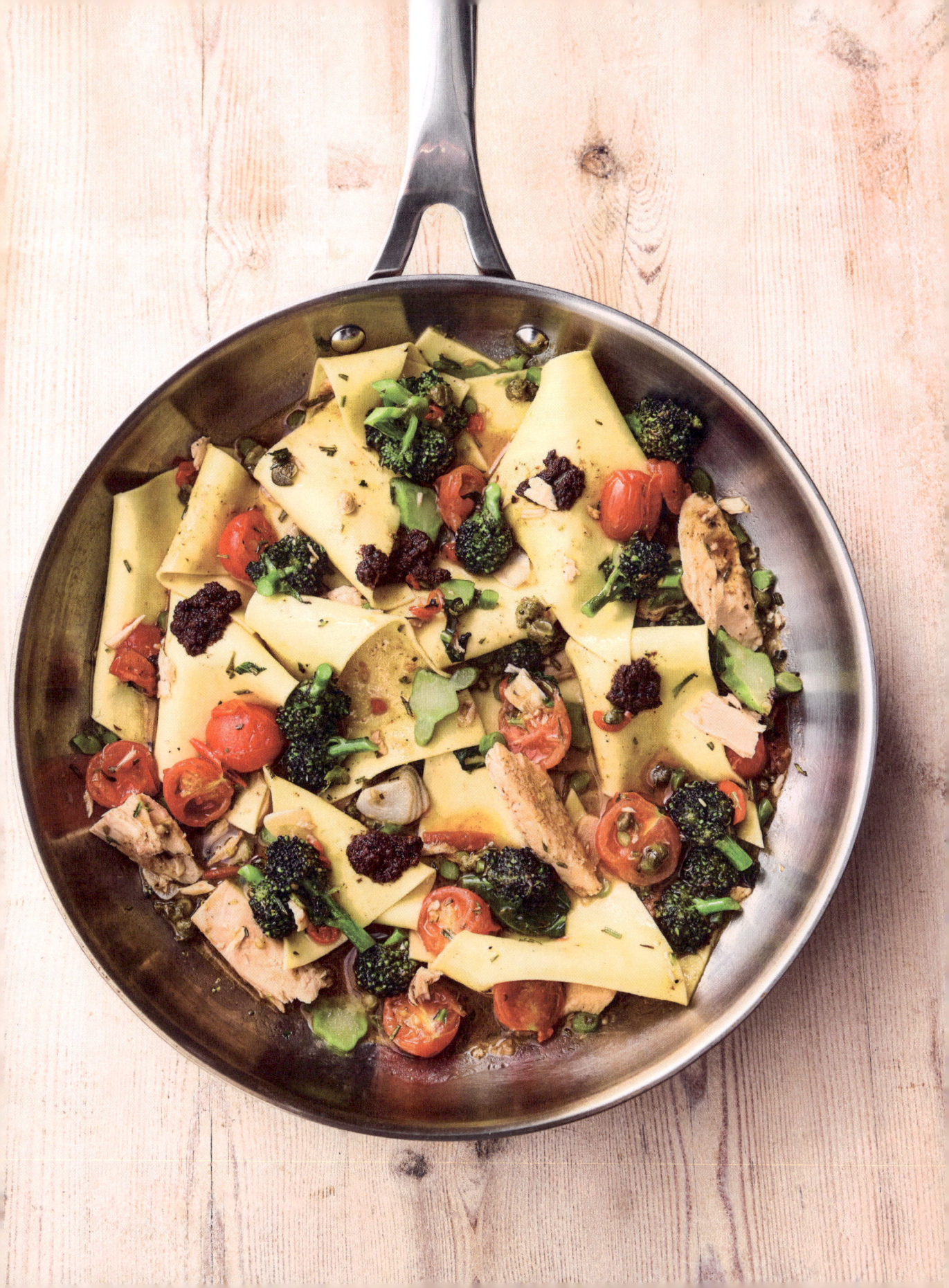

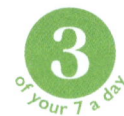

Avo & black bean omelette

Cooked avocado teamed with spice, black beans and caramelized tomatoes will make you smile

SERVES 2
18 MINUTES

2 wholemeal tortillas

1 small ripe avocado (160g)

4 spring onions

160g ripe tomatoes

1 x 400g tin of black beans

4 eggs

1 teaspoon smoked paprika

50g cottage cheese

1 tablespoon jarred sliced jalapeños

4 sprigs of coriander

1. Preheat the oven to 180°C. Put a large non-stick ovenproof frying pan on a high heat, briefly toasting the tortillas as it heats up, then remove. Halve, destone and peel the avocado, then cut into quarters. Trim the spring onions. Halve the tomatoes.

2. Drain the beans and tip them into the hot pan to char and pop, then remove and set aside. Spritz the pan with olive oil, add the avo, spring onions and tomatoes, cut side down, and season with sea salt and black pepper. Cook for 5 minutes, or until starting to char, turning as you go.

3. Crack the eggs into a bowl, add the paprika and a pinch of salt, and beat well. Return half the popped beans to the pan, pour the eggs in and around the veg, then scatter over the remaining beans. Bomb over spoonfuls of cottage cheese, scatter over most of the jalapeños, then transfer to the oven for 5 minutes, or until the eggs are cooked to your liking.

4. Finely chop the remaining jalapeños, pick the coriander leaves, and sprinkle over the omelette, before serving with the tortillas. Heaven.

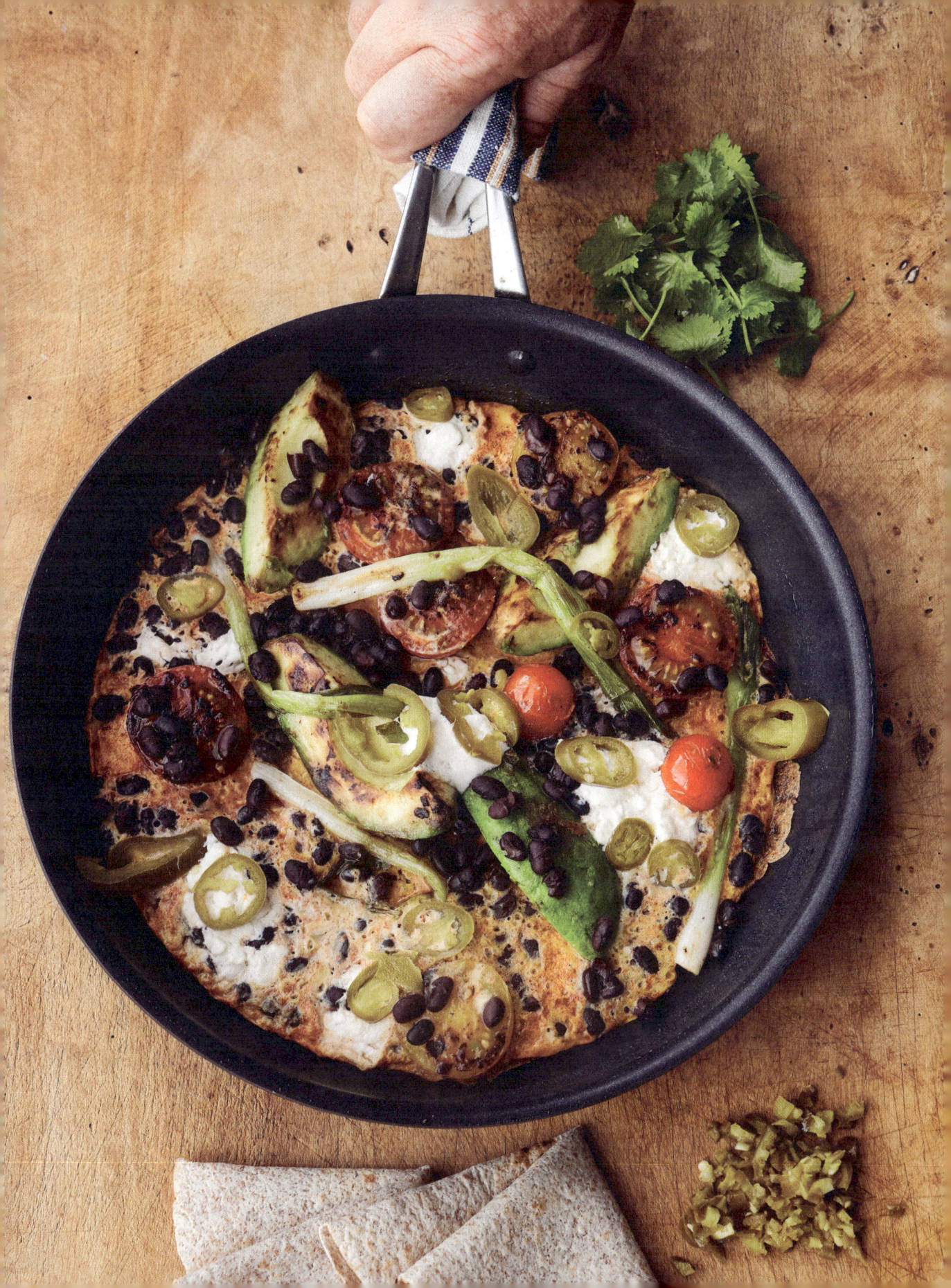

Carrot & sweet potato fritters

A celebration of colour with orange veg flavouring the fritters, and a fun spinach-green houmous

SERVES 2
20 MINUTES

1 small sweet potato (160g)

2 carrots (160g)

1 x 400g tin of chickpeas

100g self-raising flour

2 teaspoons ras el hanout, plus extra to serve

3 large eggs

160g baby spinach

1 tablespoon tahini

1 lemon

20g feta cheese

1 Wash and coarsely grate the sweet potato and carrot, then scrunch with a pinch of sea salt. Drain the chickpeas, tip half into a large bowl and lightly mash. Squeeze the grated veg to remove excess moisture, then add to the bowl with the flour, ras el hanout, 1 egg and a pinch of black pepper. Scrunch and mix well, then divide equally into 6 and shape into rough balls.

2 Put a large non-stick frying pan on a medium heat, spritz with olive oil, and add the balls, squashing them with a fish slice into fritters about 1½cm thick. Cook for 7 minutes on each side, or until golden and cooked through, then stack the fritters up at one side of the pan. Spritz the space with oil, crack in the 2 remaining eggs and fry them to your liking.

3 Tip the rest of the chickpeas into a food processor with the spinach, tahini and an ice cube, if you have it. Squeeze in half the lemon juice and blitz until smooth, then season to perfection and spoon across your plates.

4 Sit the golden fritters and fried eggs alongside, add an extra pinch of ras el hanout, crumble over the feta, and serve with lemon wedges.

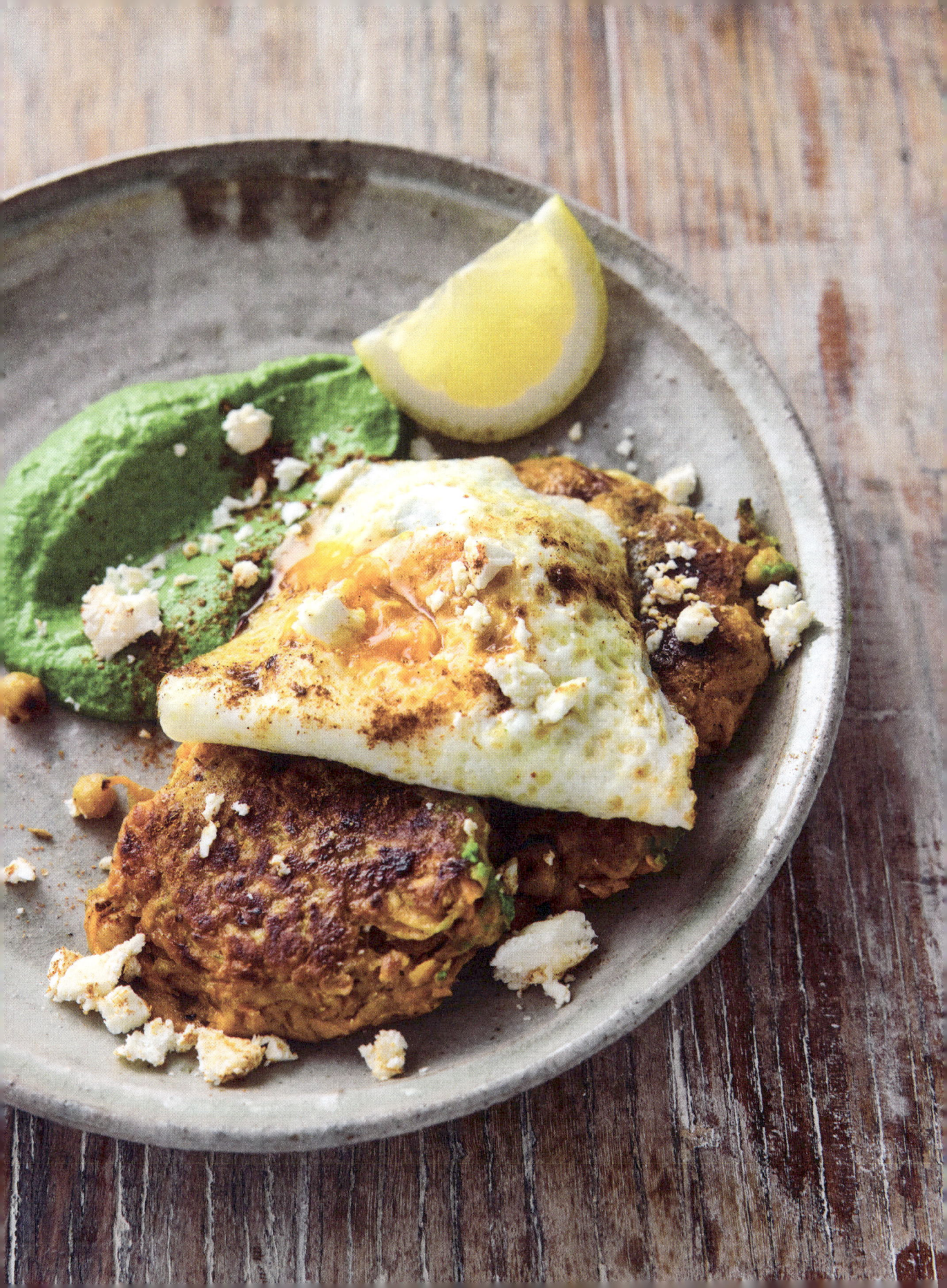

Crispy mackerel buns

An exceptional sandwich to help you celebrate super-fresh mackerel, sardines or trout

SERVES 2
20 MINUTES

1 large carrot (160g)

1 eating apple (160g)

1 spring onion

½ a bunch of flat-leaf parsley (15g)

1 gherkin

1 lemon

3 heaped tablespoons Greek yoghurt

2 heaped teaspoons jarred grated horseradish

2 x 90g boneless mackerel fillets

2 seeded wholemeal buns

1 To make a slaw, peel the carrot and coarsely grate with the apple. Trim and finely slice the spring onion. Finely chop the parsley, stalks and all, and the gherkin, finely grate the zest of half the lemon, then toss it all with the yoghurt, horseradish, and half the lemon juice, and season to perfection.

2 Season the mackerel fillets with a little sea salt and black pepper, then either cook on a hot barbecue or put into a cold non-stick frying pan and place on a medium-high heat. Cook for 4 minutes on the skin side, flipping over for just 1 minute on the flesh side, or until cooked through and the skin is crispy.

3 Split and toast the buns, and load up with slaw. Break the crispy mackerel fillets on top, squeeze a little lemon juice over each one, then pop the tops on and you're good to go. Serve any extra slaw on the side.

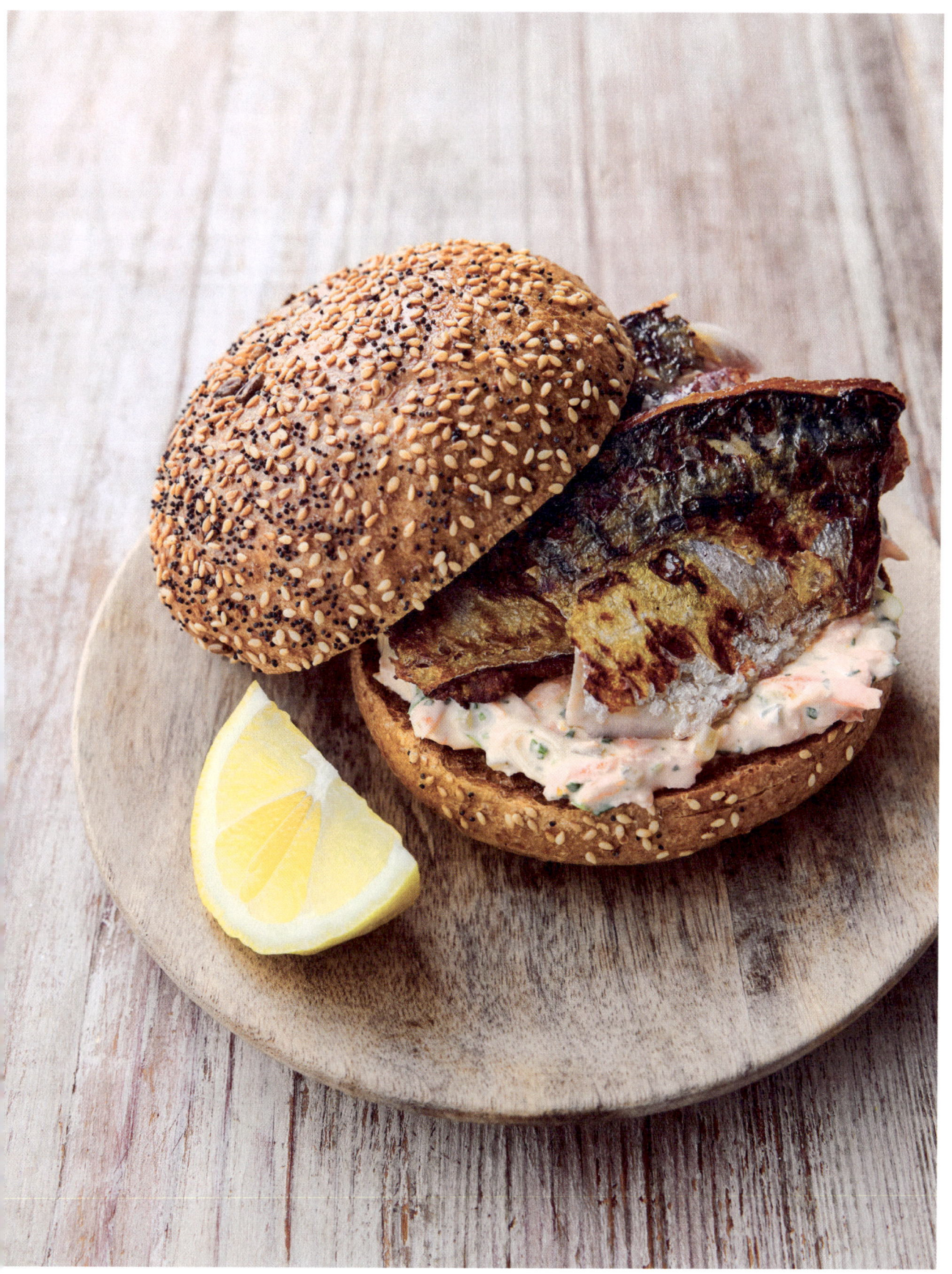

Dinner

Smashed flatbread burger

A fun evolution of the smash burger, giving both crispy, gnarly bits and soft, juicy bits, too

SERVES 1
8 MINUTES

1 sprig of basil

100g pork or beef mince

80g tinned cannellini beans

5g Parmesan cheese

1 small flatbread (80g)

80g ripe mixed-colour cherry tomatoes

1 tablespoon pesto

1 Put a non-stick frying pan on a high heat. Quickly pick the basil leaves and set aside, finely chop the stalk and scrunch with the mince, drained beans, a grating of Parmesan and a pinch of sea salt and black pepper, breaking up the beans as you go, then shape into a rough ball.

2 Spritz the pan with olive oil, add the mince mixture, then place the flatbread on top, smashing and flattening the meat. Cook for 4 to 5 minutes, or until gnarly and cooked through. Meanwhile, quarter and season the tomatoes, dressing them with a few drips of red wine vinegar.

3 Flip the flatbread burger on to your plate, spoon over the pesto, scatter over the dressed tomatoes and reserved basil leaves, finely grate over the last bit of Parmesan, then pick up and devour.

GO VEGGIE

Simply ditch the mince and use 180g of drained beans.

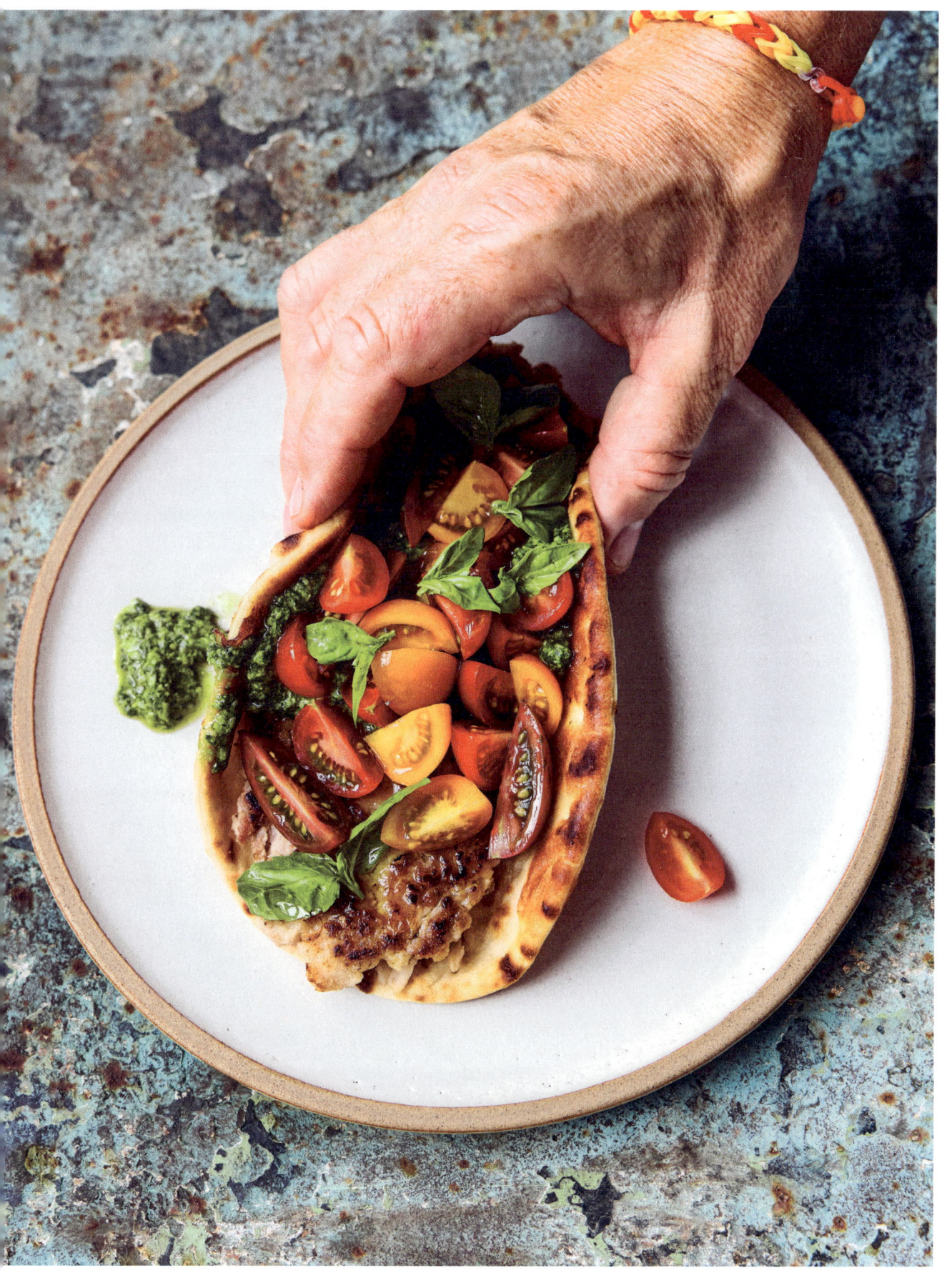

Super-green stir-fry

SERVES 1 | 10 MINUTES

80g each
asparagus, baby corn, mangetout, peas, mixed mushrooms, tenderstem broccoli, beansprouts

10g unsalted cashew nuts

1 clove of garlic

3cm piece of ginger

½–1 fresh red chilli

2 oranges

1 teaspoon low-salt soy sauce

Trim any veg that needs it, halving the corn, larger mushrooms and any thick broccoli stalks. Toast the cashews in a large non-stick frying pan on a high heat for 1 minute, then remove. Dry fry all the veg for 4 minutes, tossing regularly, while you peel the garlic and ginger, then finely grate them into a bowl with the chilli and the zest of 1 orange. Squeeze in all the orange juice, add the soy, mix well, then pour into the pan. Toss until reduced and glazed, then season to perfection. Finely chop and sprinkle over the cashews, to serve. Lovely as it is, or with wholegrain rice or noodles, if you fancy.

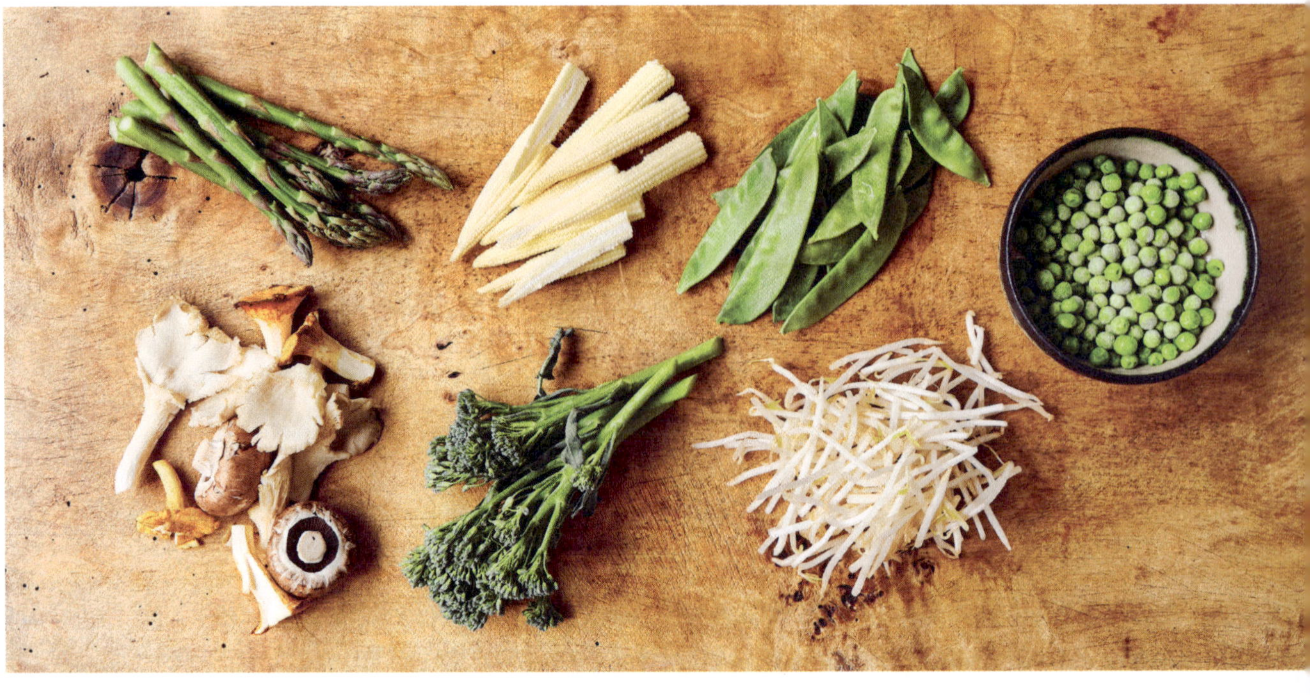

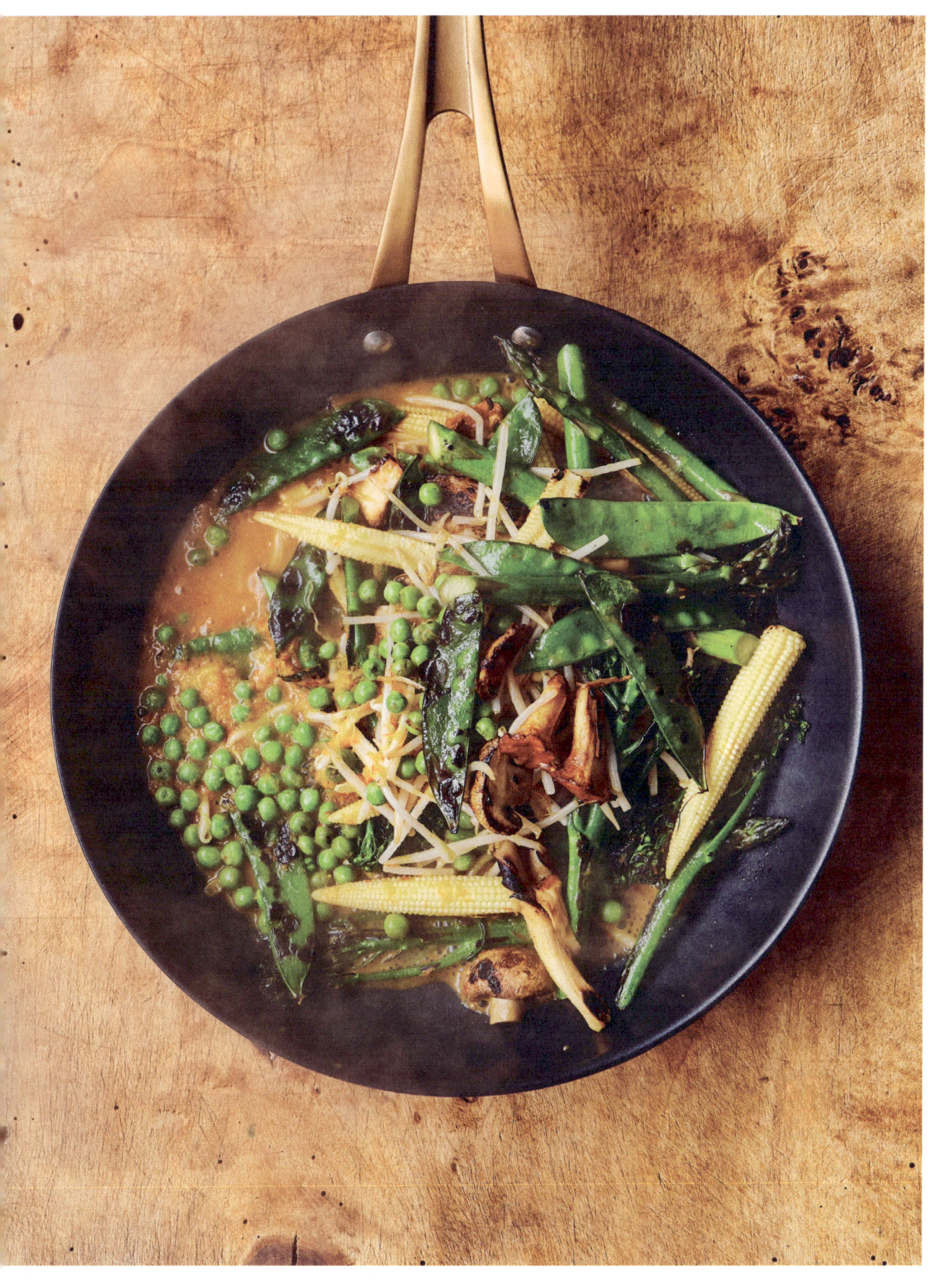

Easy prawn curry

Popular prawns cook very quickly, so they're perfect for this quick, speedy, fragrant curry

SERVES 2
10 MINUTES

1 onion (160g)

250g ripe cherry tomatoes

1 x 50g sachet of creamed coconut

1 x 400g tin of chickpeas

1 bunch of coriander (30g)

2 tablespoons of your favourite curry paste

250g frozen mango

165g raw peeled king prawns

1 x 250g packet of cooked wholegrain basmati rice

30g Bombay mix

1. Put a large non-stick frying pan on a high heat. Peel and very finely slice the onion and place in the pan to dry fry with the tomatoes, tossing regularly for 4 minutes, while you put the coconut cream in a blender with half the chickpeas and all their juice, half the coriander leaves and all the stalks, and a splash of water. Tip in half the onions and tomatoes from the pan and blitz until smooth to make a sauce.

2. Stir the curry paste and ½ a tablespoon of olive oil into the pan, followed a minute later by the frozen mango and remaining chickpeas, then the sauce. Toss over a medium heat for 2 minutes, then add the prawns and let it bubble away until the prawns are just cooked, loosening with splashes of water, if needed. Season to perfection.

3. Cook the rice according to the packet instructions, then divide between plates. Chop and stir most of the remaining coriander leaves into the curry, spoon it on top of the rice, then scatter over the last few coriander leaves. Crush and crumble over the Bombay mix for added crunch, to finish.

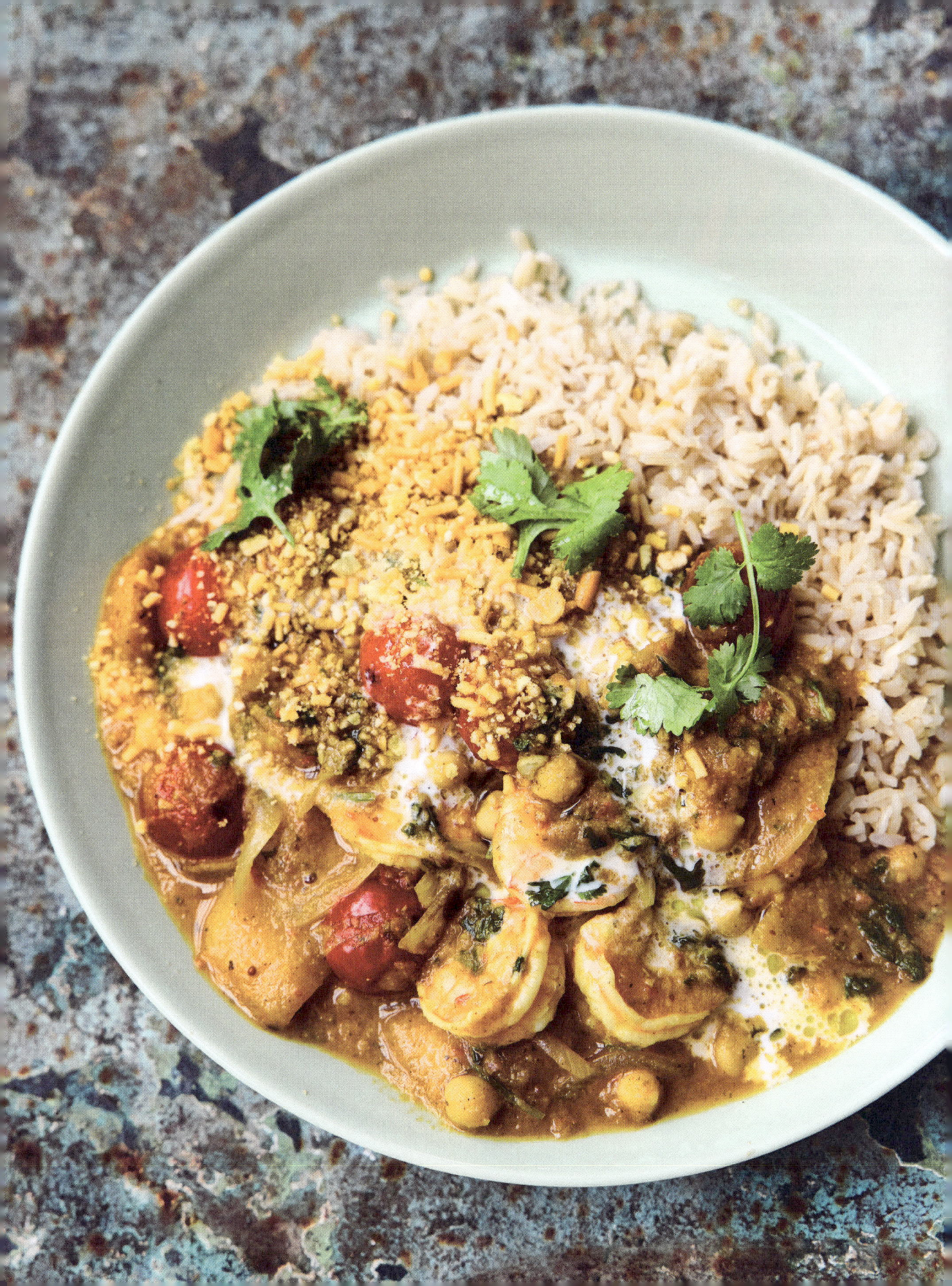

Creamy peanut chicken

Quick cooked peppers and chicken hit with a creamy, nutty sauce equals a delicious dinner, fast

SERVES 2
10 MINUTES

2 mixed-colour peppers (320g)

2 × 150g skinless chicken breasts

2 cloves of garlic

6cm piece of ginger

2 limes

1 tablespoon low-salt soy sauce

2 heaped tablespoons peanut butter

½ a bunch of coriander (15g)

160g sugar snap peas

60g dried mango

1 Put a large non-stick frying pan on a high heat. Cut the peppers into 1cm-thick slices, discarding the seeds. Dry fry for 2 minutes, tossing regularly.

2 Slice the chicken lengthways into 1cm strips, season with sea salt and a generous pinch of black pepper, then add to the pan, spritz it all with olive oil, and cook for 4 minutes, or until golden, tossing regularly.

3 Meanwhile, roughly peel the garlic and ginger, and place in a blender with the juice of 1 lime, the soy, peanut butter, coriander stalks, reserving the leaves, and 250ml of water. Blitz until smooth, then season to perfection.

4 Toss the sugar snaps and dried mango into the pan, followed by the sauce. Let it bubble vigorously for 2 minutes, then plate up. Scatter over the coriander leaves, and serve with lime wedges. Great with rice or noodles.

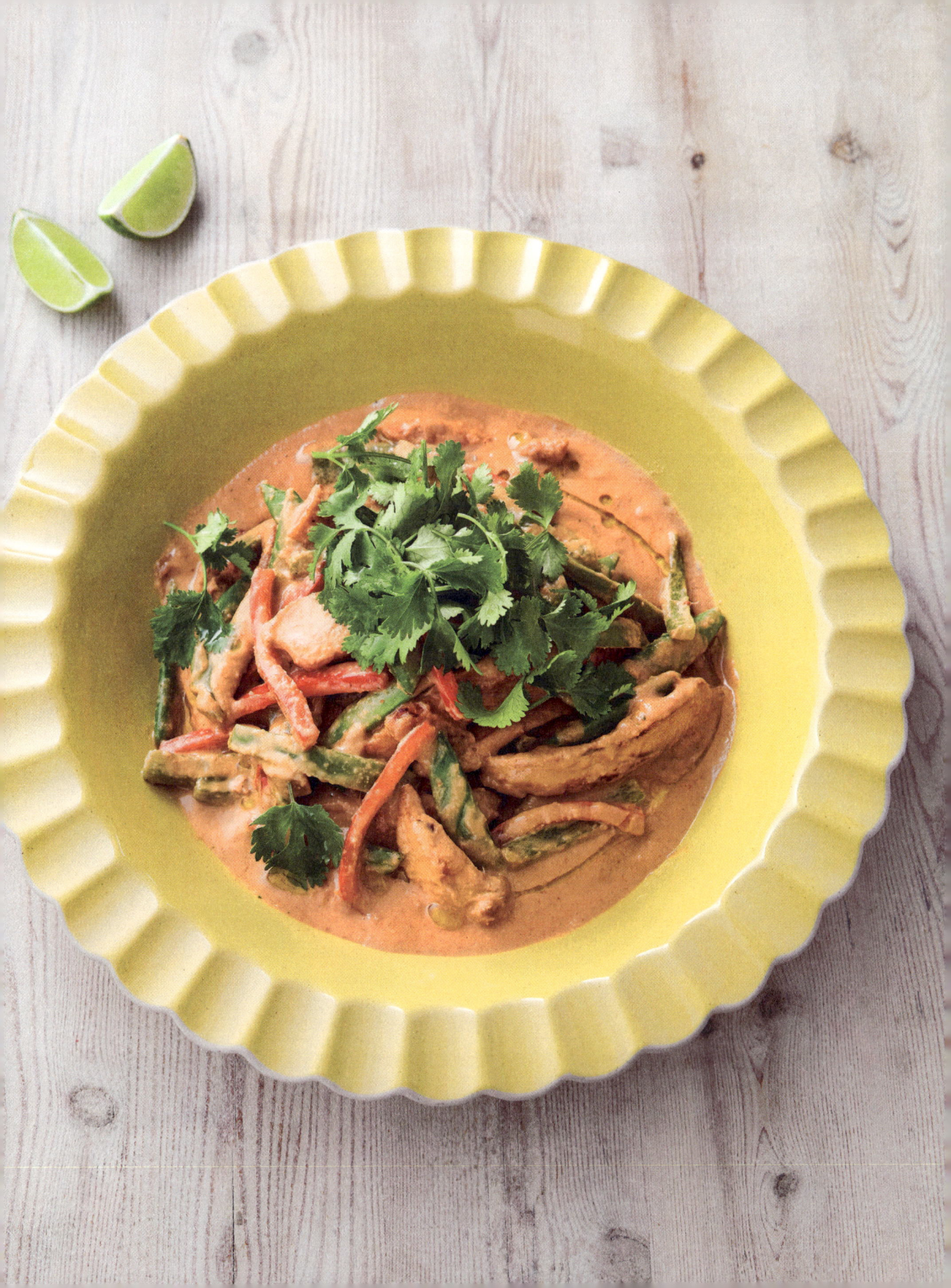

Sweet & sour prawns

A super-simple, utterly delicious sauce that clings to everything beautifully. This really is fast food

SERVES 2
10 MINUTES

320g mixed crunchy stir-fry veg, such as baby corn, sugar snap peas, mangetout

1 x 227g tin of pineapple rings in juice

300g straight-to-wok udon noodles

160g white cabbage

1 lime

1 teaspoon cornflour

1 tablespoon low-salt soy sauce, plus extra to serve

1 tablespoon sweet chilli dipping sauce

165g raw peeled king prawns

½ a bunch of basil (15g)

1 Boil the kettle. Put the crunchy veg into a large dry non-stick frying pan on a high heat. Scoop the pineapple out of the tin, reserving the juice, quarter the rings and add to the pan, tossing regularly.

2 In a large bowl, cover the noodles with boiling kettle water, then very finely slice or speed-peel the cabbage and add to the bowl.

3 Finely grate the lime zest into the tin of reserved pineapple juice, mix in the cornflour, soy and sweet chilli sauce, then top the tin up with water and pour into the pan. Add the prawns and cook for 4 minutes, or until the prawns are cooked through and the sauce has reduced and thickened.

4 Drain the noodles and cabbage and divide between your bowls. Tear the basil leaves into the pan, squeeze in the lime juice, then portion up. Toss together and tuck in, enjoying with an extra drizzle of soy, if you like.

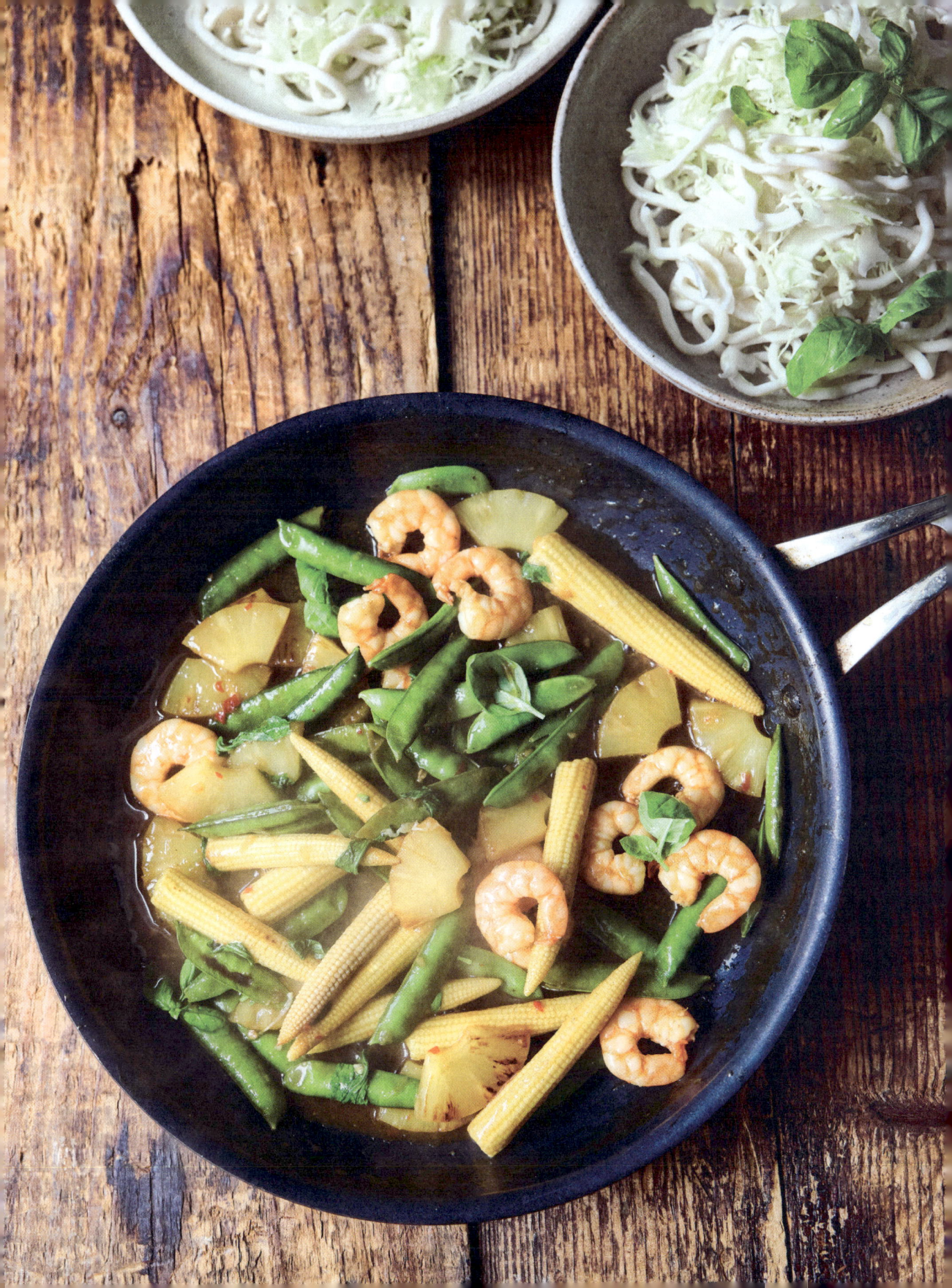

Thai-style fish curry

A great example of just how quickly you can create a tasty, steaming bowl of goodness

SERVES 4
10 MINUTES

4 long frozen white fish fillets (400g total)

320g frozen edamame beans

320g sugar snap peas

½ a bunch of coriander (15g)

1 x 120g jar of pickled ginger

1 heaped tablespoon Thai green curry paste

1 x 400g tin of light coconut milk

4 nests of instant vermicelli rice noodles (180g total)

1 fresh red chilli

1 lime

1. Boil the kettle. Put a large non-stick frying pan on a high heat, then go in with the frozen fish, frozen edamame and sugar snaps.

2. Tear the coriander, stalks and all, into a blender, reserving a few leaves for garnish. Add the pickled ginger, juice and all, curry paste and coconut milk. Blitz until smooth, then pour into the pan, cover and simmer for 7 minutes, or until the fish is nicely cooked through.

3. In a bowl, cover the noodles with boiling kettle water and leave to rehydrate, then drain and divide between warm serving bowls. Finely slice the chilli.

4. Season the curry to perfection and divide up, then sprinkle over the chilli and the reserved coriander leaves. Serve with lime wedges.

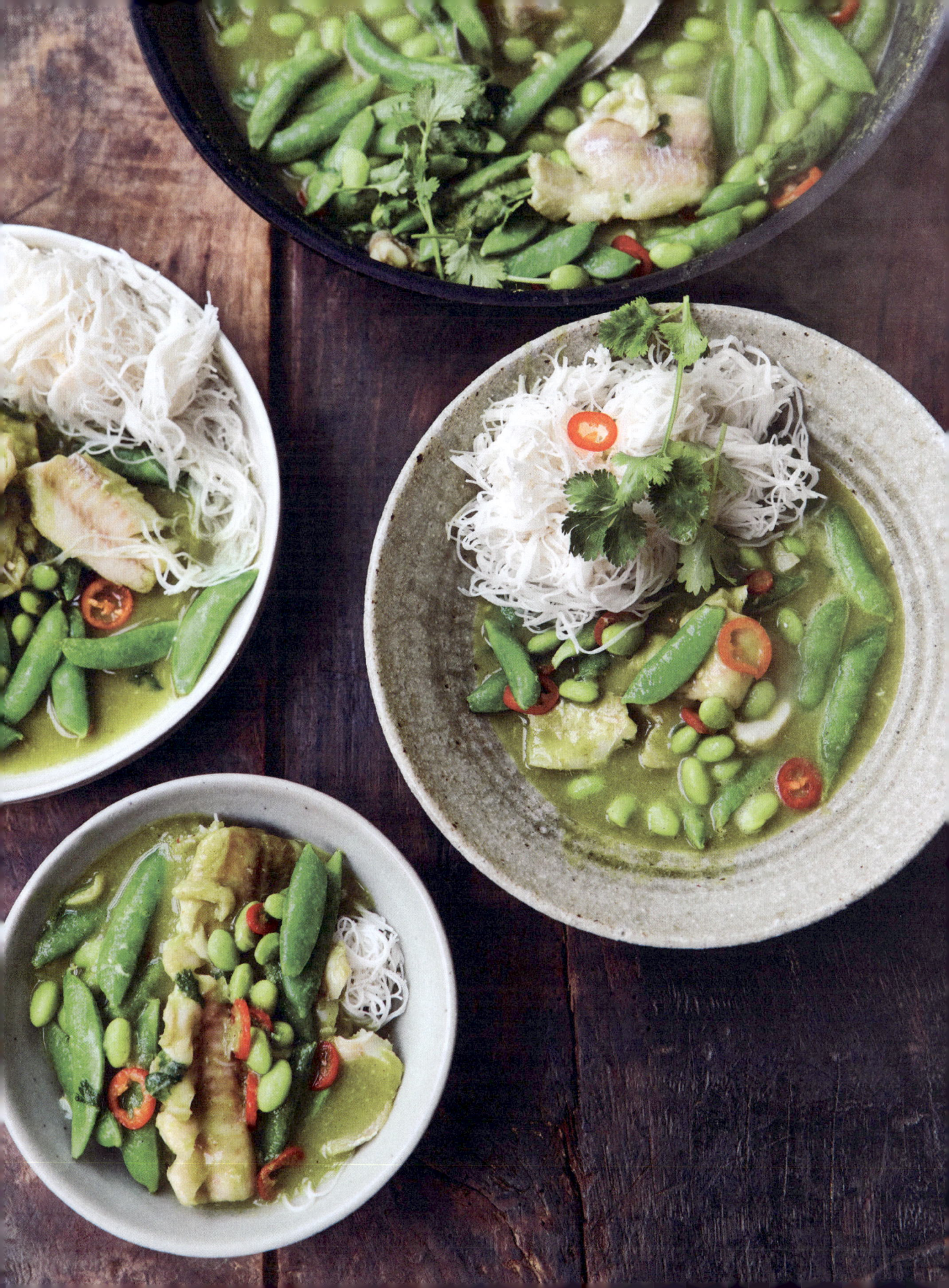

Green veg megamix

SERVES 1 | 11 MINUTES

80g each
Brussels sprouts, frozen edamame beans, pak choi, sweetheart cabbage, asparagus, broccoli, mangetout

2 cloves of garlic

1 tablespoon hoisin sauce

1 teaspoon English mustard

½–1 lemon

Soften the peeled garlic cloves for 2 minutes in a large pan of boiling salted water, then remove to a pestle and mortar. Trim the veg, as needed, then halve the Brussels sprouts, cut the cabbage into thin wedges and cut the broccoli into florets. Blanch all the veg for 3 minutes, so it retains its vibrancy. Pound the garlic into a paste, muddle in the hoisin and mustard, then squeeze in lemon juice to taste, and season to perfection. Drain the veg well, dress, and serve. Good as it is, or with noodles or mixed grains on the side.

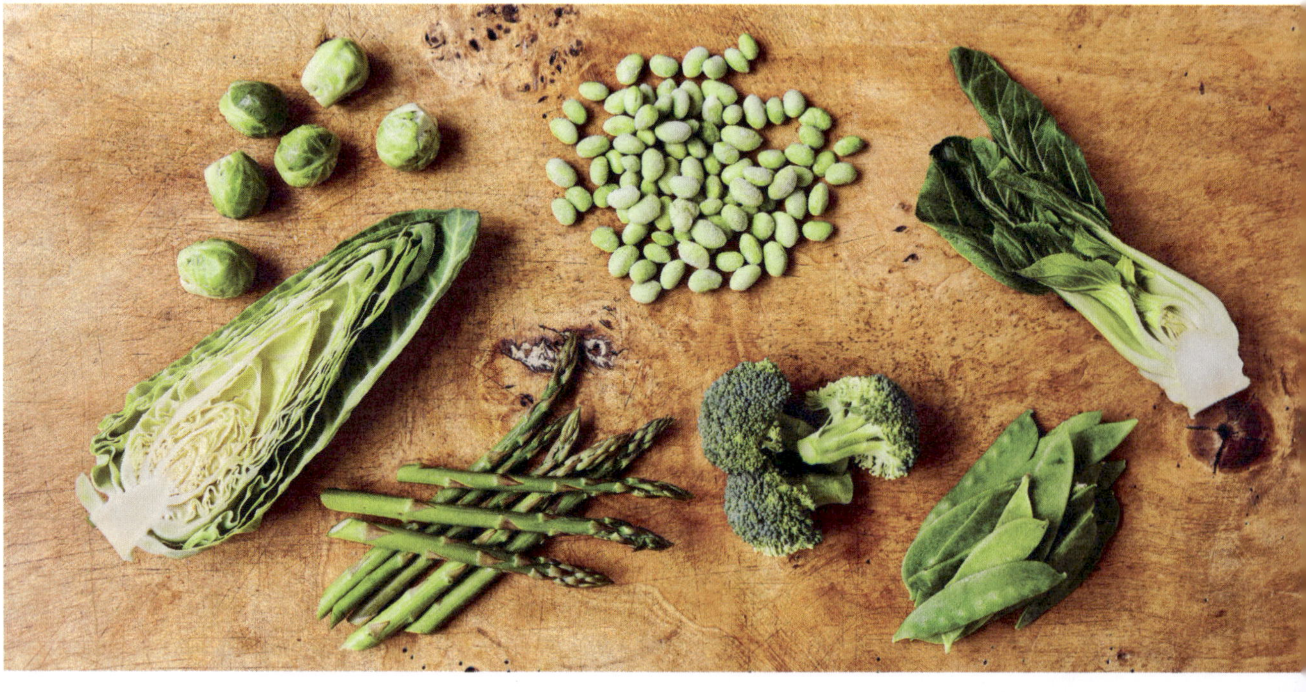

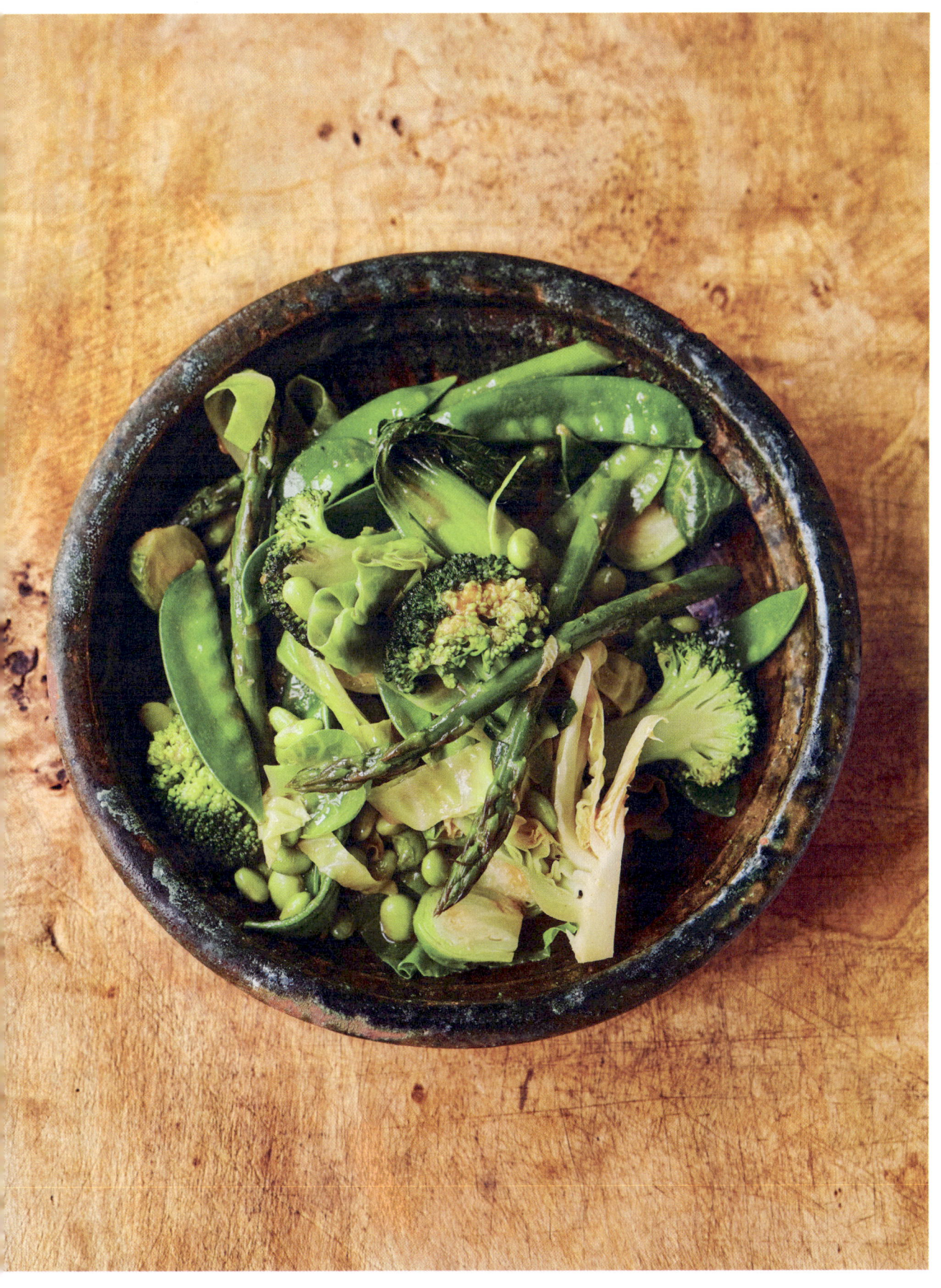

Tahini mushroom noodles

Hot, cold, crunchy, soft, fresh and comforting, this is a bowl of joyful contrast

SERVES 2
11 MINUTES

200g mixed mushrooms

2 tablespoons tahini

2 tablespoons low-salt soy sauce

2 tablespoons mirin

2 cloves of garlic

2 limes

160g radishes

2 little gem or round lettuces

300g straight-to-wok udon noodles

160g fresh or frozen edamame beans

1 Boil the kettle. Put a large dry non-stick frying pan on a high heat with the mushrooms, tearing any larger ones. Toss occasionally until starting to char while, in a bowl, you mix the tahini with the soy and 1½ tablespoons of mirin, then peel and finely grate in the garlic and the zest of 1 lime. Add 100ml of boiling kettle water and mix until combined.

2 Finely slice the radishes, toss with any small fresh radish leaves, the juice of 1 lime and a small pinch of sea salt. Click apart the lettuces, toss with the remaining mirin and the juice of ½ a lime, and arrange in two serving bowls.

3 Toss the noodles and edamame in the pan of mushrooms for 1 minute, then pour in the tahini mixture. Let it sizzle, bubble and reduce for 1 more minute, season to perfection, then divide between your bowls. Sprinkle over the dressed radishes and serve with lime wedges.

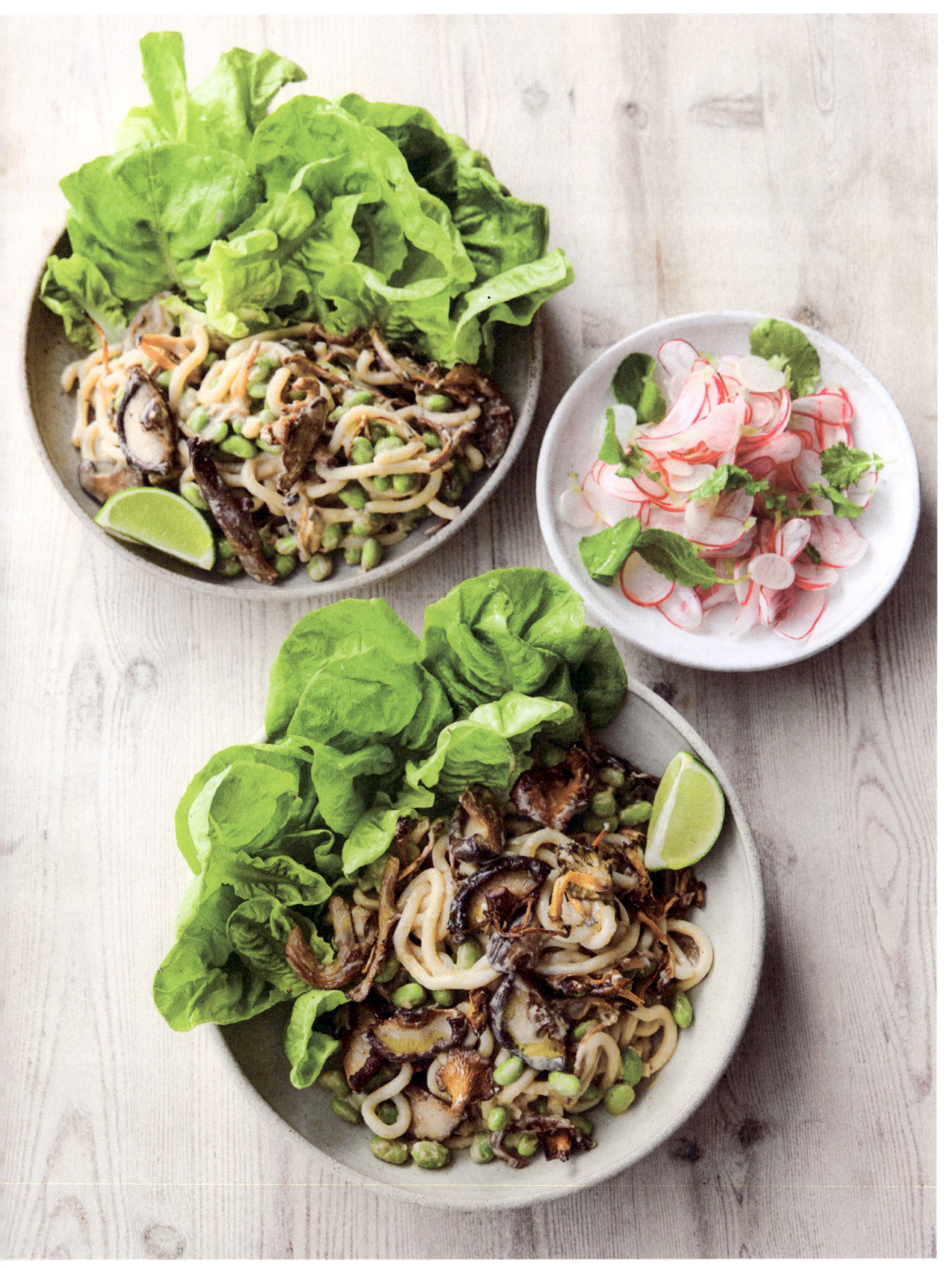

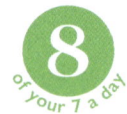

Charred Mexican salad

SERVES 1 | 12 MINUTES

80g each
jarred roasted red peppers, sweetheart cabbage, ripe tomato, spring onions, ripe avocado, cucumber, tinned black beans, tinned sweetcorn

1 tablespoon jarred sliced jalapeños

½ a bunch of coriander (15g)

1 lime

15g feta cheese

Trim the spring onions and cabbage, then dry fry in a large non-stick frying pan on a high heat with the tomato and cucumber, until starting to char. Drain and add the beans and corn until they start to pop, then tip it all on to a large board and clank up with the peppers. In a small food processor, blitz the peeled, destoned avo with the jalapeños and 1 tablespoon of their liquor, a splash of water, most of the coriander, stalks and all, and the lime juice, then season to perfection and pour on to your plate. Pile the charred chopped veg on top, crumble over the feta and pick over the remaining coriander leaves. A delight as it is, or delicious with rice of your choice on the side.

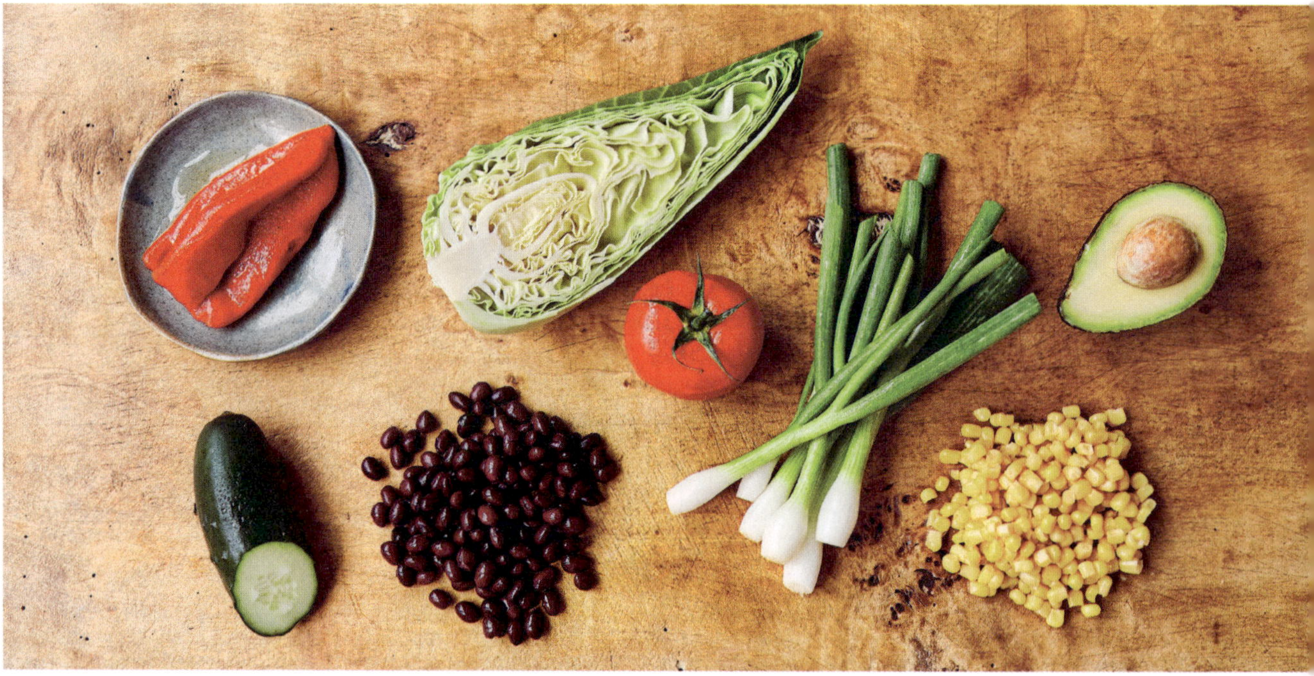

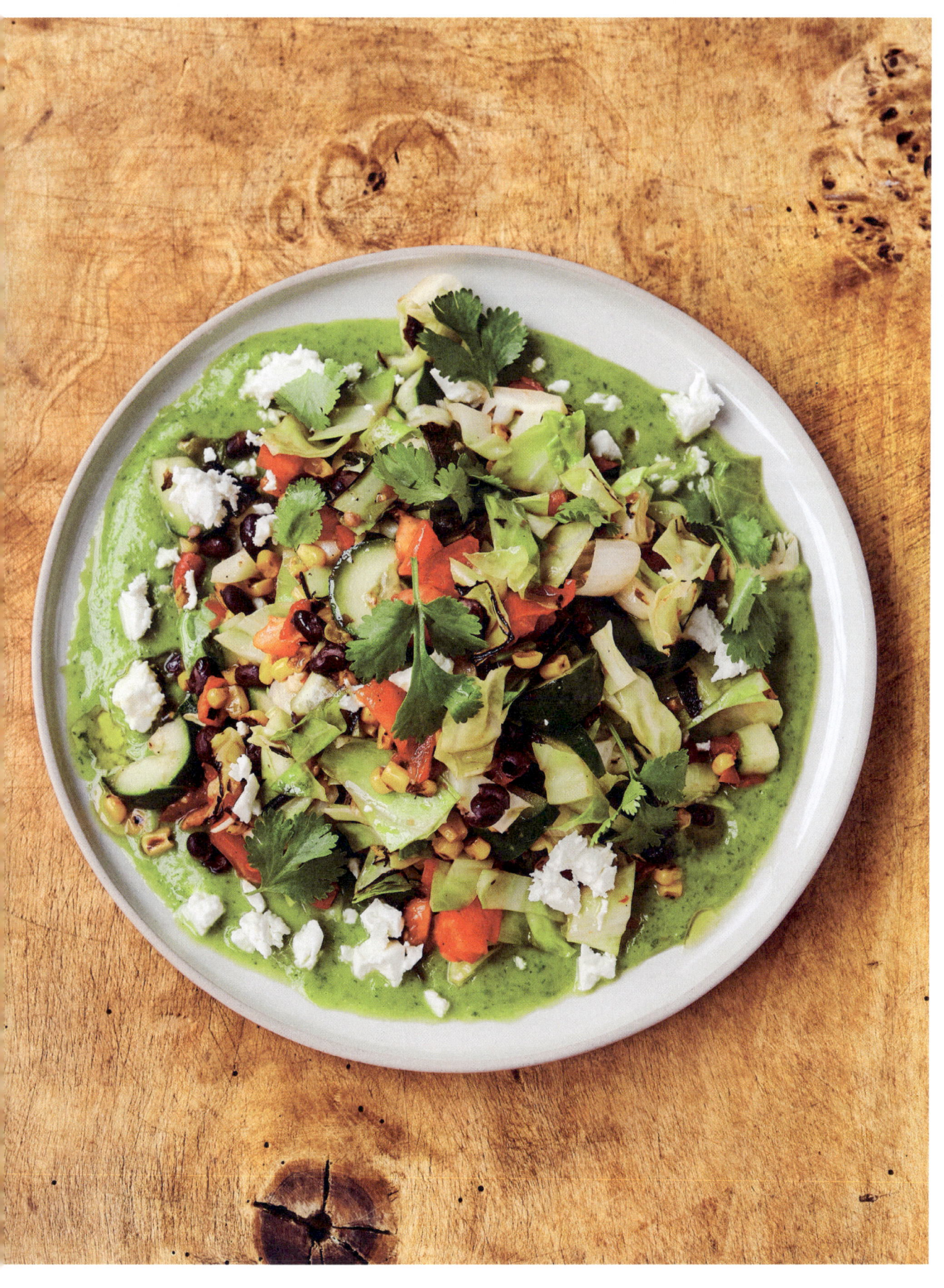

Tasty salmon couscous

This recipe is all about wholesome ingredients, put together in a delicious way

SERVES 1
12 MINUTES

1 x 130g salmon fillet, skin on, scaled, pin-boned

½ a small courgette (80g)

80g frozen broad beans

75g wholewheat couscous

½ a lemon

80g ripe mixed-colour cherry tomatoes

1 fresh red chilli

2 spring onions

2 sprigs of basil

2 heaped tablespoons natural yoghurt

1 Put a dry non-stick frying pan on a medium-high heat. Starting on the flesh side, cook the salmon for 1½ minutes on each of its four sides, or until just cooked through, then pull off the skin and crisp up on the underside, removing each once done. Halve and finely slice the courgette, add to the pan of rendered fish oil with the beans and cook for 2 minutes, tossing regularly.

2 Meanwhile, boil the kettle. Put the couscous into a bowl, finely grate in the lemon zest, season with sea salt and black pepper, just cover with boiling kettle water, cover the bowl with your serving plate and leave aside.

3 Squeeze the lemon juice into another bowl. Quarter and add the tomatoes, finely slice and add the chilli. Trim and finely slice the spring onions, tossing the whites with the tomatoes and putting the greens into a pestle and mortar. Add most of the basil leaves to the pestle and mortar with a pinch of salt, pound into a paste, then muddle in the yoghurt.

4 Fluff up the couscous and spoon on to your plate, then scatter over the courgettes, beans and dressed tomatoes. Flake over the salmon and crispy skin, dollop over the yoghurt, and finish with the remaining basil leaves. Nice with a few drips of extra virgin olive oil, if you like.

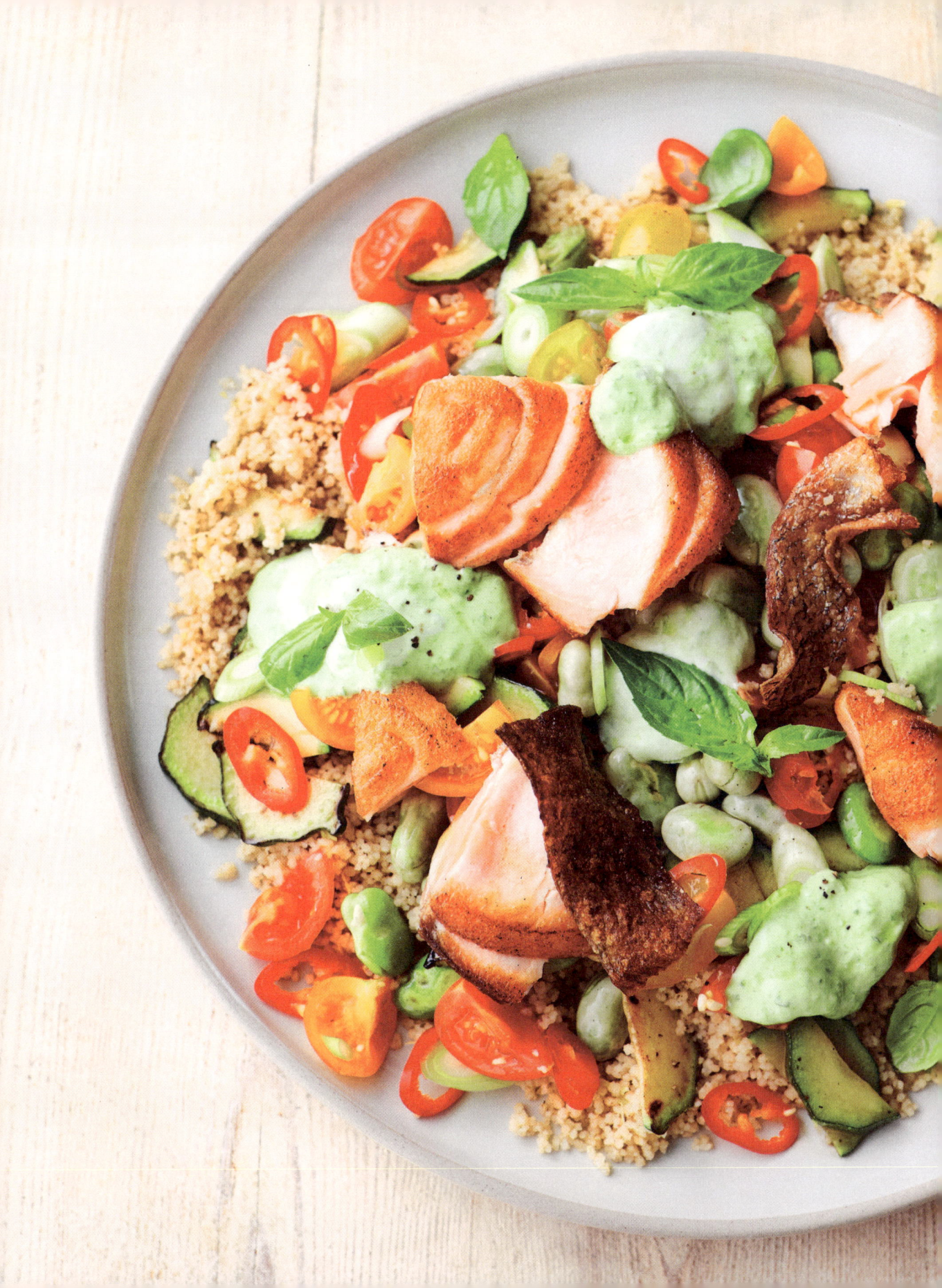

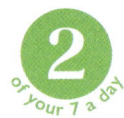

Crispy pork noodle broth

Curling up on the sofa for a good old slurp from a bowl of spicy noodle broth is a real joy

SERVES 1
12 MINUTES

100g pork mince

80g mixed mushrooms

1 nest of instant vermicelli rice noodles (45g)

2 spring onions

80g cucumber

80g frozen edamame beans

1 heaped teaspoon white miso

2 teaspoons tahini

1 teaspoon crunchy peanut & sesame chilli oil, plus extra to serve

1 clove of garlic

1 Boil the kettle. Put a non-stick frying pan on a high heat and go in with the mince, mushrooms, tearing any larger ones, and a generous pinch of black pepper. Cook until the mince is lightly golden, stirring regularly.

2 Meanwhile, put the noodles in a serving bowl, just cover with boiling kettle water and leave to rehydrate for a few minutes, while you trim and finely slice the spring onions and matchstick the cucumber.

3 Stir the frozen edamame into the pan and cook for 2 more minutes, or until hot through and the mince is dark golden. Drain the noodles. Put the miso, tahini and chilli oil into the bowl, peel and finely grate in the garlic, cover with 150ml of boiling kettle water and whisk to dissolve.

4 Add the drained noodles to the bowl of broth, sprinkle the contents of the pan on top, pile on the cucumber and spring onions, then mix and enjoy!

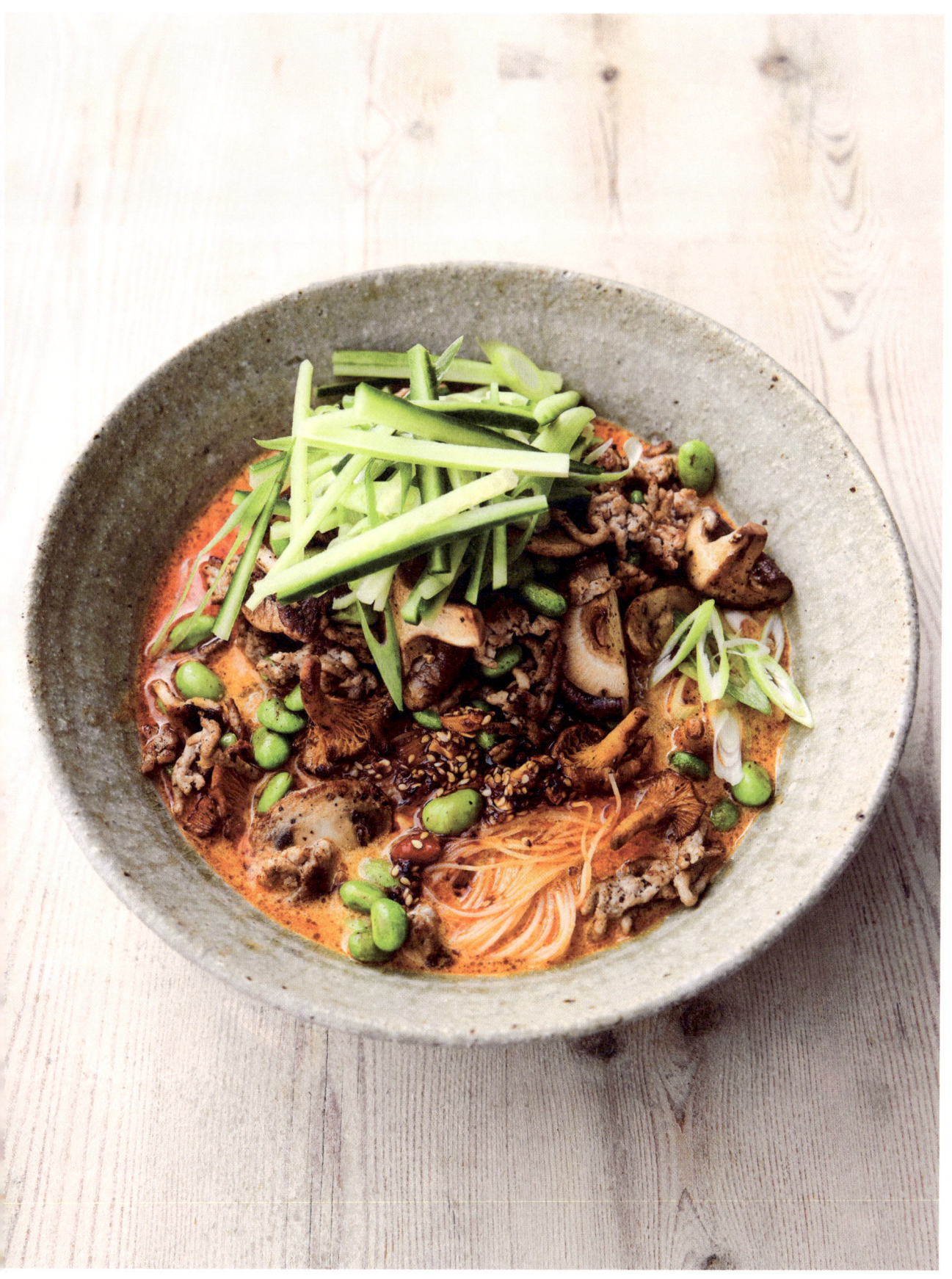

Silken tofu & black beans

Tinned beans and black bean sauce unite to create incredible depth of flavour in this rich panful

SERVES 2
13 MINUTES

1 red onion (160g)

6cm piece of ginger

2 cloves of garlic

1 fresh red chilli

½ a bunch of coriander (15g)

2 tablespoons black bean sauce

1 x 400g tin of black beans

300g silken tofu

160g pak choi

30g roasted unsalted peanuts

1 Peel and finely chop the red onion, ginger and garlic, and place in a large frying pan on a high heat with 1 tablespoon of olive oil. Finely slice the chilli, add half to the pan, then cook it all for 5 minutes, stirring regularly.

2 Meanwhile, finely chop the coriander stalks, reserving the leaves. Stir the stalks into the pan with the black bean sauce and a splash of red wine vinegar. Let it bubble and reduce, then pour in the beans, juice and all, mashing half of them with a fork for a creamier texture. Season to perfection.

3 Slice the tofu into 8 equal pieces and fan them on top of the beans. Quarter the pak choi lengthways and place around the edge of the pan. Cover and cook for 5 minutes, or until the pak choi is just cooked.

4 Scatter over the reserved coriander leaves and chilli, crush and scatter over the peanuts, and serve. Nice with wholegrain rice.

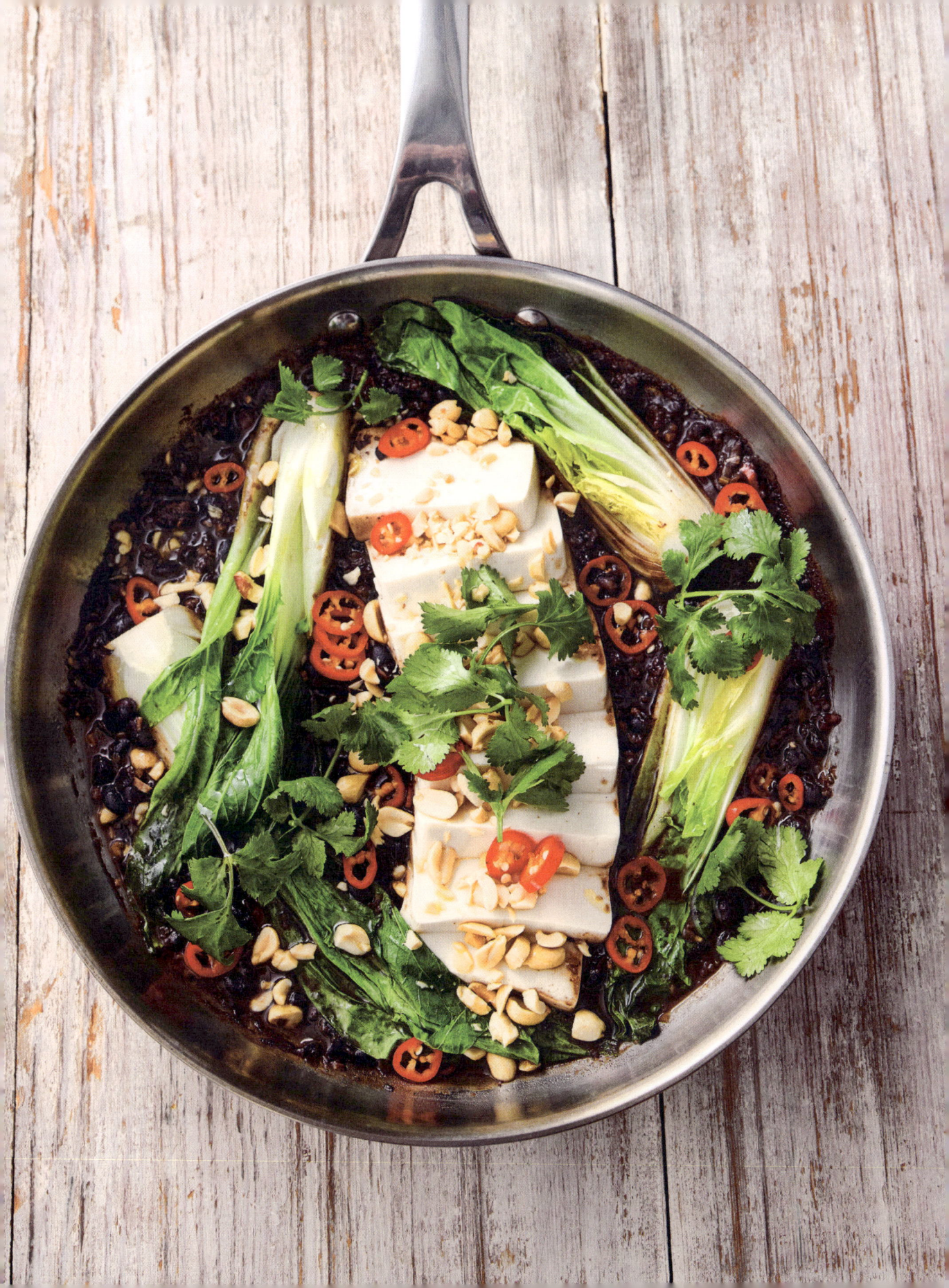

3 of your 7 a day

Chicken fajitas

These fajitas are fast and furious, but our friend the griddle pan does most of the heavy lifting

SERVES 2
13 MINUTES

1 red pepper (160g)

1 red onion (160g)

2 x 150g skinless chicken breasts

160g ripe cherry tomatoes

1 teaspoon Cajun seasoning

1 teaspoon runny honey

1 teaspoon wholegrain mustard

2 large or 4 small wholemeal tortillas

4 tablespoons natural yoghurt

½ a bunch of coriander (15g)

1 Boil the kettle. Put a griddle pan on a high heat. Deseed the pepper, peel the onion, and finely slice both. Slice the chicken lengthways into 1cm-thick strips. In a bowl, toss it all with the tomatoes, 1 tablespoon each of red wine vinegar and olive oil, the Cajun seasoning and a pinch of black pepper.

2 Scatter the contents of the bowl into the hot griddle pan and cook for 6 minutes, or until gnarly and cooked through, tossing regularly.

3 Meanwhile, in a mug, mix the honey and mustard with 2 tablespoons of boiling kettle water. Briefly warm the tortillas, over the griddle pan or directly over the flame of a gas hob, and place on your plates.

4 Pour the honey mixture into the griddle pan, mix with the chicken and veg, let it sizzle and reduce for a few seconds to a saucy consistency, then divide between the tortillas. Spoon over the yoghurt and pick over the coriander.

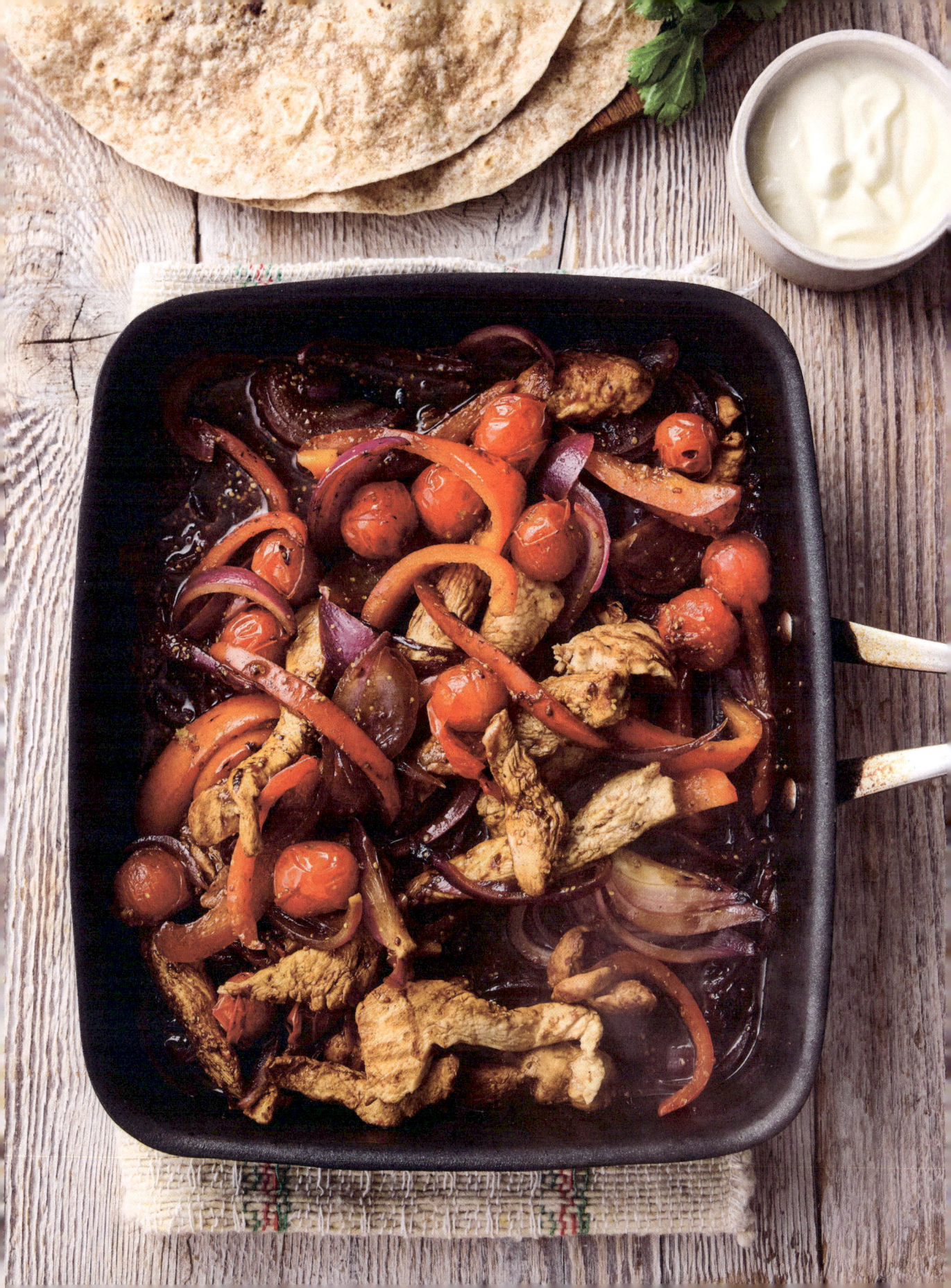

Seared tuna kimchi bowl

A colourful bowl of delicious things that complement each other just beautifully

SERVES 2
13 MINUTES

- 3 heaped tablespoons natural yoghurt
- 3 heaped tablespoons kimchi (70g)
- 1 x 250g packet of cooked wholegrain rice
- 2 carrots (160g)
- 160g frozen broad beans or peas
- 2 x 150g super-fresh tuna steaks, ideally 1½cm thick
- 2 tablespoons sesame seeds
- ½ a cucumber (160g)
- 1 lemon
- 1 tablespoon low-salt soy sauce

1. In a small food processor, blitz the yoghurt with the kimchi until smooth.

2. Put a large non-stick frying pan on a medium-high heat, spritz with olive oil, then tip in the rice. Wash, coarsely grate and stir in the carrot, along with the broad beans and a splash of water. Heat through for 2 minutes, then season to perfection. Divide between serving bowls or, I like to use a small oil-spritzed bowl to compact half the rice at a time, turning out in a mound.

3. Wipe out the pan, spritz the tuna steaks with oil, season with a small pinch of sea salt and black pepper, sear in the hot pan for 1 minute on each side, so they're still blushing in the middle – trust me – then remove.

4. Wipe out the pan and toast the sesame seeds until golden, tossing regularly, while you squash along the length of the cucumber with the heel of your hand, then roughly chop it. Toss with the lemon zest and juice, and the soy.

5. Add the kimchi yoghurt to the bowls with the dressed cucumber, slice and add the tuna, scatter over the hot toasted sesame seeds, toss and tuck in.

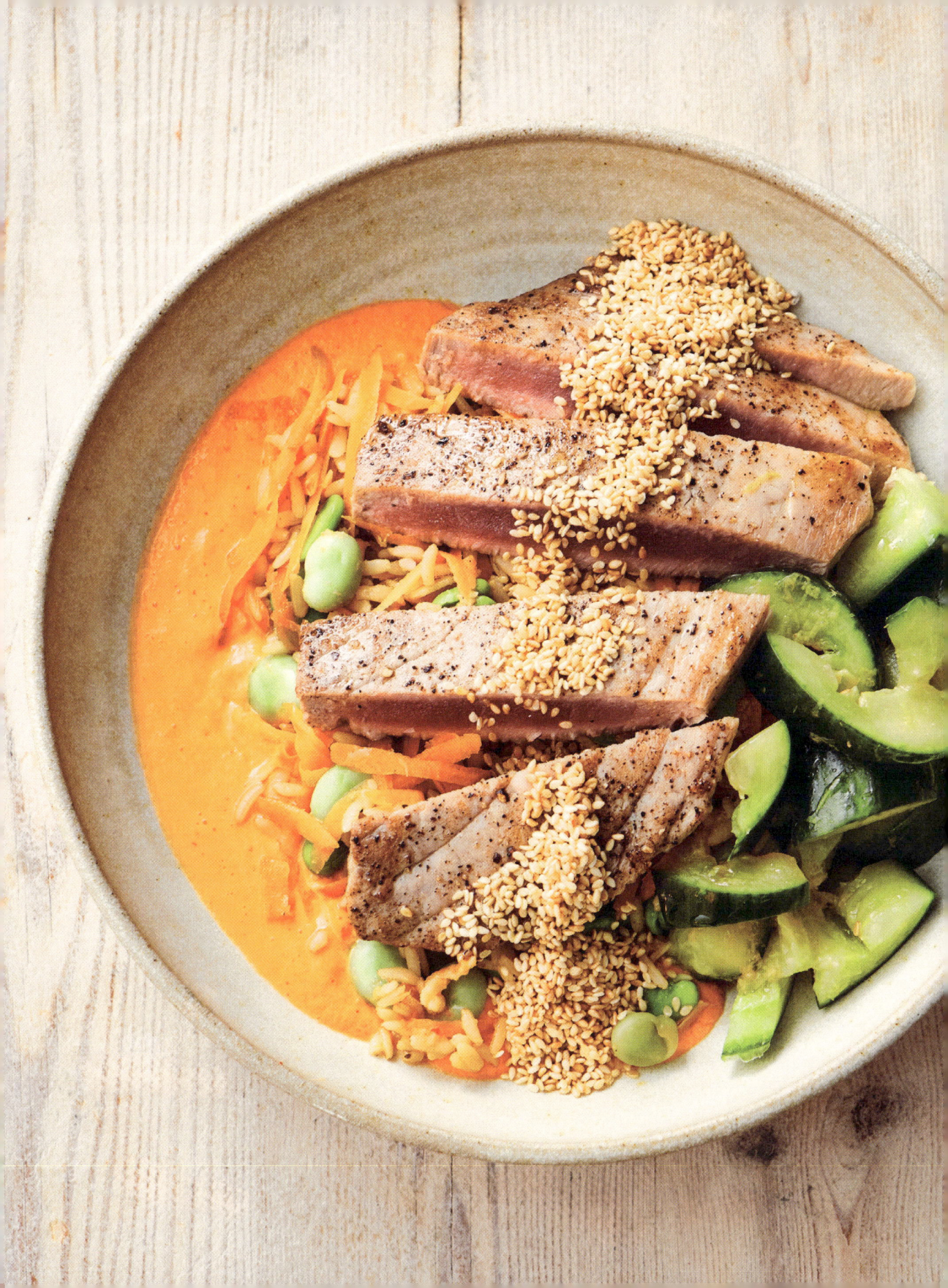

Lemon tahini chicken & grains

Here we're jazzing up a handy grain packet, meaning you get big flavour, fast

SERVES 2
13 MINUTES

160g tenderstem broccoli

2 x 150g skinless chicken breasts

1 x 460g jar of roasted red peppers

2 cloves of garlic

½ a bunch of basil (15g)

30g black olives, stone in

1 lemon

2 tablespoons tahini

1 x 250g packet of cooked mixed grains

1 x 400g tin of cannellini beans

1 Put a large shallow non-stick casserole pan on a high heat. Trim the broccoli, halve any thicker stalks lengthways, and dry fry while you score deeply across the chicken breasts at 1cm intervals. Spritz with olive oil, rub with sea salt and black pepper, and cook for 3 minutes on each side, or until the chicken is golden and cooked through and the broccoli is lightly charred.

2 Meanwhile, tip the peppers into a blender, juice and all, then peel and add the garlic. Add the basil, stalks and all, reserving a few nice leaves, and blitz until smooth. Squash, destone and finely chop the olives. Finely grate and reserve the lemon zest. Squeeze the juice into a bowl with the tahini, which will thicken it, then loosen with splashes of water and season to perfection.

3 Move the chicken to a board to rest with the broccoli. Pour the pepper sauce into the pan with the grains. Drain and add the beans, mix together, boil for a couple of minutes, or until reduced, then season to perfection and divide between plates. Scatter over the broccoli, slice and add the chicken, spoon over the lemon tahini sauce, then sprinkle with the olives, lemon zest and reserved basil leaves.

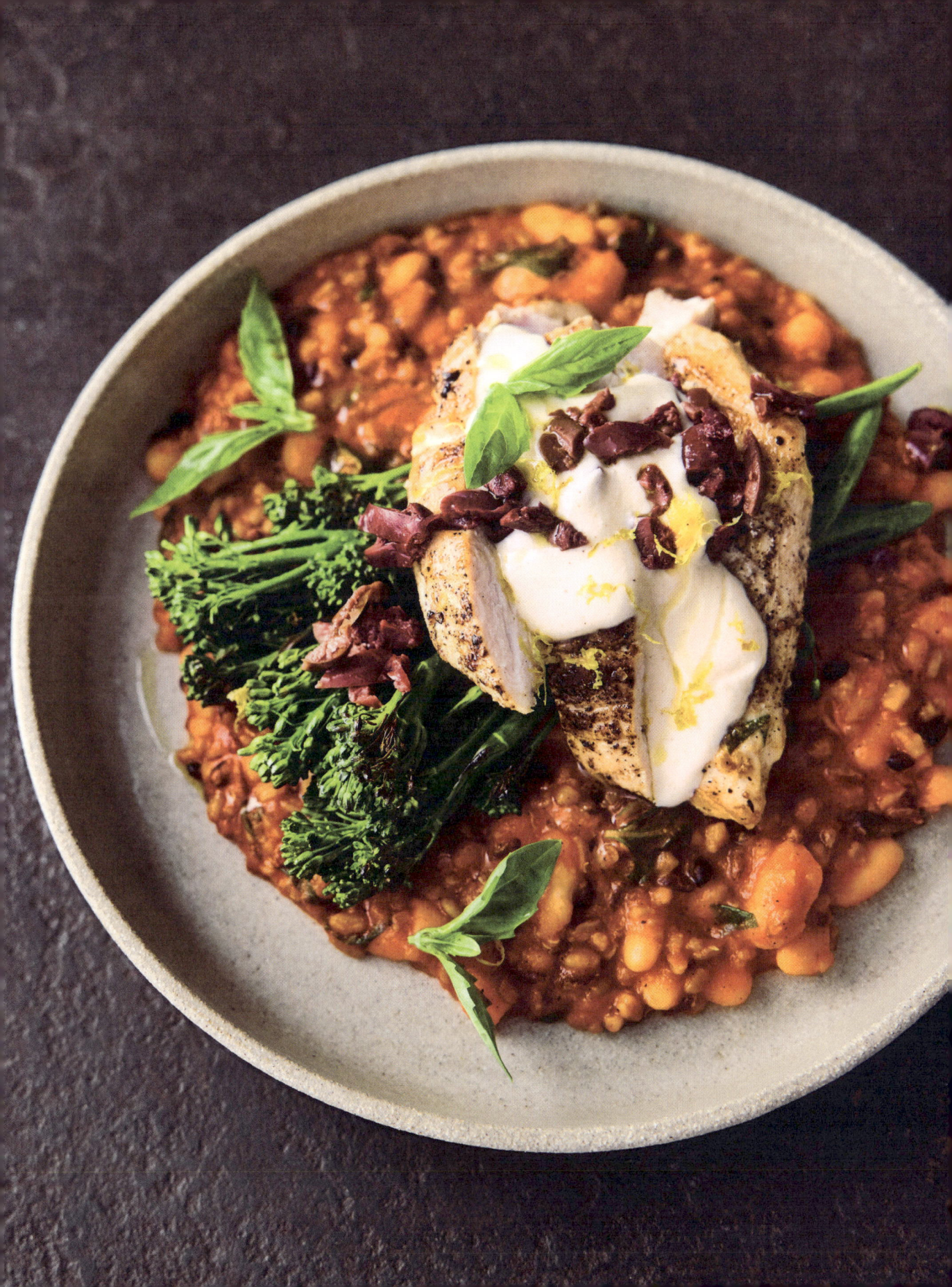

Golden chicken, peppers & rice

This is my perfect kind of midweek meal – fast, sizzling, flavoursome and fun

SERVES 2
14 MINUTES

160g kale

½ a head of broccoli (160g)

1 red pepper (160g)

2 x 150g skinless chicken breasts

1 x 250g packet of cooked wholegrain rice

1 tablespoon harissa paste, plus extra to serve

1 lemon

30g feta cheese

2 heaped tablespoons houmous

1 Put a large non-stick frying pan on a high heat and tear in the kale, discarding any tough stalks, to wilt and lightly char as the pan heats up. Meanwhile, cut the broccoli into small florets. Cut the pepper into 1cm-thick slices, discarding the seeds. Cut the chicken lengthways into 1cm-thick strips.

2 Once the kale has wilted, tip the rice into the pan, add the harissa, squeeze in half the lemon juice, then toss over the heat for 2 minutes until the rice is hot through, season to perfection and divide between your plates.

3 Put 1 tablespoon of olive oil into the hot pan, then add the chicken, peppers and broccoli. Season with sea salt and black pepper, and cook for 5 minutes, or until everything is dark golden and cooked through, tossing regularly.

4 Divide up the chicken, peppers and broccoli, crumble over the feta, and spoon over the houmous and a little extra harissa. Serve with lemon wedges.

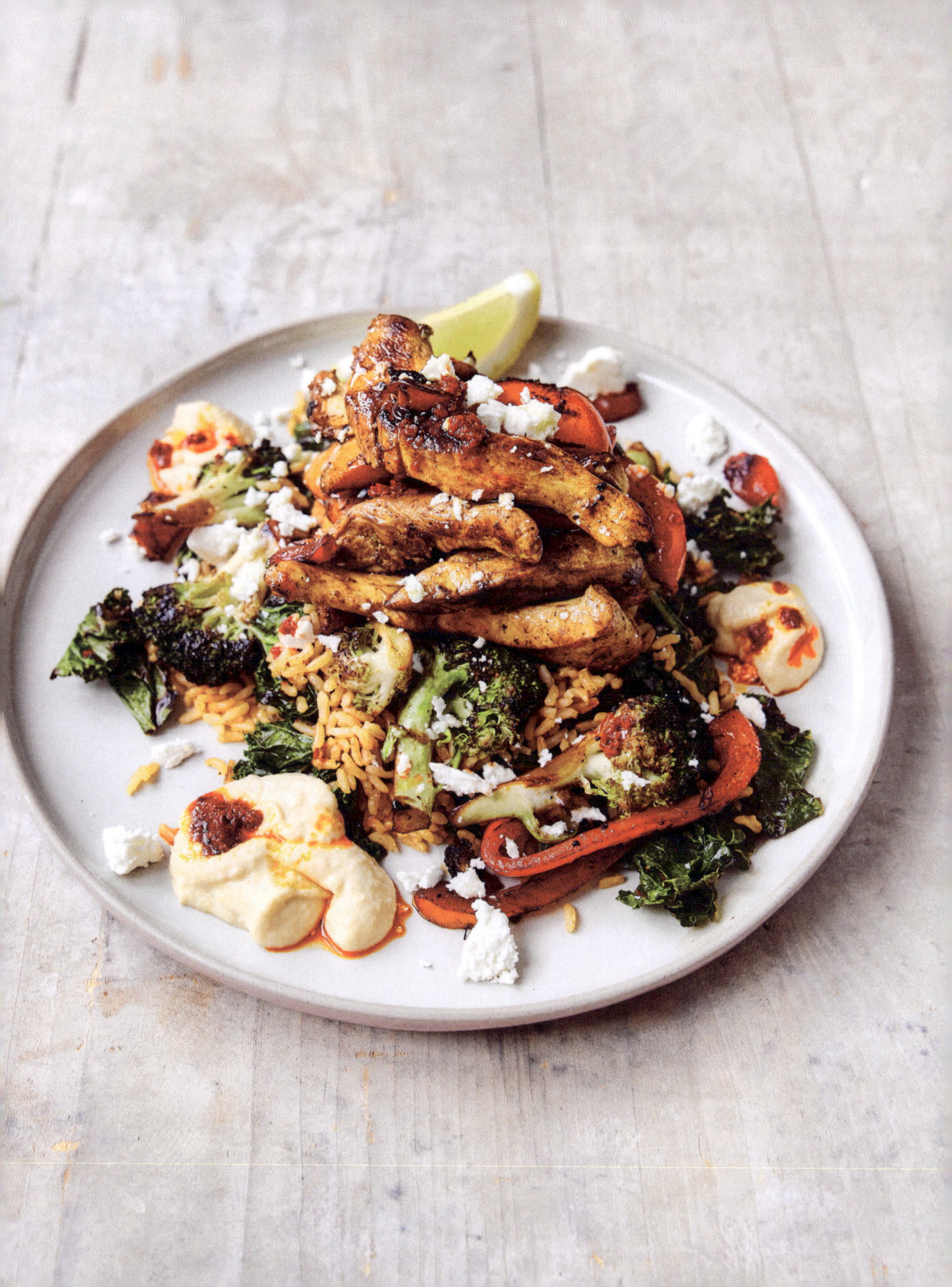

Crispy black bean beef

Quick, easy and full of flavour, this one-pan stir-fry is a total cracker, delivering big on all fronts

SERVES 1
15 MINUTES

100g beef mince

80g shiitake mushrooms

2cm piece of ginger

2 sprigs of coriander or mint

½–1 fresh red chilli

150g straight-to-wok udon noodles

80g mangetout

80g fresh or frozen edamame beans

80g sliced water chestnuts

2 tablespoons black bean sauce

1. Put a large frying pan on a high heat, spritz with olive oil, and add the mince, breaking it up with your spoon, then the mushrooms, halving any larger ones. Peel, finely chop and add the ginger, along with the coriander stalks, if using. Fry for 5 minutes, or until the beef is crispy, stirring regularly.

2. Finely slice and add the chilli, tear in the noodles and add the mangetout, edamame and water chestnuts, with a splash of their juice, continuing to stir.

3. In a bowl, loosen the black bean sauce with 1 tablespoon of red wine vinegar and 4 tablespoons of water, toss into the pan until well coated, and serve right away, sprinkled with the coriander leaves.

EASY SWAPS

Use your favourite mushrooms, or swap in other crunchy green veg.

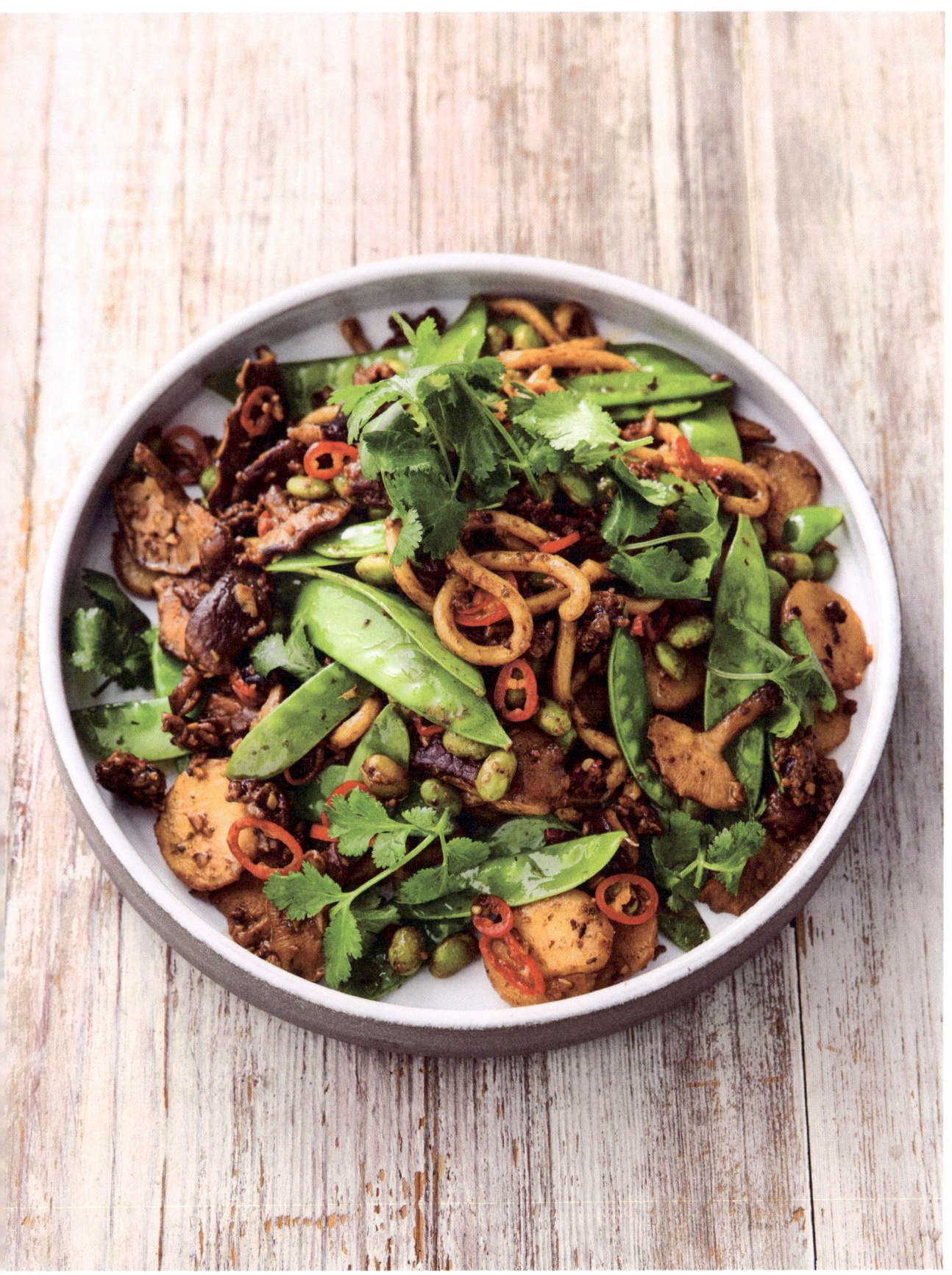

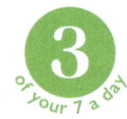

Chicken cup salad

Here we're using gem lettuce as a receptacle for hot, cold, sweet, salty and sour ingredients

SERVES 2
16 MINUTES

2 gem lettuces

½ a bunch of tarragon (10g)

1 nest of instant vermicelli rice noodles (45g)

2 x 150g skinless chicken breasts

1 red onion (160g)

4cm piece of ginger

2 cloves of garlic

160g frozen mango

2 tablespoons sweet chilli dipping sauce, plus extra to serve

2 limes

1 Boil the kettle. Click the outer leaves off the lettuces and arrange on a serving platter like cups. Finely shred the rest of the lettuce, place in a large bowl, and pick in the tarragon. In another bowl, cover the noodles with boiling kettle water, leave to rehydrate for a few minutes, then drain.

2 Put a large non-stick frying pan on a medium-high heat and spritz with olive oil. Chop the chicken breasts into 2cm chunks and add to the pan. Peel the red onion, cut into eighths and break into petals, peel and matchstick the ginger and garlic, add to the pan with the frozen mango and cook it all for 5 minutes, or until the chicken is golden and cooked through, tossing regularly.

3 Loosen the sweet chilli sauce with the juice of 1 lime, add to the pan and toss over the heat for 1 minute, while you divide the shredded lettuce and noodles between the lettuce cups. Season the chicken to perfection and portion up with the veg. Serve with lime wedges.

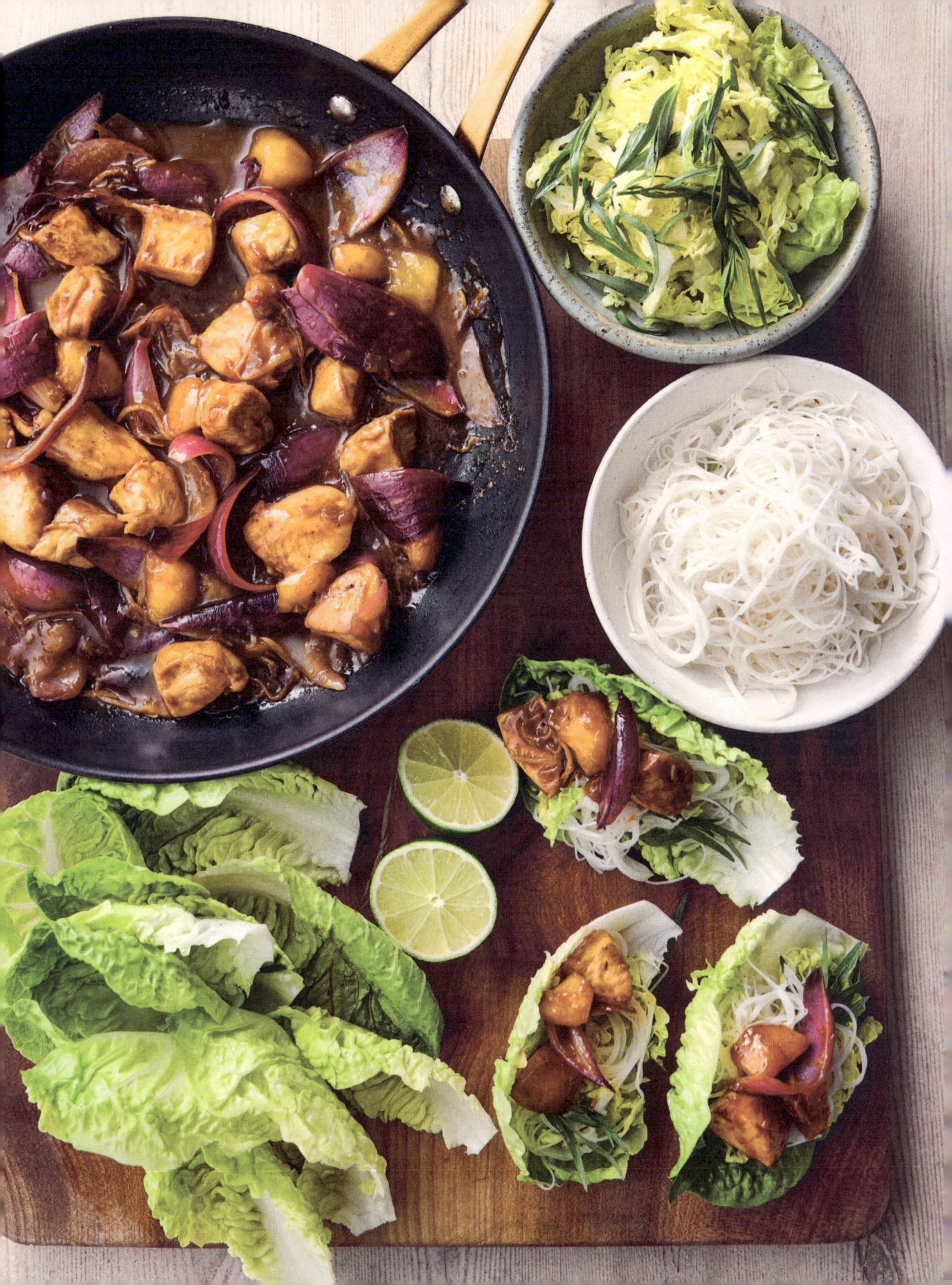

Steak & sticky aubergine salad

Fast, fun and full of flavour, this warming steak dish is a real favourite of mine

SERVES 2
18 MINUTES

1 aubergine (250g)

2 nests of instant vermicelli rice noodles (90g total)

1 x 200g sirloin steak

8cm piece of ginger

160g asparagus

2 cloves of garlic

1 lime

1 tablespoon gochujang paste

½ a cucumber (160g)

½ a bunch of coriander (15g)

1 Boil the kettle. Quarter the aubergine lengthways and microwave at 800W for 6 minutes, or until soft. In a bowl, cover the noodles with boiling kettle water and leave to rehydrate for a few minutes, then drain and arrange on a nice serving platter.

2 Put a large non-stick frying pan on a medium-high heat. Cut any fat off the steak, finely chop the fat, then place it in the pan to render. Peel, finely chop and add the ginger, fry for 2 minutes, tossing regularly, then remove the crispy bits to a bowl, leaving the rendered fat in the pan. Cut off the sinew, season the steak, sear for 90 seconds on each side so it's still blushing in the centre, then remove to rest.

3 Put the soft aubergine in the pan, trim the woody ends off the asparagus, then add the spears to the pan and let it all char and catch for a couple of minutes. Meanwhile, peel the garlic, finely grate it into the bowl of crispy bits with the lime zest, squeeze in half the juice, then stir in the gochujang and 5 tablespoons of boiling kettle water.

4 Toss the sauce mixture into the pan and let it sizzle away, then arrange the gochujang veg on the platter, drizzling over any remaining sauce. Finely slice the cucumber, finely chop most of the coriander, reserving a few leaves, then toss both with the remaining lime juice and a pinch of sea salt and black pepper. Slice the steak and add to the platter, top with the dressed cucumber, and finish with the last few coriander leaves.

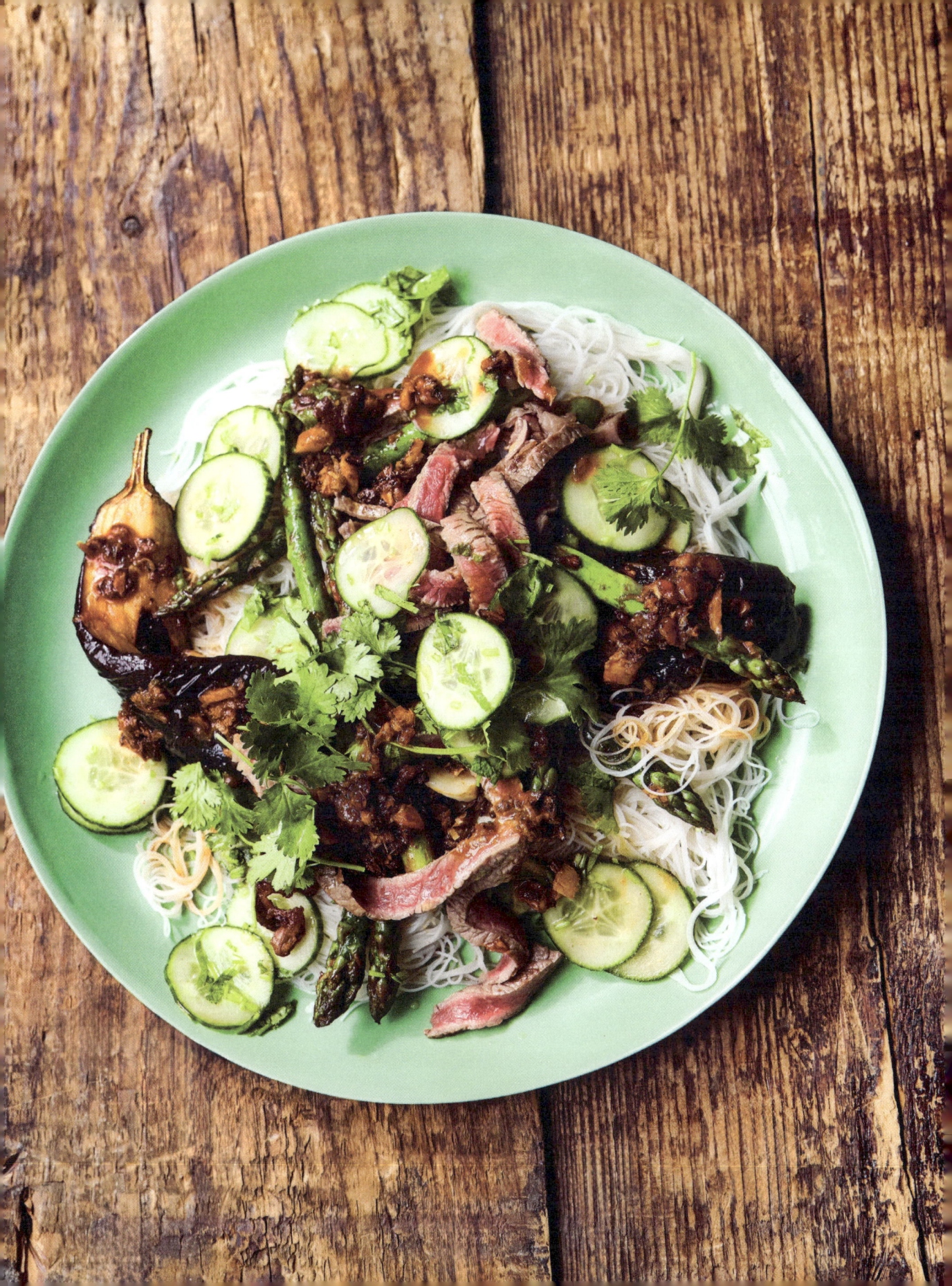

Chicken balls & rainbow broth

Satisfying to both make and eat, these fragrant balls are fresh and super-tasty

SERVES 4
18 MINUTES

2 fresh red chillies

4 cloves of garlic

2 x 150g skinless chicken breasts

1 x 250g packet of cooked wholegrain rice

2 tablespoons white miso

100g pickled ginger

1 bunch of coriander (30g)

2 limes

1.5 litres chicken stock

2 x 320g packets of mixed stir-fry veg

1 Boil the kettle. Deseed the chillies, peel the garlic and place both in a food processor with the chicken, rice, half the miso and the pickled ginger, reserving the juice. Add most of the coriander, stalks and all, reserving a few nice leaves. Finely grate in the lime zest, and pulse until combined. Divide the mixture into 16 equal-sized pieces and, with wet hands, shape into balls.

2 Place a large deep pan on a medium-high heat. Pour in the stock, add the remaining miso and bring to the boil. Gently drop in the balls, cover and poach for 3 minutes, then add all the stir-fry veg and cook for another 3 minutes, or until the balls are cooked through.

3 Taste the broth and season to perfection with lime juice, a little pickled ginger juice, if you like, and sea salt and black pepper. Divide between serving bowls with the reserved coriander leaves, and serve with lime wedges.

EMBELLISH IT

For extra flavour, make your own stock! Use chicken or beef bones (ask your butcher!) with offcuts or peelings of onion, carrot and celery, plus any leftover herbs. Dried mushrooms add great depth, too. Cover with water and let it tick away for 3 to 4 hours, skimming occasionally, then strain, season to perfection, and fridge or freezer stash till needed.

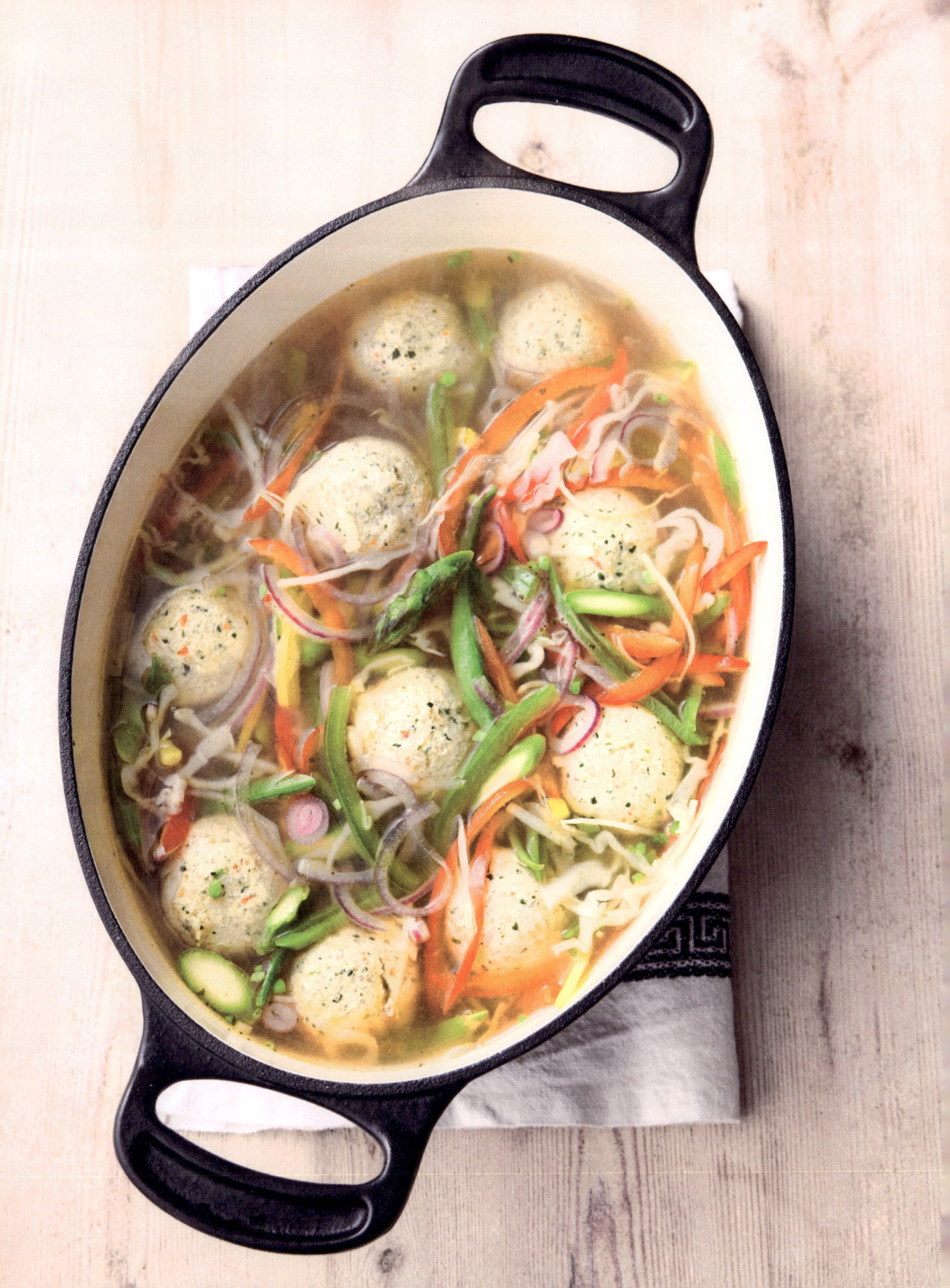

Spinach & lentil fritter salad

From the ruby dressing to the flavoursome fritters, this is a scrumptious salad with bells on

SERVES 2
19 MINUTES

1 x 400g tin of lentils

160g baby spinach

1 bunch of chives (20g)

2 slices of wholemeal sourdough bread (100g)

1 large egg

160g raspberries

1 teaspoon English mustard

50g rinded goat's cheese

20g walnut halves

200g mixed salad leaves

1 Drain the lentils and place in a food processor with the spinach and most of the chives. Tear in the bread and crack in the egg. Add a pinch of sea salt and black pepper and blitz until well combined.

2 Put a large non-stick frying pan on a medium heat with a spritz of olive oil. Working in batches, cook heaped tablespoons of the mixture for 3 minutes on each side, or until golden and crispy, then remove to a board.

3 Meanwhile, for the dressing, use a fork to crush half the raspberries in a bowl, mix in the mustard and ½ a tablespoon each of red wine vinegar and extra virgin olive oil, and season to perfection.

4 When all the fritters are done, very finely slice the goat's cheese and lay it in the pan to crisp up for a couple of minutes, crumbling the walnuts on top.

5 Divide the salad leaves between your plates, finely chop and scatter over the remaining chives, then plate up the fritters, goat's cheese and walnuts. Add the remaining raspberries and drizzle over the ruby dressing, to serve.

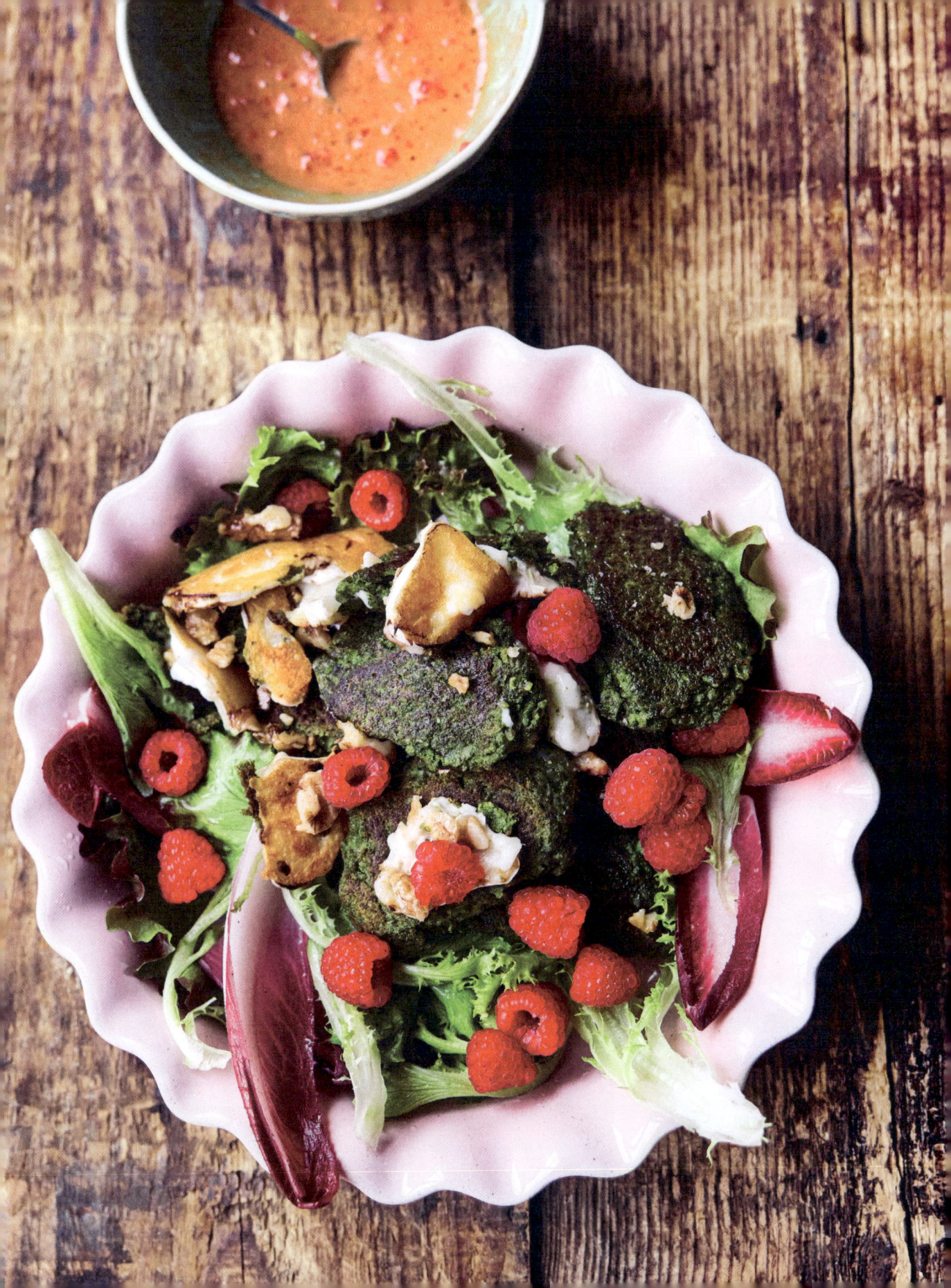

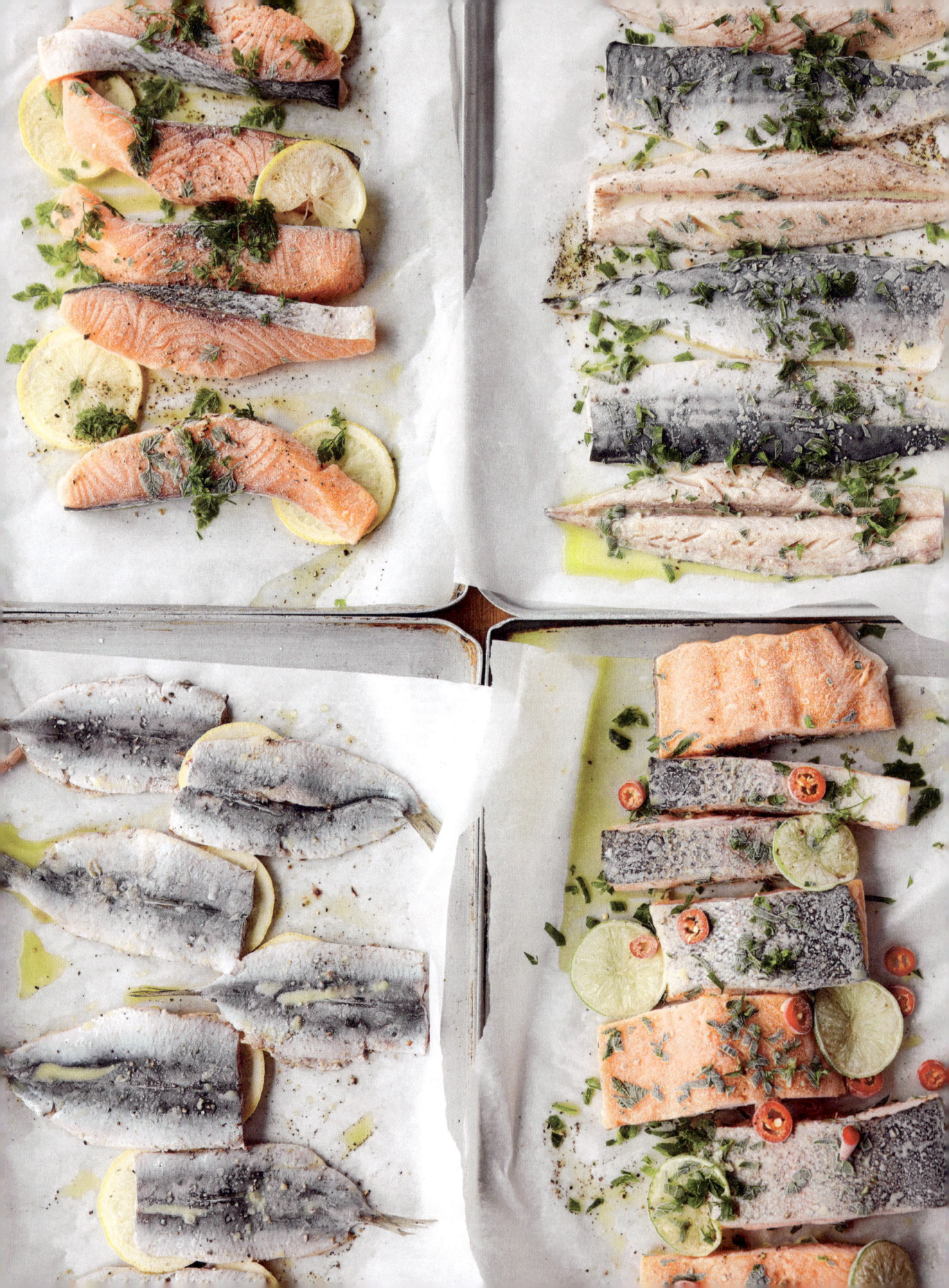

BONUS HACK

Freeze your fish

Most of us aren't eating enough fish, especially oily fish, which is a great source of omega-3s. The problem with fish is that as soon as it comes out of the water, it starts deteriorating in quality, so you need to get it fresh. Now, as much as it would be lovely to buy it straight from the fisherfolk that caught it, that's not very realistic for most of us! So every Saturday, I visit my local mobile fishmonger, Dan Eastwood, and see what fish he'd recommend that day. We always have fish for Saturday lunch, as you can really taste the difference in terms of flavour, texture and freshness by eating fish the day you buy it. I also buy extra fish for the week ahead, marinate it, and freeze it, ready to cook when I need it.

But my big hack is to use kitchen paper to pat the fish really dry first, removing as much moisture as possible, and this applies to whole fish, fillets or smaller slices and portions. Fishy smells come from ammonia created by moisture, so ironically, water is not a fish's friend when it's on land. By freezing it, you catch it at its best. I like to spritz it with olive oil, and often I add a little lemon zest, sliced chilli, a few fennel seeds or some soft fresh herbs. I either place it on a greaseproof-paper-lined tray, cover and freeze, then transfer to little bags for efficient storage, or I divide it up between small enamel roasting tins, meaning they can go straight from the freezer to a hot oven as desired. Cook until hot through and flaky.

Of course, if you don't have a local fishmonger, you can utilize your local supermarket. It's always worth looking for offers, particularly on a side of fish, which you can portion up as you want it. Just try and chat to the staff before you buy to see what came in that day, so you can be sure you're going for the freshest option.

Seared salmon rice

One-pan, quick cooking, big flavour and texture, and a nutritious result – happy days

SERVES 2
19 MINUTES

2 x 130g salmon fillets, skin on, scaled, pin-boned

1 x 250g packet of cooked wholegrain rice

1 tablespoon sesame seeds

160g frozen peas

30g pickled ginger

2 tablespoons low-salt soy sauce, plus extra to serve

1 egg

1 lemon

160g jarred roasted red peppers

4 spring onions

1 Spritz a cold 30cm non-stick frying pan with olive oil, then carefully slice each salmon fillet in half lengthways and lay in the pan.

2 Tip the rice into a bowl with the sesame seeds, peas, pickled ginger and soy. Crack in the egg, and finely grate in the lemon zest. Chop and add the peppers, with a splash of their juice. Trim the spring onions, finely slice the green tops, add to the bowl and mix well, reserving the white halves.

3 Tip the rice mixture over the salmon in an even layer, pat it down, cover, and cook on a medium-high heat for 8 minutes, or until the salmon is golden and the rice is hot through. Meanwhile, finely slice the reserved white spring onions lengthways and pop them in a bowl of cold water to curl up.

4 Carefully and confidently turn out the salmon rice as one on to a board or platter, then drain and sprinkle over the crisp white spring onions. Serve with lemon wedges and an extra drizzle of soy, if you like.

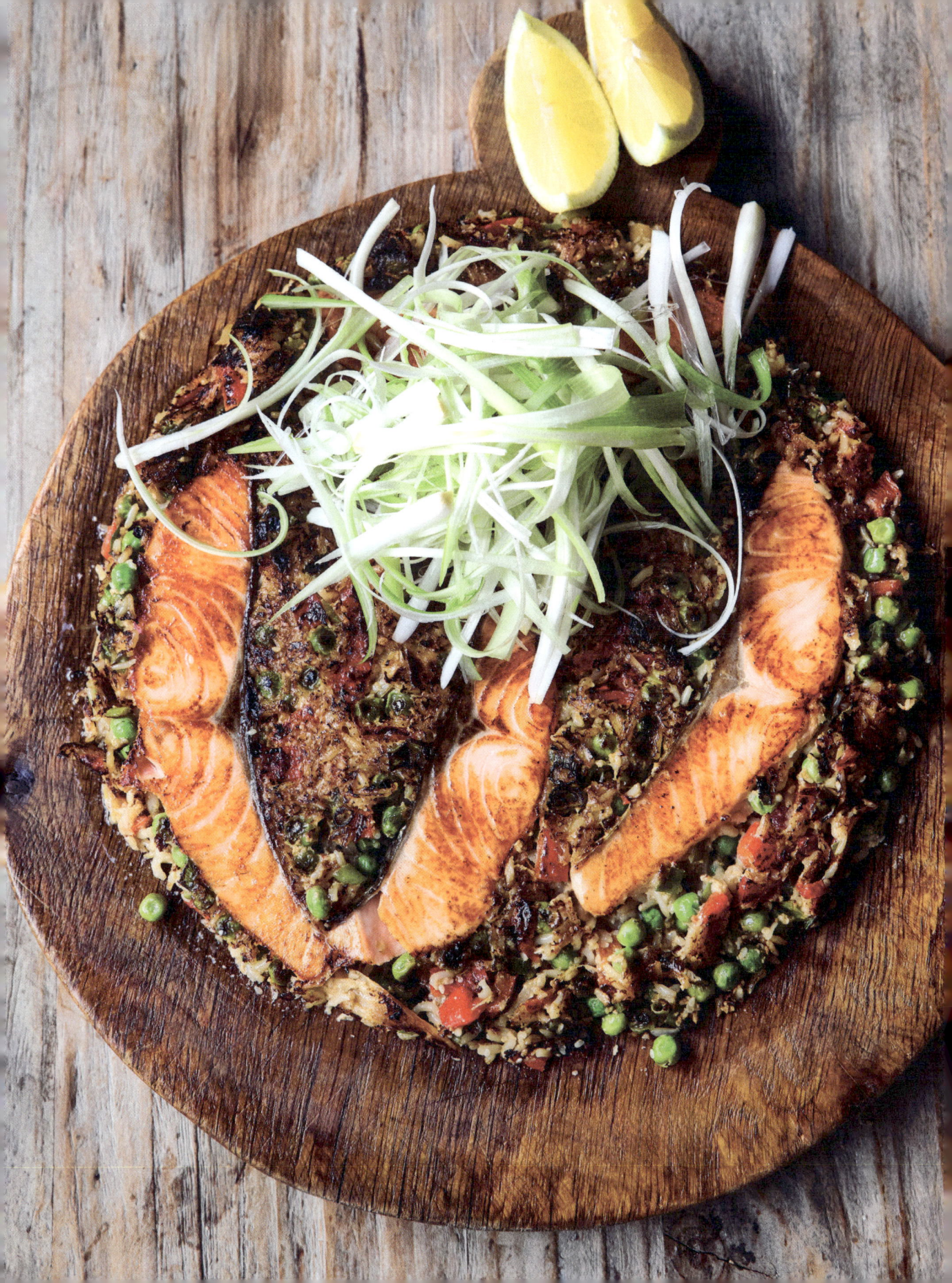

Chicken in milk

A simple one-pan dish for those days when you need a hug in a bowl

SERVES 2
20 MINUTES

800ml semi-skimmed milk

2 x 150g skinless chicken breasts

½ a small cauliflower (160g)

2 cloves of garlic

½ a bunch of sage (10g)

160g mixed mushrooms

2 heaped teaspoons English mustard

1 lemon

2 nests of instant vermicelli rice noodles (90g total)

160g baby spinach

1 Put a large deep pan on a high heat, pour in the milk, season with sea salt and black pepper, and add the chicken. Simmer vigorously for 5 minutes, while you cut the cauliflower into florets, and peel and finely slice the garlic.

2 Add the cauliflower, garlic and sage to the pan, then tear in the mushrooms and add the mustard. Cook for 5 more minutes, or until the chicken is cooked through, while you use a speed-peeler to strip in the lemon peel, then squeeze in the juice. It will split the milk, but that's the vibe.

3 Transfer the cooked chicken to a board, and remove and discard the sage. Add the noodles to the pan, followed by the spinach. Cook for a final 3 minutes so the noodles rehydrate and the spinach wilts, then stir well, season to perfection, and divide the veg and noodles between serving bowls. Slice the chicken and place on top, spooning over the liquor.

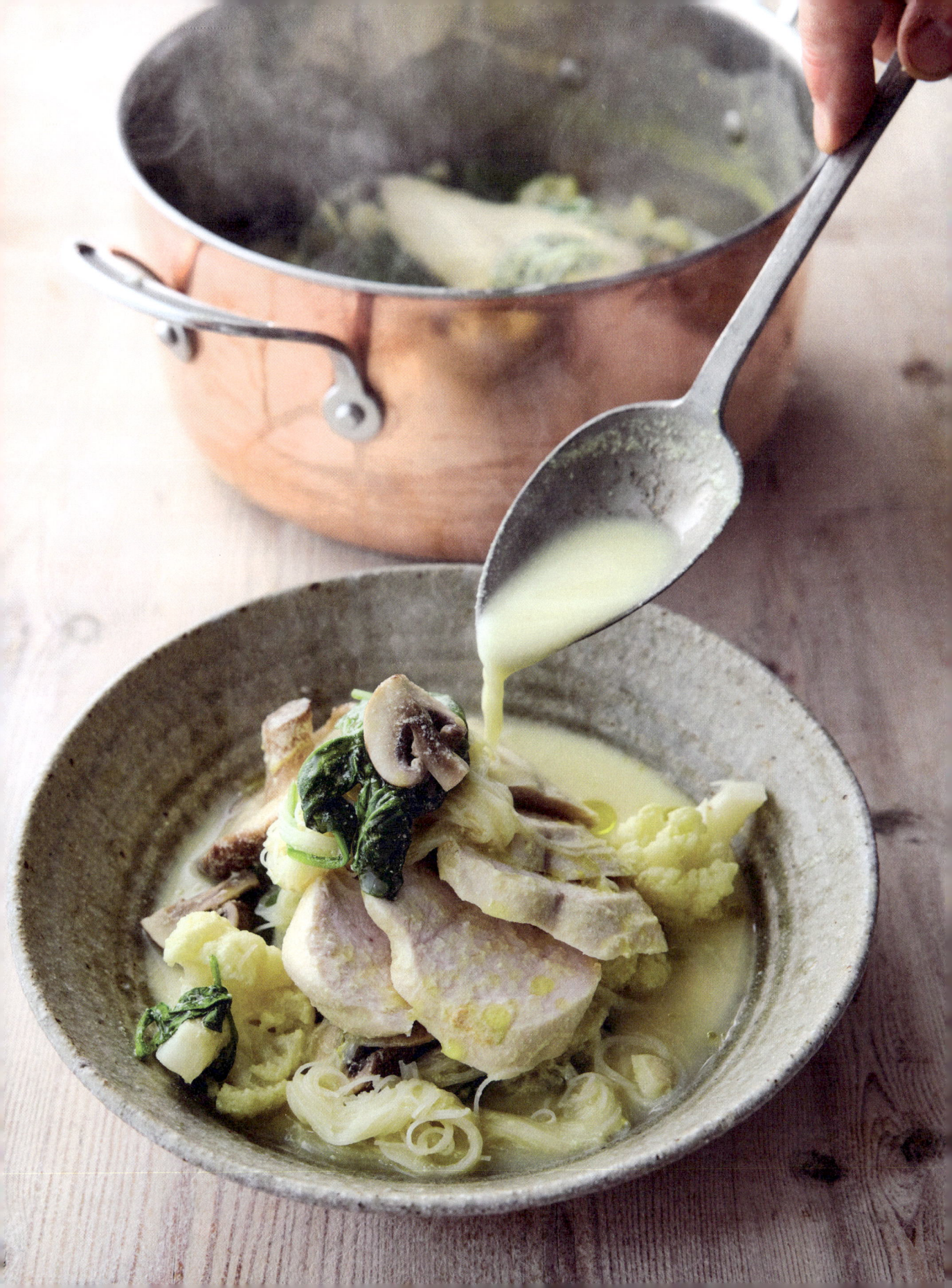

Crispy steamy parcels

These golden veg-packed parcels are super-fun to make and eat – chewy, crunchy, moreish, yum!

SERVES 2
21 MINUTES

14 rice paper wrappers

2 tablespoons sesame seeds

1 x 225g tin of sliced water chestnuts

1 x 320g packet of mixed stir-fry veg

1 bunch of coriander (30g)

165g raw peeled king prawns

1 x 120g jar of pickled ginger

2 tablespoons low-salt soy sauce

2 tablespoons sweet chilli dipping sauce

1 lime

1 One by one, dunk the rice paper wrappers into a large bowl of cold water, then lay them out on a clean olive oil-spritzed work surface, to soften.

2 Spritz a large cold non-stick frying pan well with oil and scatter the sesame seeds across the base. Drain the water chestnuts and place on a board with the stir-fry veg and half the coriander, stalks and all. Roughly chop it all together, then divide evenly between the papers. Bring in the sides of each paper to make little parcels, sitting them in the pan as you go – there's no need to be neat about it and please don't worry if they tear.

3 Place the pan on a high heat. Once it starts to sizzle, poke the prawns in between the parcels, cover, and cook for 4 minutes, or until the parcels are nicely golden on the bottom and the prawns are cooked through.

4 Meanwhile, reserving a few nice leaves, place the rest of the coriander in a blender, stalks and all. Add the pickled ginger, juice and all. Blitz until smooth, then pour into a bowl for dunking. Decant the soy and chilli sauces.

5 Carefully and confidently turn the parcels and prawns out on to a board and sprinkle with the reserved coriander leaves. Serve with lime wedges and the three sauces, stashing excess green sauce in the fridge for future meals. Dunk the prawns and parcels – once, twice or thrice, it's up to you!

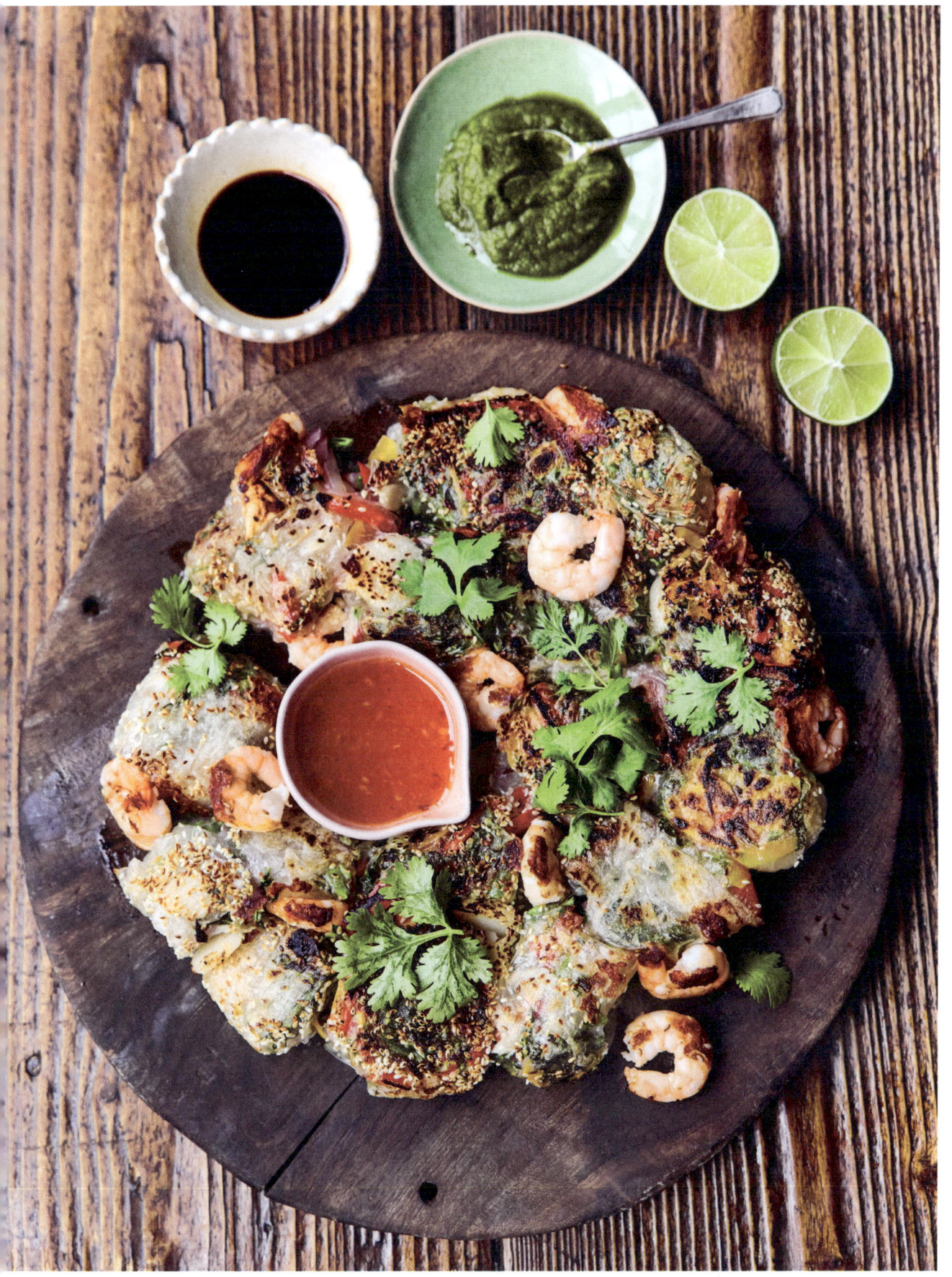

Peasto chicken salad

Here we utilize green veg in two tasty ways to elevate juicy, golden chicken

SERVES 2
21 MINUTES

160g frozen peas

160g frozen broad beans

1 lemon

20g Parmesan cheese

1 bunch of basil (30g)

2 x 150g skinless chicken breasts

160g asparagus

2 cloves of garlic

2 tablespoons pine nuts

2 heaped tablespoons cottage cheese

1. Put a large non-stick frying pan on a medium-high heat with the peas and broad beans. Cover with 100ml of water and boil for 2 minutes.

2. Put half the peas and broad beans into a blender with a good splash of the water, then drain the rest. Use a speed-peeler to strip the lemon peel, and reserve. Squeeze half the juice into the blender, add most of the Parmesan, and most of the basil, stalks and all, reserving the smaller leaves for garnish. Add 1 tablespoon of extra virgin olive oil and blitz until smooth, then season to perfection and divide between serving plates.

3. Season the chicken breasts with sea salt and black pepper, and place in the pan with a spritz of olive oil. Fry on medium-high for 7 minutes, or until cooked through, turning them halfway. Trim and add the asparagus spears and reserved lemon peel when you turn the chicken, shaking regularly.

4. With a minute to go, use a garlic crusher to crush the garlic over the chicken, add the pine nuts and the remaining peas and broad beans, squeeze over the remaining lemon juice, toss together and turn the heat off. Leave to rest for 3 minutes in the pan, then slice the chicken and pile everything on top of the peasto. Scatter over the reserved basil leaves, spoon over the cottage cheese and shave over the remaining Parmesan. Nice with bread.

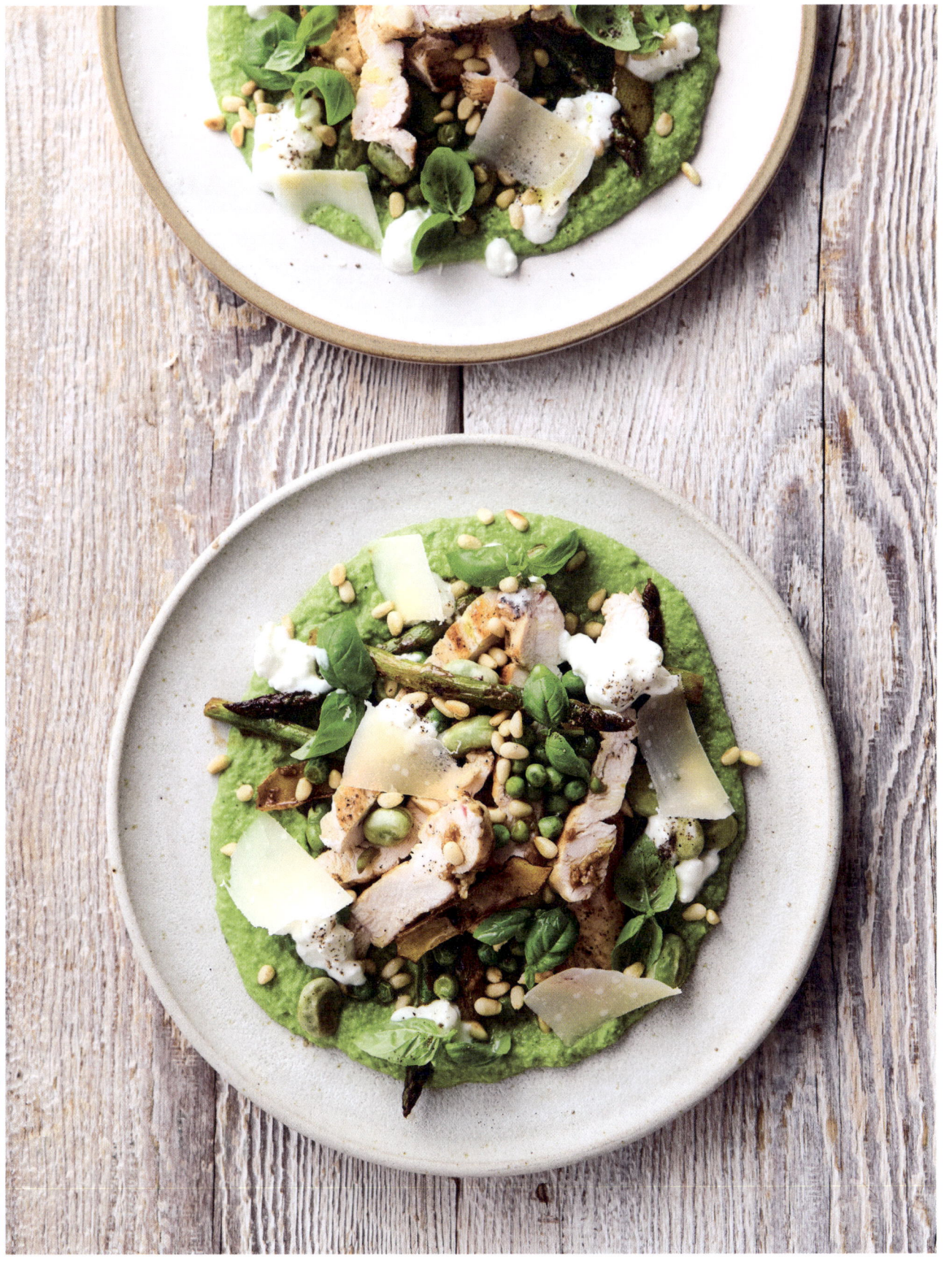

Chicken & berry grain bowl

Blistered blueberries amplify the deliciousness in this beautiful warm chicken salad

SERVES 2
21 MINUTES

2 x 150g skinless chicken breasts

1 teaspoon ras el hanout, plus extra to serve

2 cloves of garlic

1 lemon

160g blueberries

1 x 250g packet of cooked mixed grains

1 x 400g tin of lentils

160g frozen peas

½ a bunch of mint (15g)

30g feta cheese

1. Lightly score the thickest part of the chicken and season with sea salt, black pepper and the ras el hanout. Place in a large non-stick frying pan on a medium-high heat with 1 tablespoon of olive oil and cook for 5 minutes, or until golden, turning halfway.

2. Peel and finely slice the garlic, use a speed-peeler to strip the lemon peel into small pieces and add both to the pan. Cook for 2 minutes, or until the garlic is golden, then move the garlic on top of the chicken and add the blueberries. Once they start to pop and the chicken is cooked through, remove it all to a board, leaving the pan on the heat.

3. Tip in the grains with the lentils, juice and all. Reduce for 2 minutes, then add the peas and cook until hot through. Squeeze in half the lemon juice, season to perfection and divide between serving bowls with the blueberries.

4. Slice and add the chicken, plus any resting juices. Pick over the mint and crumble over the feta. Serve with lemon wedges and extra ras el hanout.

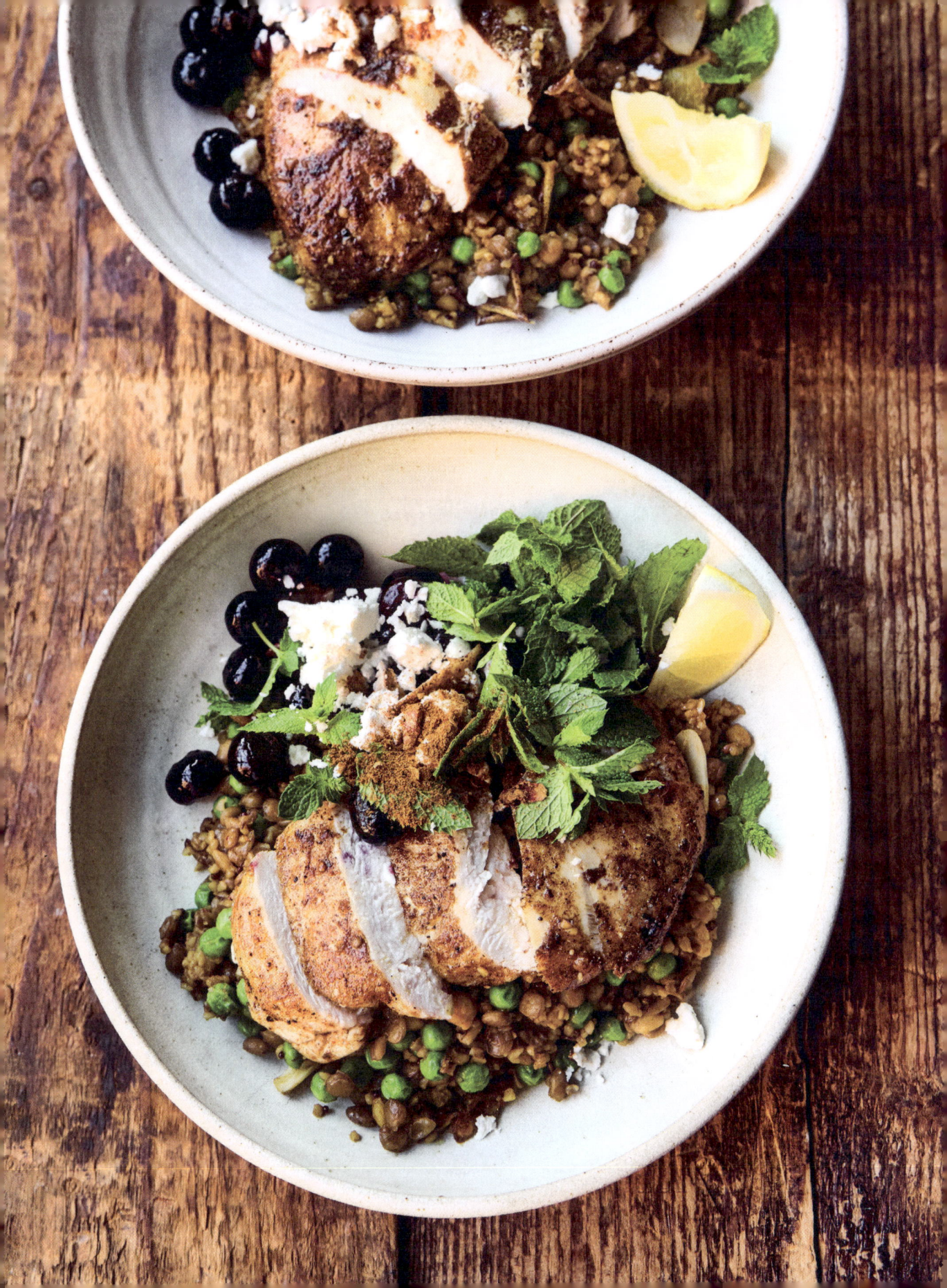

Crab spaghetti

Tasty, elegant and a little bit posh, this pasta dish has lovely contrasting flavours and textures

SERVES 2
21 MINUTES

2 cloves of garlic

1 red onion (160g)

1 sprig of rosemary

½ a teaspoon dried red chilli flakes

150g dried wholewheat spaghetti

1 x 400g tin of plum tomatoes

160g asparagus

1 lemon

200g white crabmeat

1 Peel and finely slice the garlic and onion. Put a large non-stick frying pan on a high heat with 1 tablespoon of olive oil and strip in the rosemary leaves. As soon as they start to sizzle, stir in the garlic, onion and chilli flakes. Cook for 5 minutes, or until softened, stirring regularly.

2 Meanwhile, cook the pasta in a pan of boiling salted water according to the packet instructions, then drain, reserving a mugful of starchy cooking water.

3 Stir the tomatoes into the frying pan, breaking them up with your spoon. Simmer for 5 minutes, while you trim the asparagus, then speed-peel the spears into a bowl. Finely grate in the lemon zest, squeeze over the juice, toss with the crab and a little extra virgin olive oil, and season to perfection.

4 Season the tomato sauce to perfection and stir in the spaghetti, loosening with a splash of reserved cooking water, if needed. Divide between plates, sprinkle over the dressed crab and asparagus, and serve.

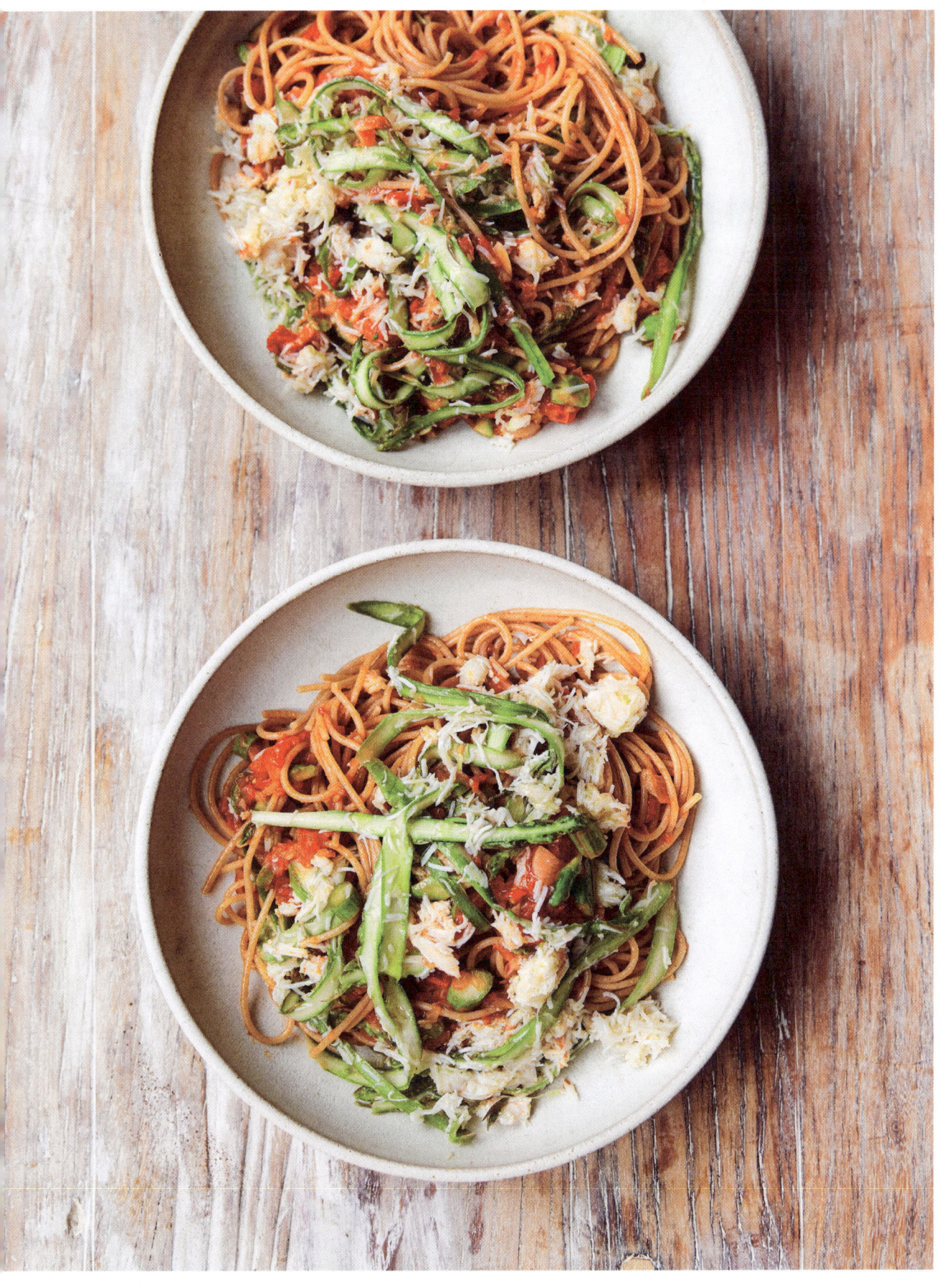

Vibrant veg & creamy bean salad

A bunch of delicious, nutritious things unite to create a bowlful of joy

SERVES 2
24 MINUTES

20g goat's cheese

2 slices of seeded sourdough bread (100g)

160g blueberries

1 x 400g tin of butter beans

1 heaped teaspoon Dijon mustard

80g baby spinach

1 small bulb of fennel (160g)

1 small ripe avocado (160g)

1 bunch of tarragon (20g)

20g walnut halves

1 If you can, a nice hack is to freeze a little log of goat's cheese the night before, so you can finely grate it into a dust of seasoning, to order.

2 Chop the bread into 1cm chunks and dry fry in a large non-stick frying pan on a medium heat, tossing regularly and removing once golden. Blister the blueberries in the pan for 1 minute, then tip into a big salad bowl. Pour the beans into the pan, juice and all, with 1 tablespoon of red wine vinegar, season and boil until thick and creamy, stirring occasionally.

3 Meanwhile, mash half the blueberries, then mix them all with the mustard, 1 tablespoon of red wine vinegar and 2 tablespoons of extra virgin olive oil, and season to perfection. Pile the spinach on top, then very finely slice the fennel, either by hand with good knife skills, or with a speed-peeler, picking over any leafy tops. Halve, destone, peel, finely slice and add the avocado, pick in the tarragon leaves, add the croutons and mix well.

4 Pour over the creamy beans. Crumble over the walnuts, and finely grate over a dusting of frozen goat's cheese, to finish.

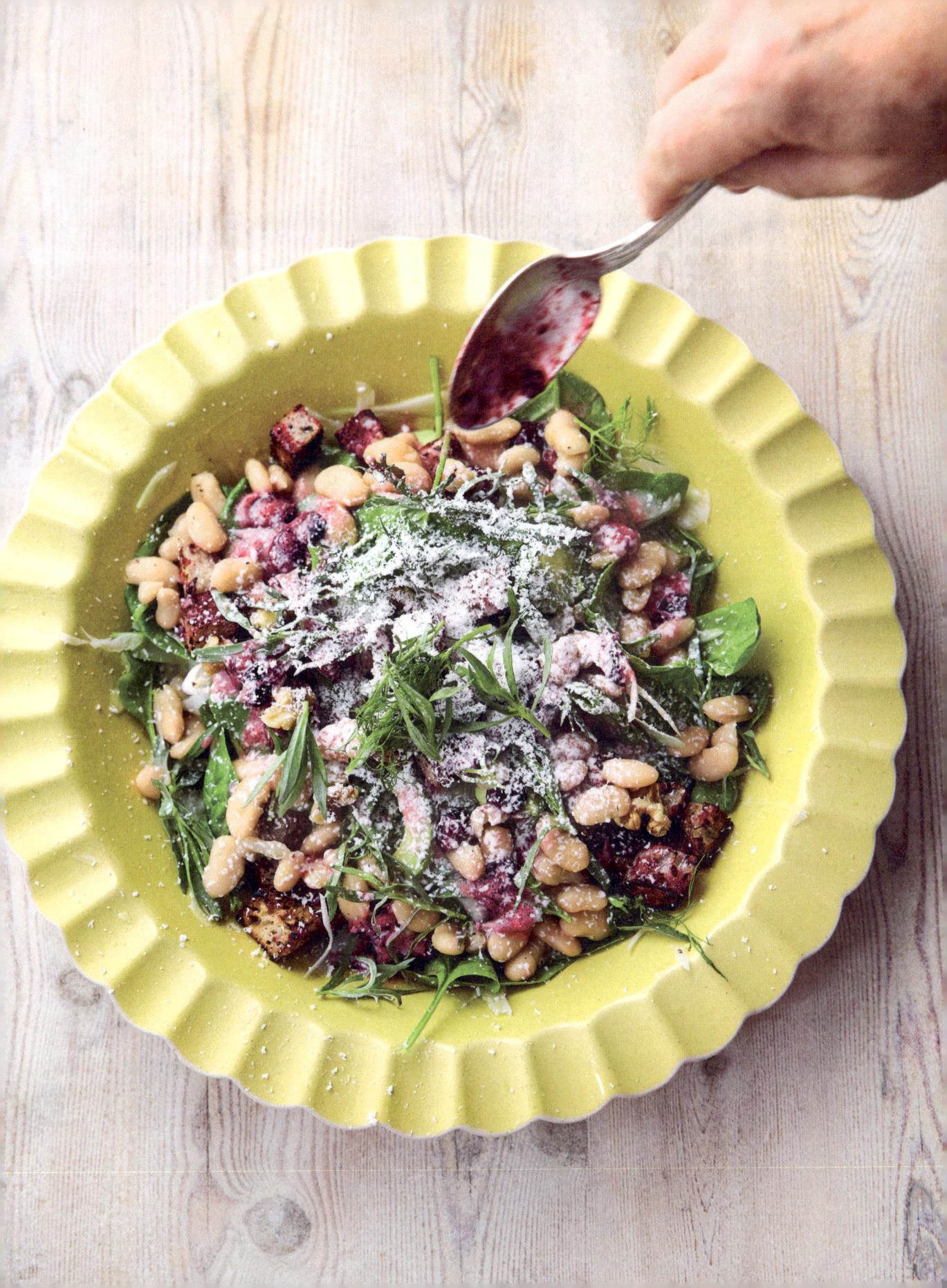

Fish in crazy water

Gently cooking whole fish in a veg sauce, or *acqua pazza* in Italian, is just lovely. Perfect for sharing

SERVES 2
24 MINUTES

4 cloves of garlic

1 fresh red chilli

1 small courgette (160g)

160g ripe mixed-colour cherry tomatoes

1 bunch of basil (30g)

1 x 400g tin of cannellini beans

160g frozen peas

1 lemon

1 x 450g whole bream, scaled, gutted, fins removed

2 slices of wholemeal sourdough bread

1 Peel the garlic and finely slice with the chilli. Halve the courgette lengthways, remove the seedy core, then finely slice. Put a large non-stick frying pan on a medium-high heat with 2 tablespoons of olive oil, the courgette, garlic, chilli and tomatoes. Tear in most of the basil leaves, reserving a few baby ones in a bowl of cold water, and fry for 2 minutes, tossing regularly.

2 Add the beans, juice and all, along with ½ a tin's worth of water, then the peas. Squeeze in half the lemon juice, bring to the boil, season to perfection, then nestle in the fish. Cover and simmer gently for 15 minutes, or until the fish is just cooked through – to check, go to the thickest part up near the head, and if the flesh pulls easily away from the bone, it's done. Remove to a plate. Leave the pan on the heat and reduce the sauce to your liking.

3 To serve, use two forks to gently coax the fillets away from the fish, removing any bones as you go. Don't worry about getting the fillets off in one piece, the more times you cook whole fish like this, the easier it will become. Cooking on the bone gives extra juiciness and flavour, so it's worth it. Serve with the beans, veg, reserved basil leaves, lemon wedges and toast.

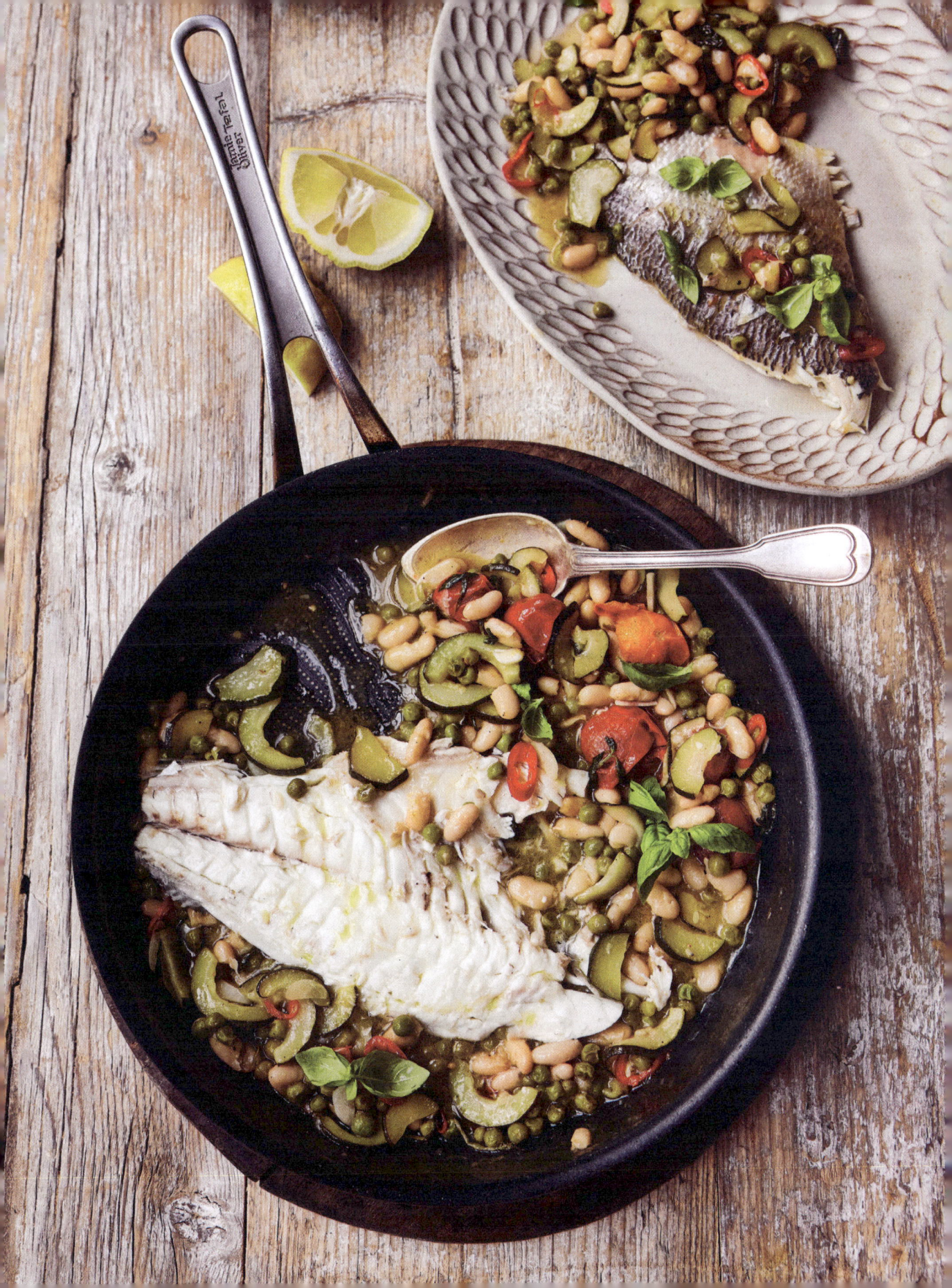

Super-green orecchiette

A mighty fine way to get more greens into your life. Embrace the greens!

SERVES 4
24 MINUTES

80g rosemary focaccia

4 cloves of garlic

1 head of broccoli (320g)

320g baby spinach

50g Parmesan cheese

1 lemon

dried red chilli flakes

300g dried orecchiette

320g frozen peas

4 tablespoons cottage cheese

1. Boil the kettle. In a blender, blitz the focaccia with a spritz of olive oil and a pinch of sea salt into fine crumbs, then toast in a large deep pan over a high heat until golden, stirring regularly. Tip into a bowl, then return the pan to the heat and half-fill with boiling salted water.

2. Peel the garlic cloves and add to the water. Cut small bite-size broccoli florets off the stalk and set aside, then trim and roughly chop the stalk and add to the water. Boil for 5 minutes, adding the spinach for the final minute.

3. Use tongs or a slotted spoon to put the broccoli stalks, spinach and garlic in the blender, gently shaking off excess water. Finely grate in the Parmesan, squeeze in the lemon juice, add a pinch of chilli flakes and 2 tablespoons of oil, blitz until smooth and season to perfection.

4. Cook the pasta in the pan of boiling salted water according to the packet instructions, topping up the water, if needed, and adding the broccoli florets and peas for the last 2 minutes, or until just tender. Drain it all, reserving a mugful of starchy cooking water, then toss with the green sauce, loosening with a little reserved water, if needed, and divide between serving bowls.

5. Spoon over the cottage cheese, and sprinkle over a pinch of chilli flakes and the crispy crumbs. Finish with a drizzle of extra virgin olive oil, if you like.

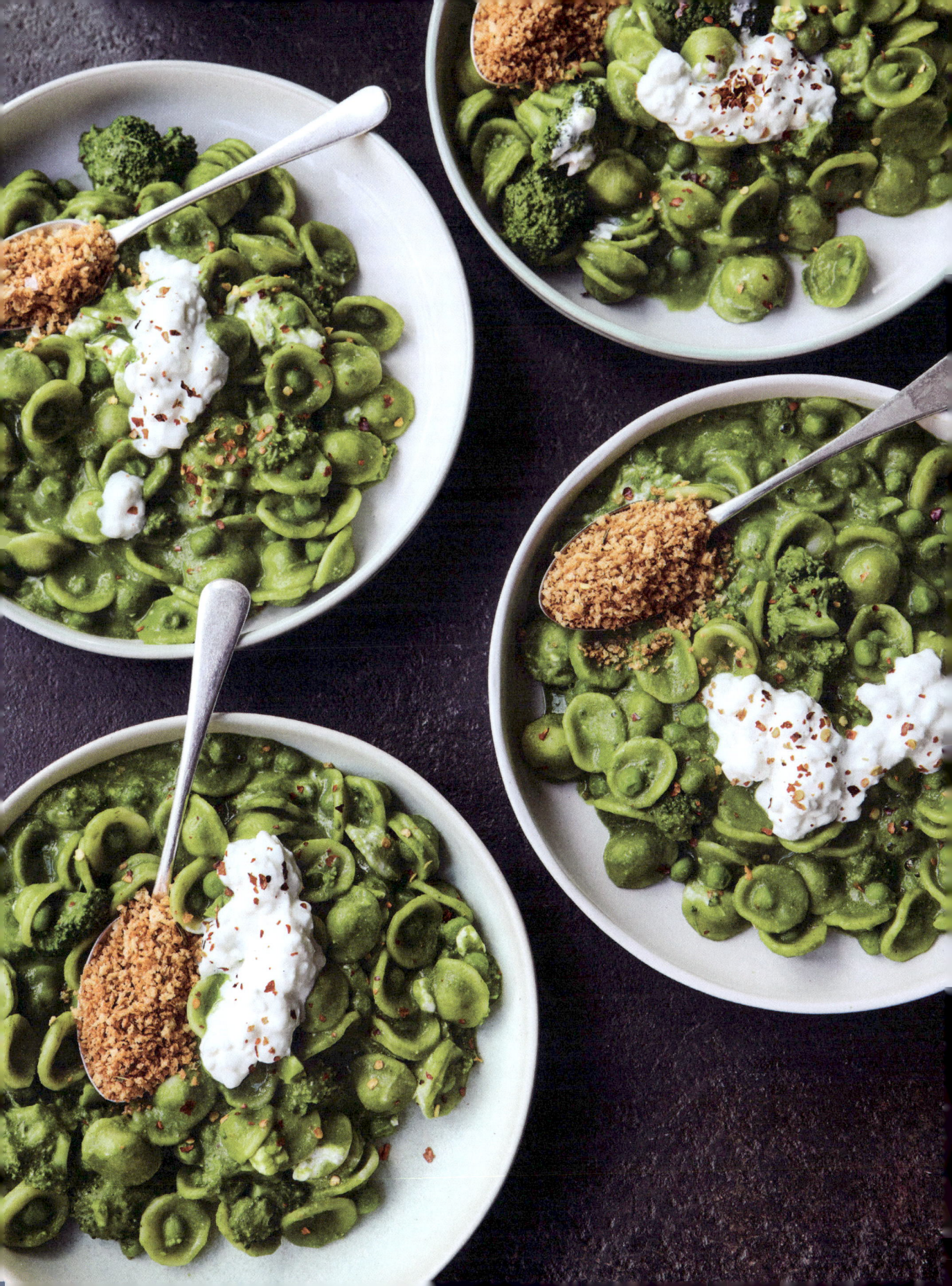

Fish parcels & tomato orzo

A really classy way to cook fish and a beautiful thing to present at the table

SERVES 2
24 MINUTES

150g dried orzo

1 x 400g tin of plum tomatoes

2 cloves of garlic

1 fresh red chilli

½ a bunch of basil (15g)

160g roasted red peppers

1 small courgette (160g)

2 x 130g chunky white fish fillets, skin on, scaled, pin-boned

1 lemon

15g Parmesan cheese

1 Boil the kettle. Put a medium pan on a high heat with the orzo. Just cover with boiling salted water and cook for 5 minutes, while you put the tomatoes into a blender. Peel and add the garlic. Halve, deseed and add the chilli, then tear in the basil stalks, reserving the leaves. Blitz until smooth, then season to perfection. Stir the sauce into the pan, finely chop and add the peppers and most of the basil leaves, reserving a few baby ones, then bring to the boil and cook on a medium heat for 5 more minutes, stirring regularly.

2 Meanwhile, use a speed-peeler to peel the courgette into long ribbons (keeping the excess for another day). Line up the ribbons, slightly overlapping, in two sets, then sit the fish fillets on top. Season, spritz with olive oil, finely grate over the lemon zest, and wrap them up. Nestle the parcels into the orzo, cover, reduce to a medium-low heat and cook for 10 minutes, or until the fish is beautifully cooked through.

3 Squeeze half the lemon juice over the fish parcels, then finely grate over the Parmesan, scatter over the reserved basil, and serve with lemon wedges.

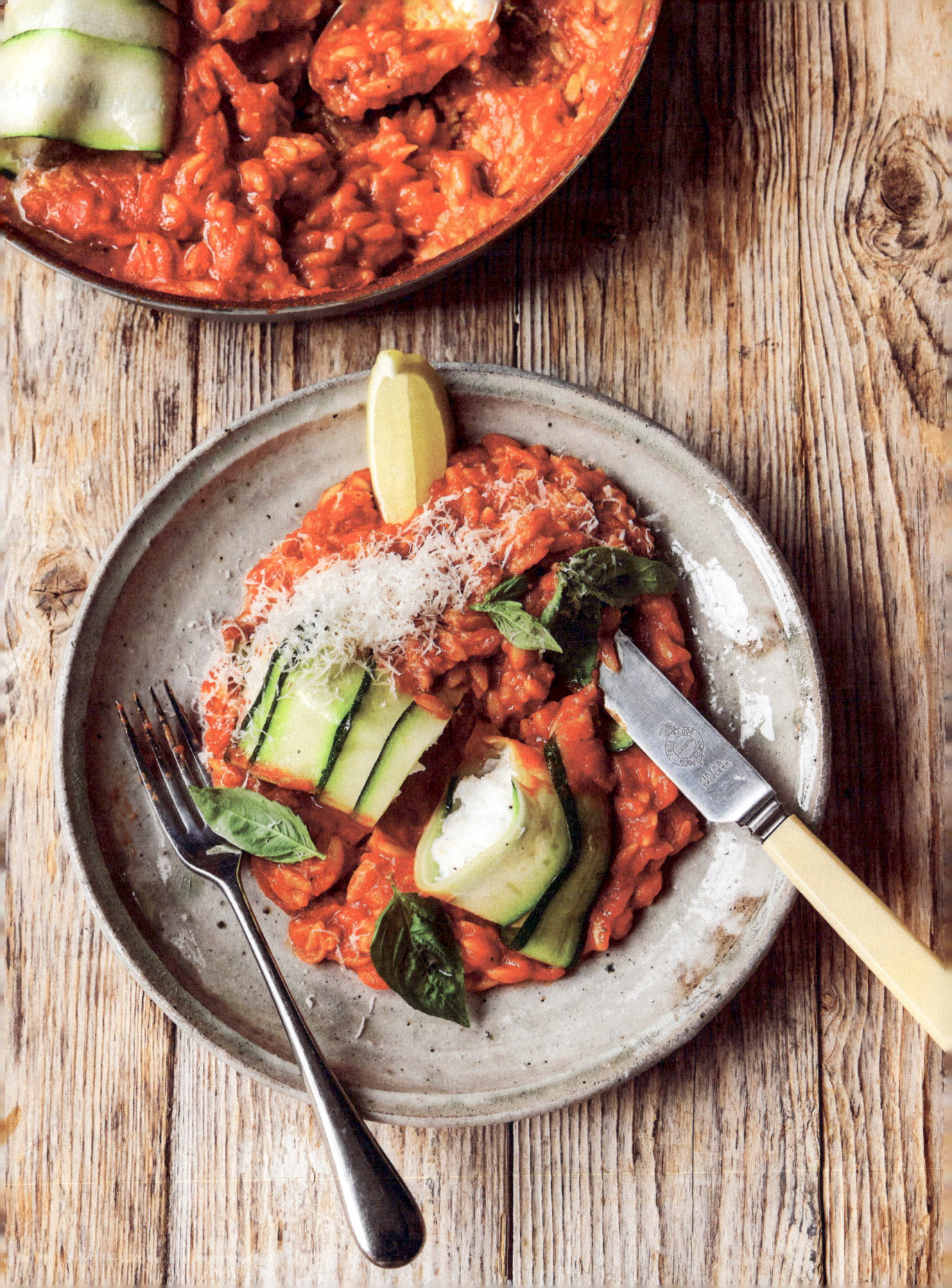

Silky aubergine flavour fest

A joy to eat and to look at, this is a glorious way to cook and celebrate aubergine

SERVES 2
28 MINUTES

2 large aubergines (400g each)

1 × 400g tin of chickpeas

1 bunch of mint (30g)

½ a bunch of coriander (15g)

4 tablespoons natural yoghurt

½ a lemon

½ a pomegranate

2 tablespoons mango chutney

30g Bombay mix

4 poppadoms

1. Boil the kettle. Halve the aubergines lengthways and place skin side up in a large shallow casserole pan with 1cm of boiling water, place on a high heat, cover, and boil for 10 minutes.

2. Uncover, let any remaining water cook away, add 1 tablespoon of olive oil, then drain and sprinkle in the chickpeas, lifting the aubergines on top. Fry until golden and sizzling, then season to perfection and pile on to a platter.

3. Reserving a few nice leaves for garnish, pick the mint and finely chop with the coriander, stalks and all. Mix with the yoghurt, add the lemon zest and juice, and season to perfection.

4. Halve the pomegranate, hold one half cut side down in your palm and bash the back with a spoon so the seeds tumble out into a bowl. Squeeze in the juice from the other half through a sieve, and stir in the mango chutney.

5. Spoon both sauces over the aubergines. Crush the Bombay mix and scatter over the platter, pick over the remaining mint leaves, and add a drizzle of extra virgin olive oil, if you like. Serve with poppadoms.

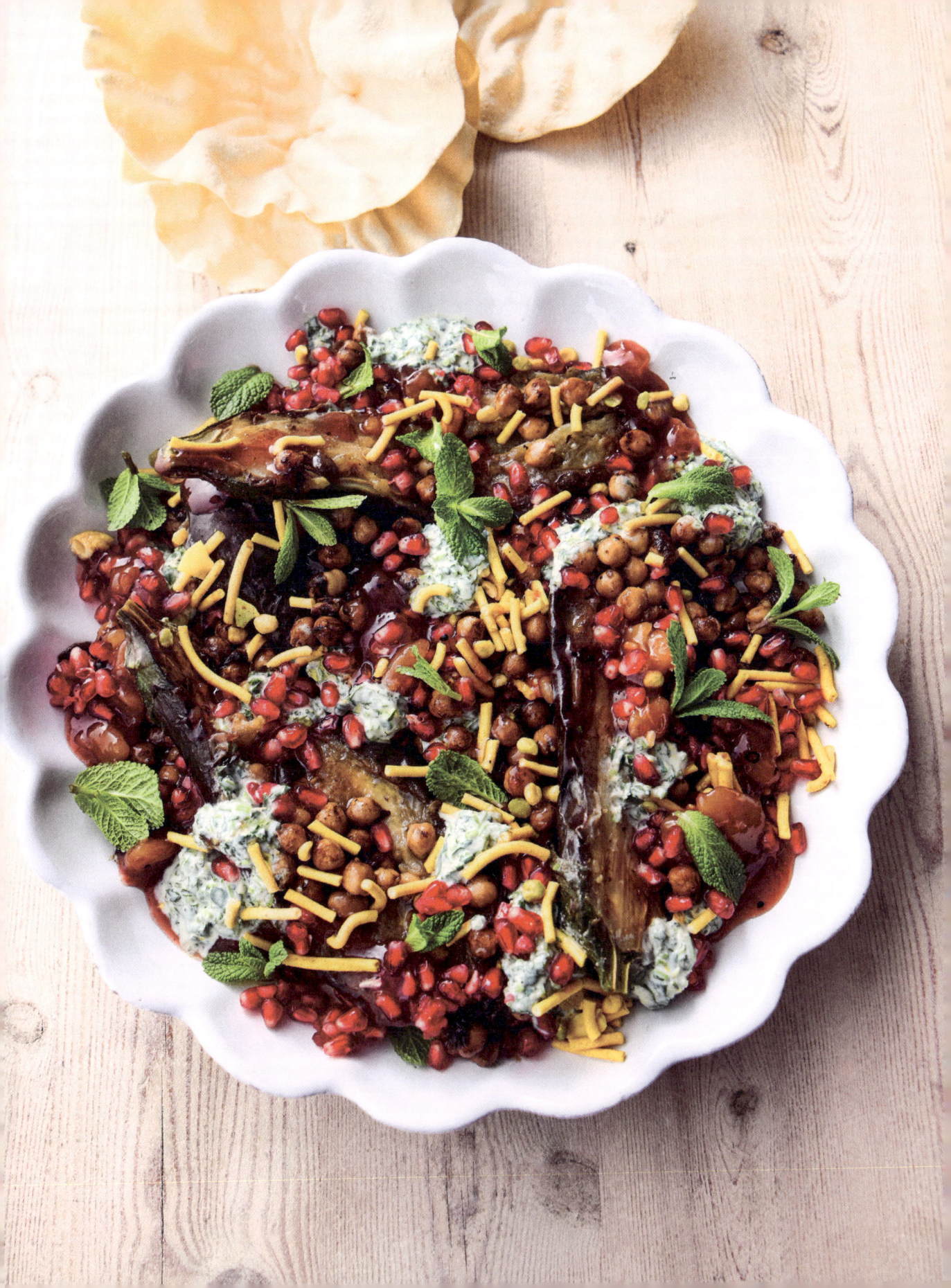

Gochujang tomato noodle soup

Wonderfully warming Korean chilli paste takes humble tomato soup to a new flavour dimension

SERVES 4
29 MINUTES

2 red onions (320g)

2 carrots (160g)

2 tablespoons gochujang paste

600g ripe tomatoes

4 sprigs of coriander

4 nests of instant vermicelli rice noodles (180g total)

300g silken tofu

1 Put a large deep non-stick pan on a high heat. Peel and roughly chop the onions and carrot, then dry fry and char for 8 minutes, stirring regularly.

2 Boil the kettle. Add 2 tablespoons of olive oil and the gochujang, then roughly chop and add the tomatoes and coriander stalks, reserving the leaves. Pour in 1 litre of boiling kettle water, cover, and boil for 10 minutes. Meanwhile, in a bowl, cover the noodles with boiling kettle water and leave to rehydrate, then drain well and divide between large warm soup bowls.

3 In batches, carefully pour most of the soup into a blender and blitz until smooth, leaving some chunky bits, then season to perfection and pour into the bowls. Cube up and scatter over the tofu, sprinkle over the coriander leaves and finish with a drizzle of extra virgin olive oil, if you like.

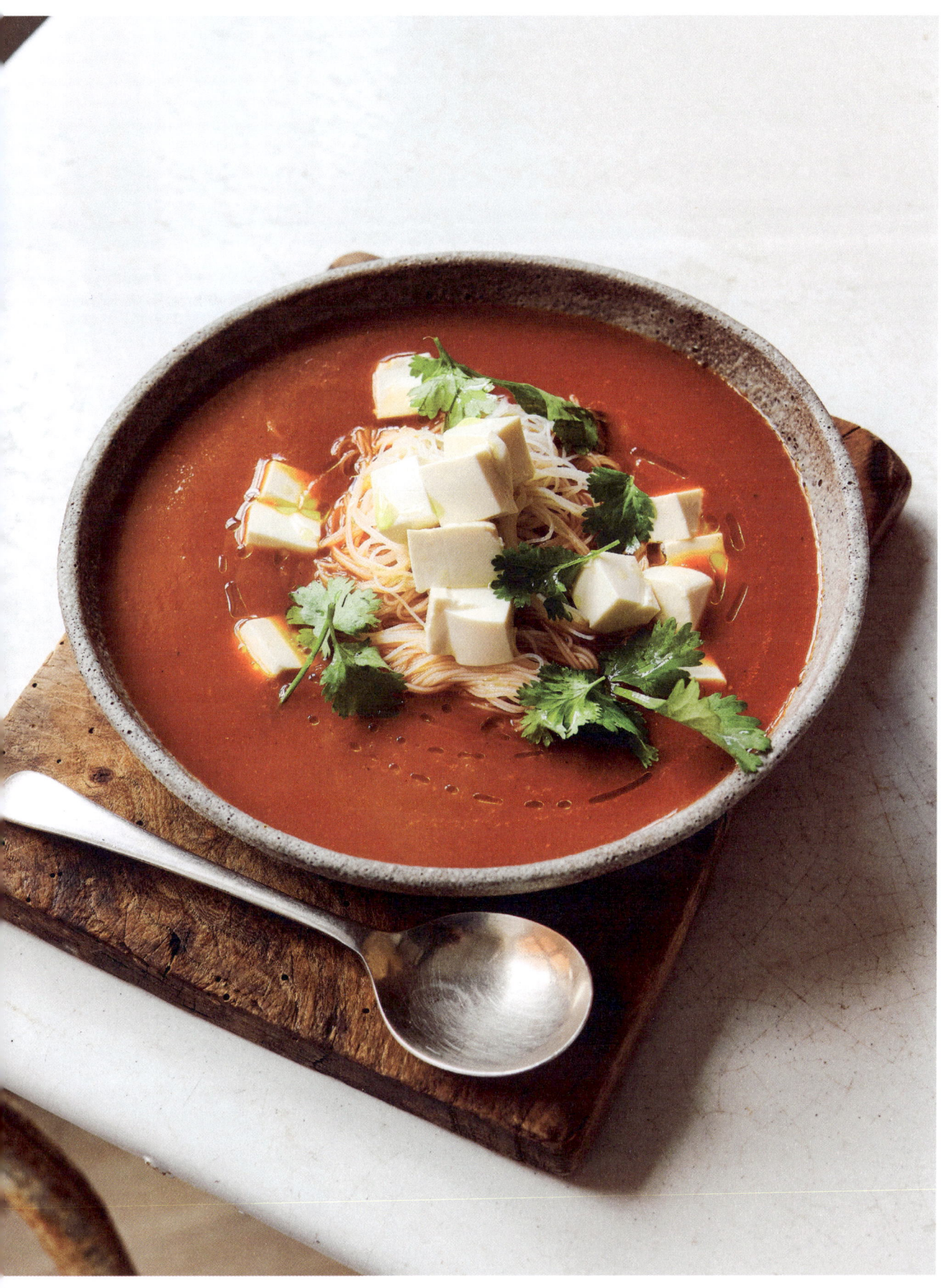

Roasted veg & chickpea smash

SERVES 1 | 30 MINUTES

80g each
- tinned chickpeas, red onion, jarred roasted red peppers, ripe tomatoes, Brussels sprouts, carrots, cauliflower, tenderstem broccoli

30g dried apricots

½ a bunch of flat-leaf parsley (15g)

1 heaped teaspoon harissa paste

2 tablespoons Greek yoghurt

½ a lemon

Preheat the oven to 200°C. Reserving the chickpeas and peppers, prep all the veg and chop into bite-size chunks. Place in a large roasting tray, toss with 1 tablespoon of olive oil and a pinch of sea salt and black pepper, and roast for 25 minutes, or until soft and golden. Very finely chop the peppers, dried apricots and parsley leaves, mash with the chickpeas, then mix in the harissa, yoghurt and lemon juice, and season to perfection. Pile the golden roasted veg on top, to serve. Nice with wholemeal bread, couscous or pasta.

AIR FRYER IT

Simply cook the veg in an air fryer for 20 minutes at 180°C, or until soft and golden, shaking halfway.

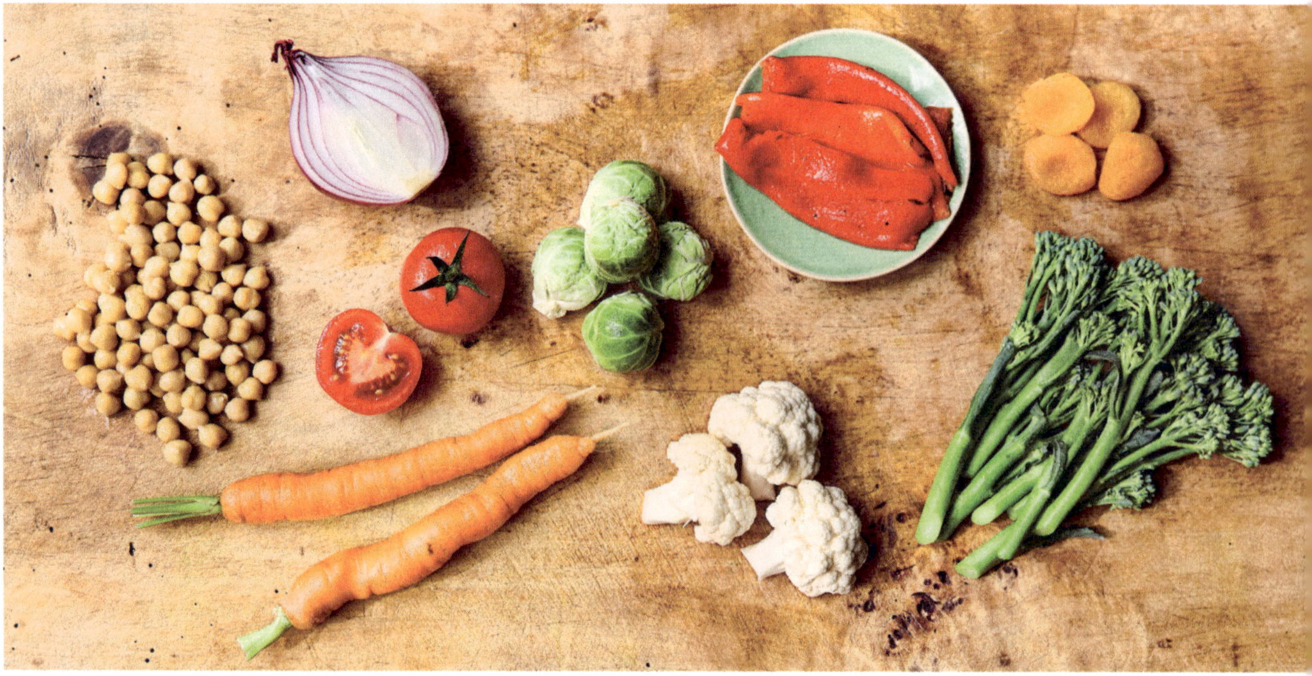

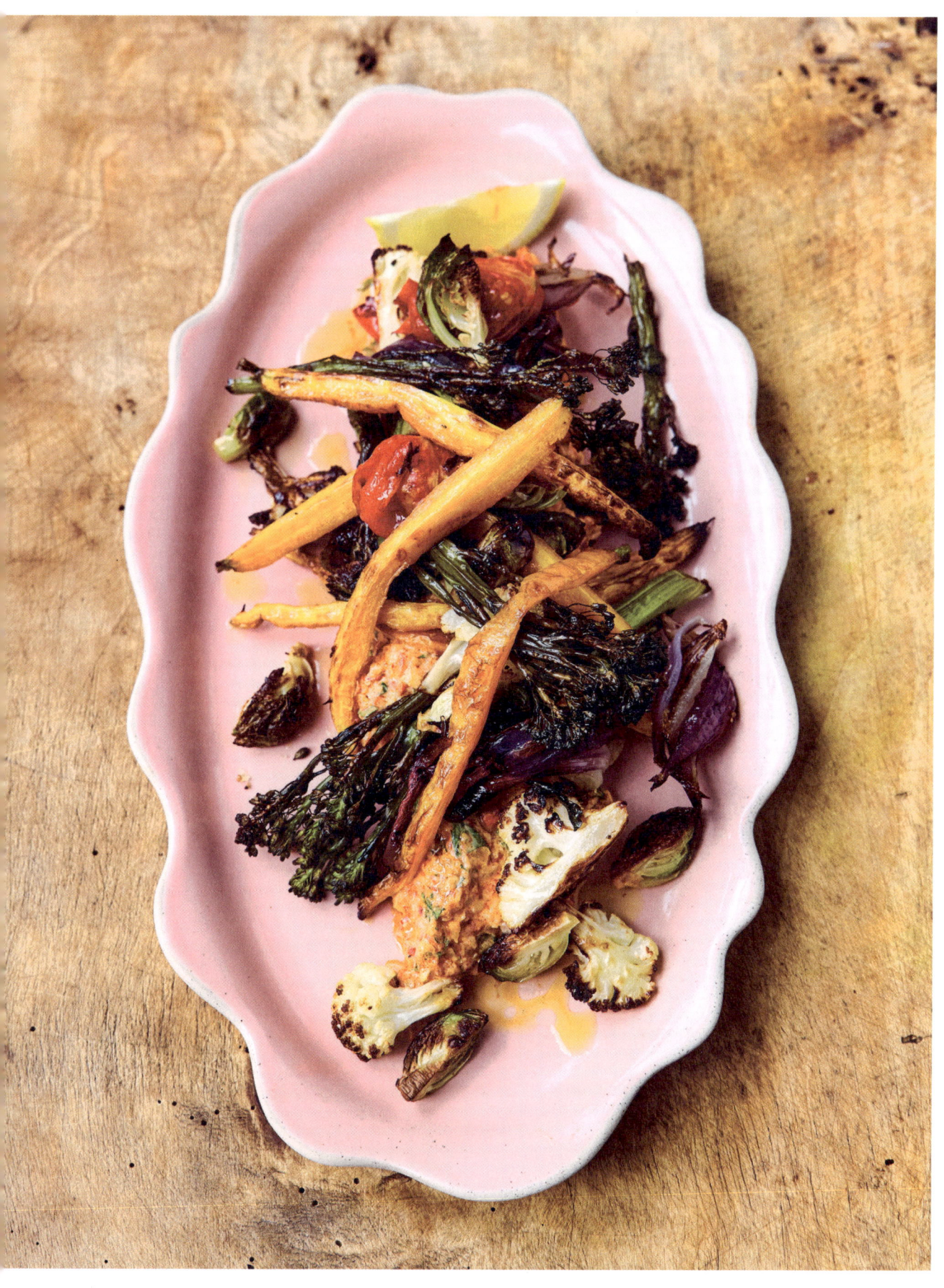

Mushroom stew

A hearty, delicious dish with deep warming gochujang flavour and fluffy dumpling vibes

SERVES 2
30 MINUTES

250g mixed mushrooms

4 spring onions

2 carrots (160g)

5cm piece of ginger

150g self-raising flour

1 x 400g tin of black beans

1 x 225g tin of sliced water chestnuts

160g beansprouts

2 tablespoons gochujang paste

150g silken tofu

1 Put a large frying pan on a high heat. Trim and go in with the mushrooms, tearing any larger ones, and leave to dry fry and get nutty while the pan heats up, removing to a plate once starting to catch.

2 Meanwhile, trim the spring onions, finely slice the green tops and put aside for later, then cut the whites into 2cm lengths. Wash the carrot and very finely slice into rounds. Peel and matchstick the ginger. When the mushrooms come out, go in with the white spring onions, carrot, ginger and 1 tablespoon of olive oil, and cook for 5 minutes, stirring regularly.

3 For the dumplings, mix 90ml of water into the flour with a small pinch of sea salt and bring it together into a ball of dough. Tear off 3cm chunks and roll into balls – you should get around 12 in total. Boil the kettle.

4 Pour the beans and water chestnuts, juice and all, into the pan, then put the mushrooms back in. Tip in the beansprouts, stir in the gochujang, cover with 500ml of boiling kettle water, then gently plop the dumplings into the stew, cover, and cook for 10 minutes, or until the dumplings are fluffy.

5 Season the stew to perfection, dice and add the tofu, and the green spring onion tops, and drizzle over a little extra virgin olive oil, if you like.

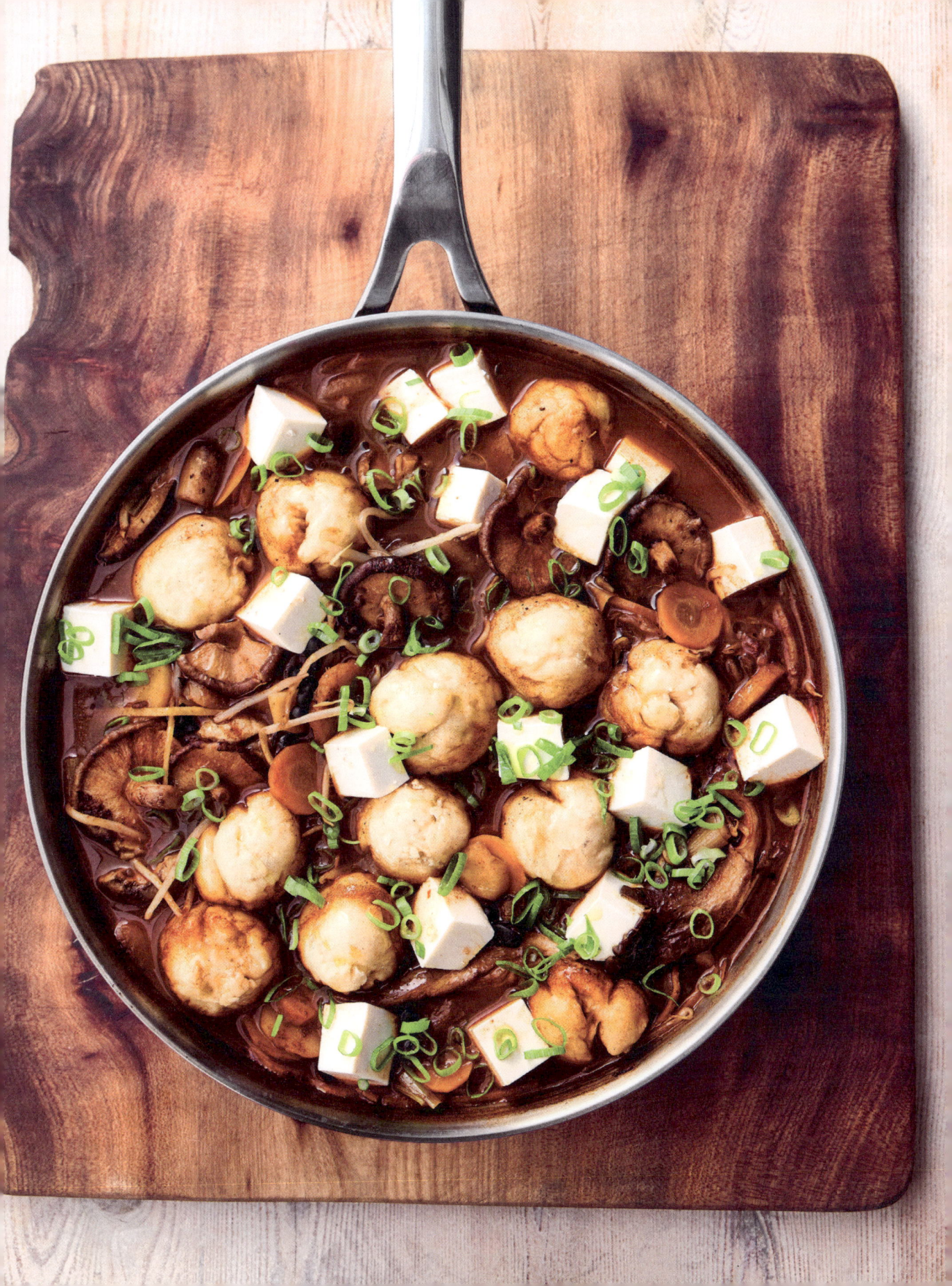

Chicken curry & chapati

A super-comforting, simple addition to your curry repertoire, with lovely, quick rustic chapatis

SERVES 2
31 MINUTES

100g wholemeal flour, plus extra for dusting

1 onion (160g)

8cm piece of ginger

1 small handful of fresh curry leaves

1 heaped tablespoon madras curry paste

2 x 150g skinless chicken breasts

2 tablespoons desiccated coconut

250g ripe cherry tomatoes

1 x 400g tin of butter beans

2 heaped tablespoons natural yoghurt

1. For the chapatis, put the flour in a bowl with a pinch of sea salt, make a well in the middle, then gradually add 60ml of warm water, mixing with a fork until it starts to come together. Bring into a ball of dough, cover and rest.

2. Peel the onion and chop into chunks the same size as a butter bean. Peel and finely chop the ginger. Put a large shallow casserole pan on a high heat, go in with 1 tablespoon of olive oil and the curry leaves, fry for 1 minute, then use a slotted spoon to remove to a plate, leaving the oil behind in the pan. Add the onion and ginger and cook for 10 minutes, stirring regularly, adding splashes of water, if needed.

3. Stir in the curry paste. Dice and add the chicken, stir in the coconut. Halve and add the tomatoes, then the beans, juice and all. Cook for 10 minutes, or until the sauce has thickened, stirring occasionally, then season to perfection.

4. Put a frying pan on a medium-high heat. Divide the dough into two and roll out each piece on a flour-dusted surface until about 2mm thick. Cook each chapati for 1 to 2 minutes per side, or until lightly charred.

5. Plate up the curry with the chapati, spoon over the yoghurt, and finish with the crispy curry leaves. Great with a fresh salad and a multitude of pickles.

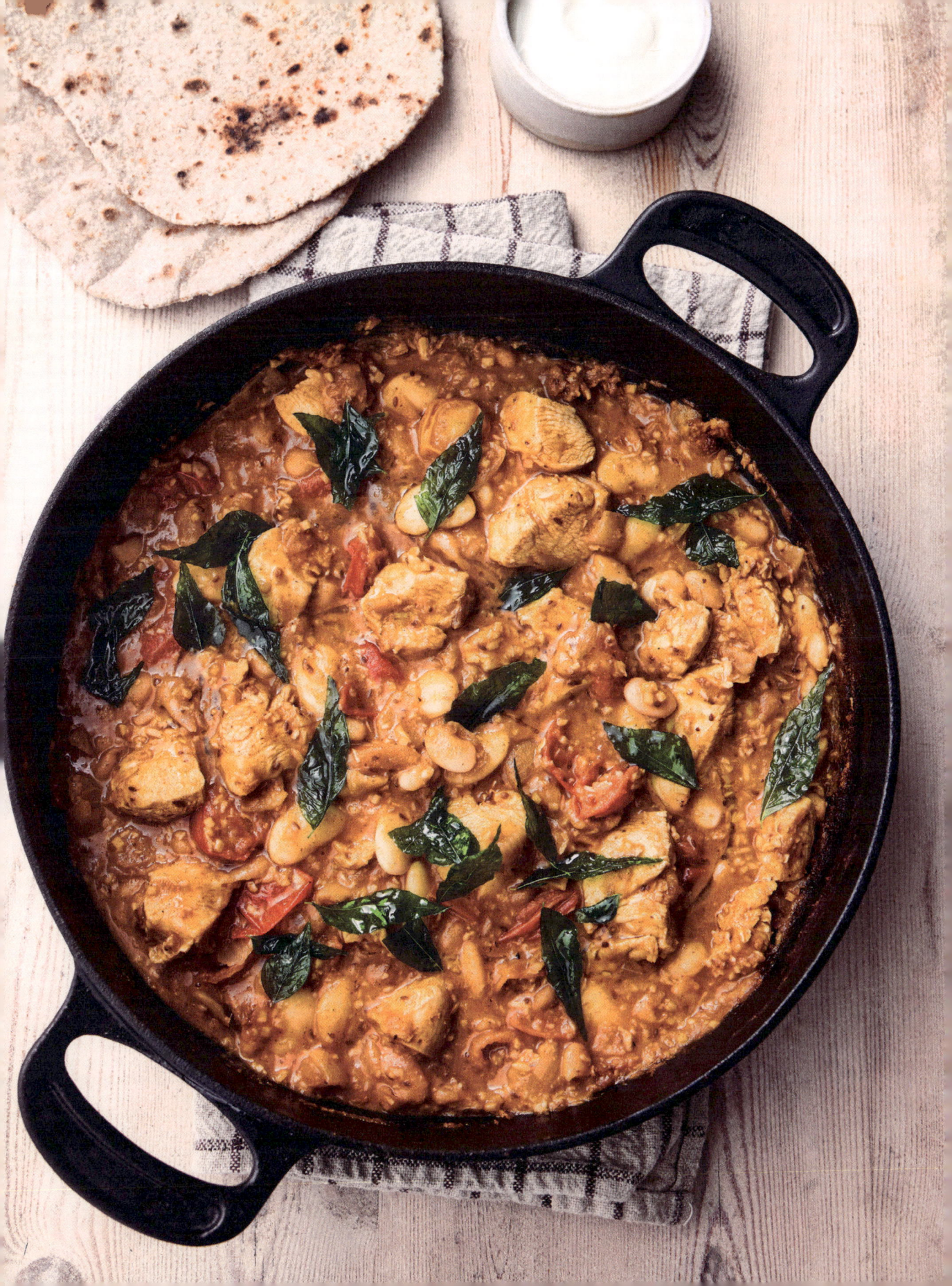

Roasted Mediterranean veg

SERVES 1 | PREP 8 MINUTES | COOK 30 MINUTES

80g each
 aubergine, ripe tomato, butternut squash, red onion, courgette, red pepper, sweet potato

1 teaspoon dried oregano

1 tablespoon thick balsamic vinegar

2 sprigs of basil

Preheat the oven to 200°C. Trim or deseed the veg, as needed, then chop it all into 2cm dice, leaving the tomato whole. Place it all in a large roasting tray, toss with 1 tablespoon of olive oil, the oregano and a pinch of sea salt and black pepper, and roast for 30 minutes, or until soft and golden. Carefully pinch off the tomato skin, then use a fork to smush up the tomato, add the balsamic to the tray, and toss it all together, scraping up any sticky bits. Season to perfection, pick over the basil leaves, and serve. Wonderful as it is, or you can try tossing with some jarred beans, adding a crumbling of feta cheese, or teaming with pasta or wholemeal bread.

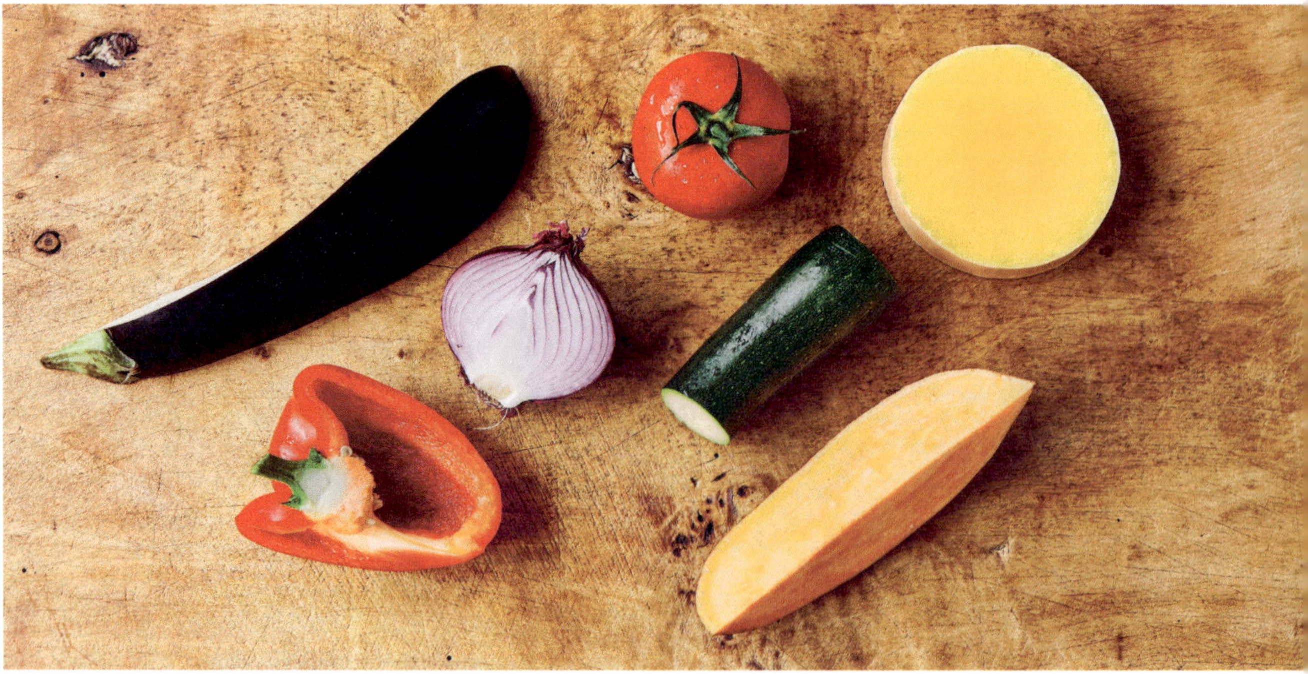

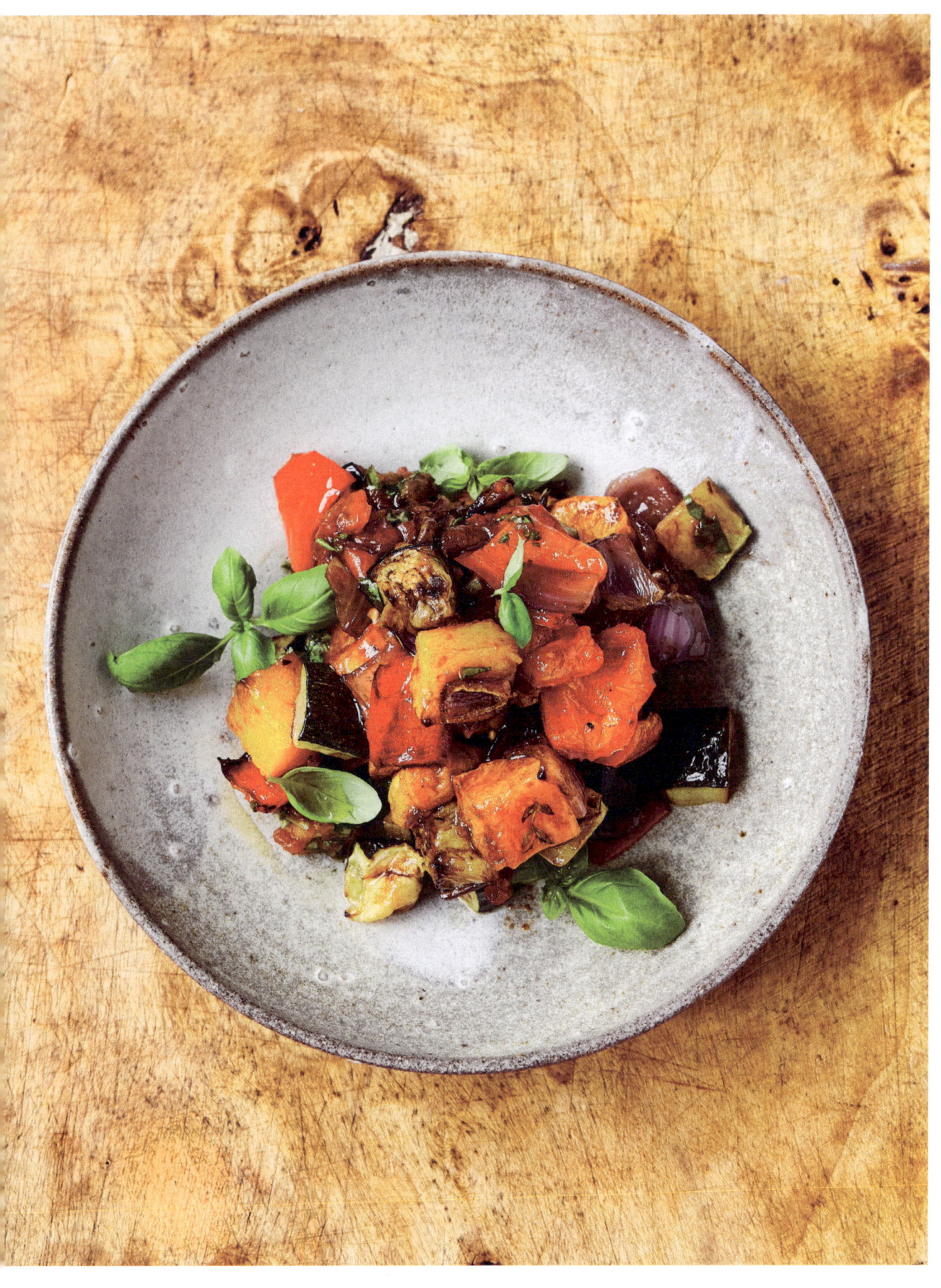

Harissa tuna bean parcels

Crispy filo parcels celebrating the combo of creamy beans, tuna, harissa and sweet dried apricots

SERVES 2
PREP 20 MINUTES
COOK 30 MINUTES

1 x 400g tin of cannellini beans

1 x 145g tin of tuna in spring water

60g dried apricots

1 lemon

1 tablespoon harissa paste, plus extra to serve

4 sheets of filo pastry

1 large carrot (160g)

½ a cucumber (160g)

2 sprigs of mint

2 tablespoons natural yoghurt

1. Preheat the oven to 200°C. Drain the beans and tuna, put into a bowl and roughly mash. Finely chop and add the apricots, finely grate in the lemon zest, add the harissa and a pinch of black pepper, then scrunch and mix it all together well and divide into 2 equal-sized portions.

2. Lay out 2 sheets of filo on a clean work surface with the short ends towards you. Spritz with olive oil, then lay the remaining 2 sheets on top. Sit a portion of filling at the base of each, fold in the sides, then fold up into parcels. Space evenly on an oil-spritzed baking tray, spritz the tops with oil, and bake for 30 minutes, or until golden and crispy.

3. Meanwhile, peel the carrot, then finely slice by hand with good knife skills, or a speed-peeler. Run a fork down the length of the cucumber, then very finely slice. Finely slice and scatter over the mint leaves, leaving the baby ones whole. Toss with the lemon juice, season to perfection and divide between your plates. Sit the golden filo parcels on top, dollop over the yoghurt, and ripple through a little extra harissa, to serve.

AIR FRYER IT

Cook in an air fryer for 15 minutes at 200°C, or until golden and crispy, working in batches, if needed.

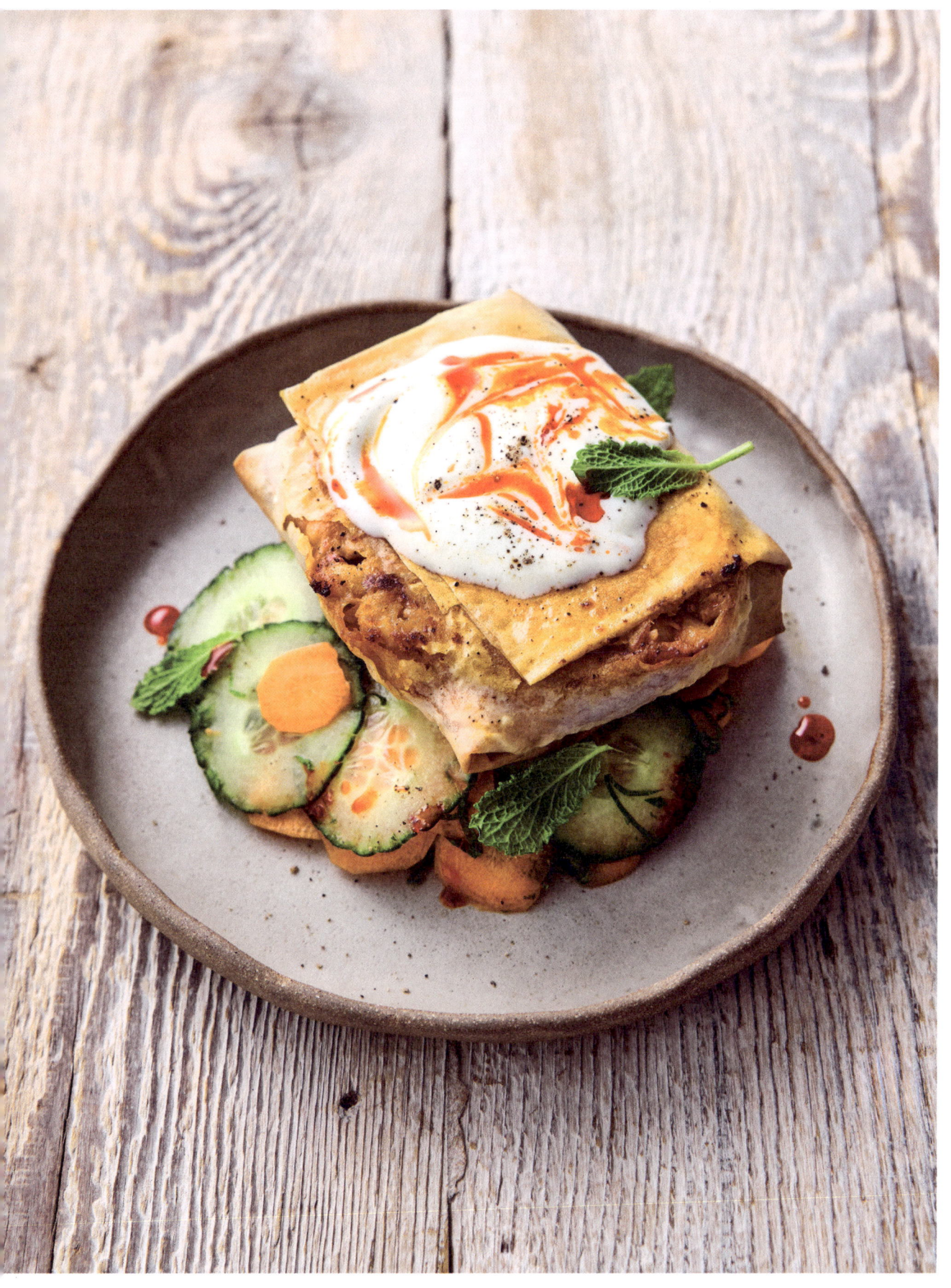

Aubergine involtini

Filled aubergines are submerged in a blipping sweet tomato sauce for a very tasty tea

SERVES 2
PREP 20 MINUTES
COOK 30 MINUTES

2 aubergines (250g each)

1 bunch of basil (30g)

1 x 400g tin of borlotti beans

100g ricotta cheese

20g Parmesan cheese

1 lemon

2 cloves of garlic

2 heaped teaspoons baby capers in brine

1 pinch of ground cinnamon

2 x 400g tins of plum tomatoes

1. Preheat the oven to 180°C. Put a large non-stick ovenproof frying pan on a high heat. Slice the aubergines lengthways 1cm thick, then dry fry and soften, in batches, for 2 minutes on each side, then remove to your board.

2. Meanwhile, pick a few nice basil leaves and reserve in a bowl of cold water, then put the rest, stalks and all, into a food processor. Drain and add the beans, add the ricotta, then finely grate in the Parmesan and lemon zest, squeeze in the juice and blitz to combine, then season to perfection.

3. Once all the aubergines are done, add 1 tablespoon of olive oil to the empty pan. Peel, finely slice and add the garlic, along with the capers and cinnamon. Fry for 2 minutes, then tip and crush in the tomatoes.

4. Divide and spread the ricotta mixture between the aubergine slices, then roll them up and nestle them into the sauce. Transfer to the oven to cook for 30 minutes, or until golden and bubbling, then scatter over the reserved basil leaves. Nice with crusty wholemeal bread for mopping up the sauce.

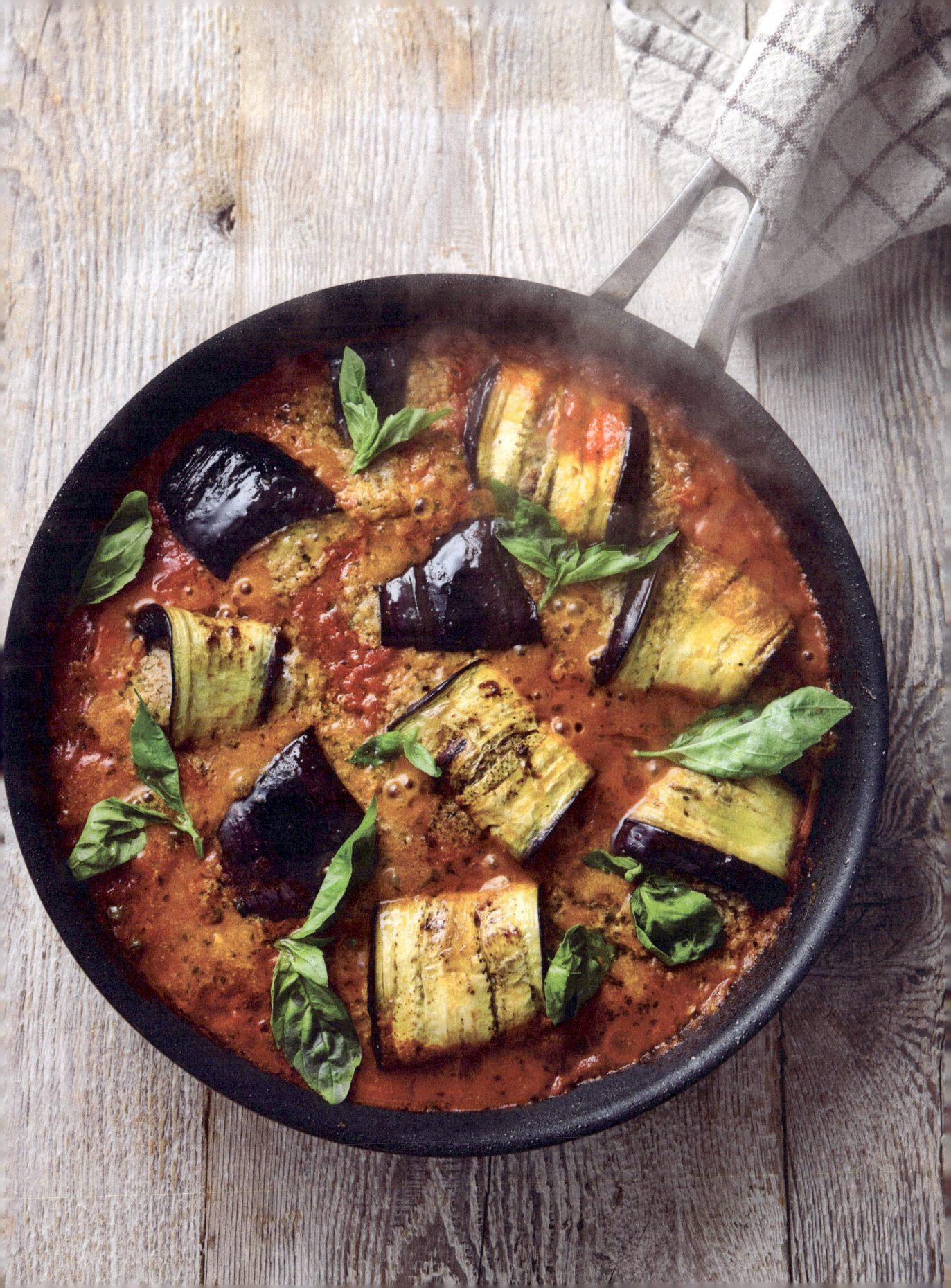

Chicken, bean & rice bake

You know where you stand with a trusty traybake, and this medley of flavours hits the spot

SERVES 4
PREP 10 MINUTES
COOK 50 MINUTES

2 red onions (320g)

320g butternut squash or pumpkin

320g celery

2 green peppers (320g)

4 large chicken thighs, skin on, bone in

2 heaped teaspoons harissa paste

2 x 250g packets of cooked wholegrain rice

2 x 400g tins of cannellini beans

1 lemon

4 tablespoons natural yoghurt

1 Preheat the oven to 180°C. Peel the onions, wash the squash and chop both into small wedges, discarding any squash seeds. Peel and roughly chop the celery, reserving any nice yellow leaves. Tear the peppers into 4cm chunks, discarding the seeds. Place it all in a 30cm x 40cm roasting tray, toss with 1 tablespoon each of red wine vinegar and olive oil, and season.

2 Spritz the chicken thighs with oil and season them, then sit them directly on the bars of the oven with the tray of veg beneath. Roast for 30 minutes.

3 Use tongs to move the chicken to your board, then remove the tray from the oven and stir in the harissa paste. Mix in the rice and the beans, juice and all, then sit the chicken on top in the tray, skin side up. Roast for another 20 minutes, or until the chicken is golden and cooked through.

4 To serve, squeeze the lemon juice over everything in the tray, then spoon over the yoghurt and scatter over any reserved celery leaves.

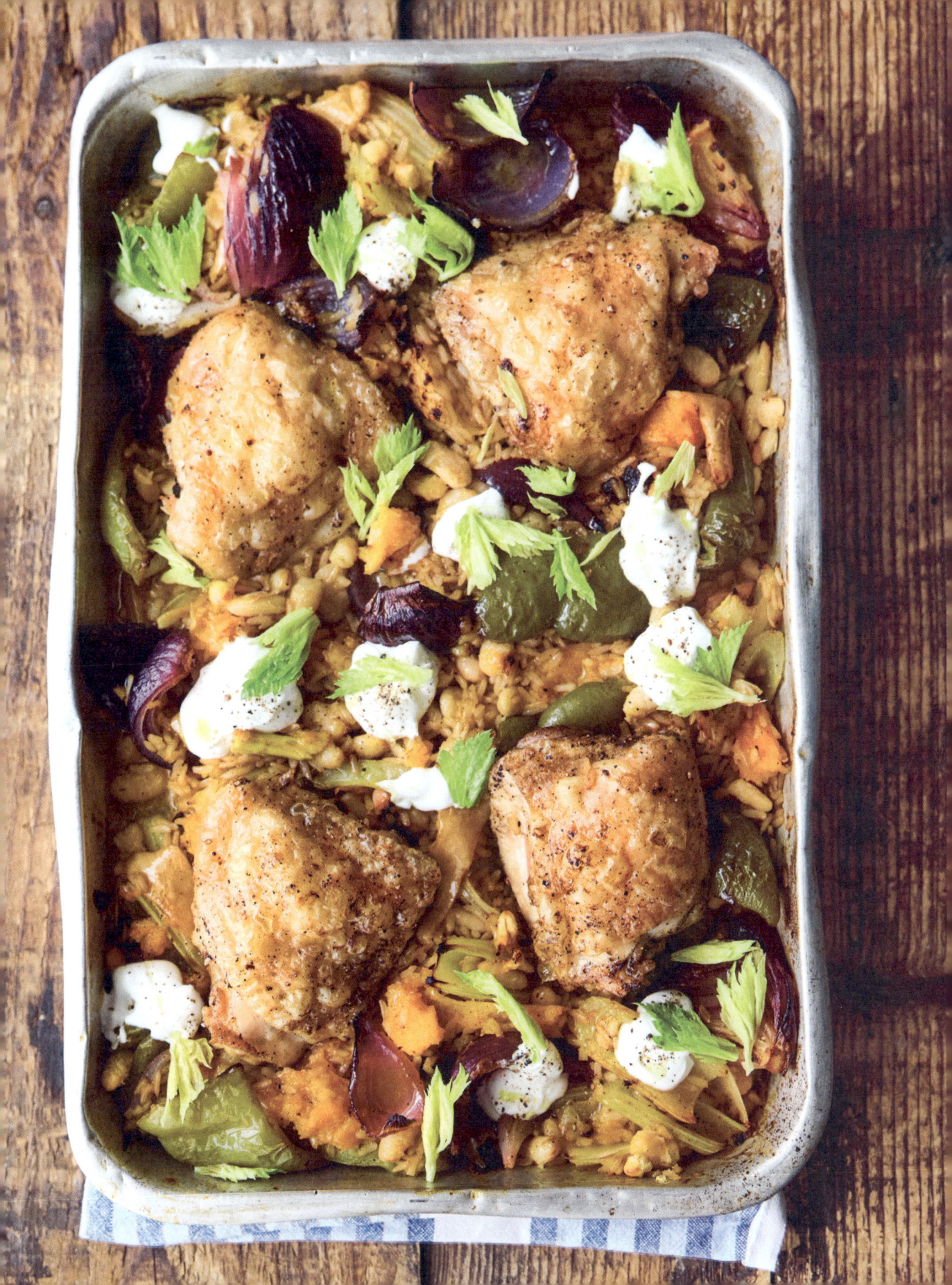

Veggie curry traybake

An utterly simple and fulfilling traybake that will really make your veggies sing

SERVES 4
PREP 10 MINUTES
COOK 55 MINUTES

2 aubergines (250g each)

1 head of cauliflower (800g)

2 onions (320g)

4 medium ripe tomatoes

1 lemon

½ a bunch of coriander (15g)

2 heaped tablespoons korma curry paste

1 jar of lime pickle

1 x 400g tin of light coconut milk

20g unsalted roasted peanuts

1. Preheat the oven to 200°C. Halve the aubergines lengthways, then finely slice across the skin three-quarters of the way through to hasselback them. Click off and discard any tatty outer cauliflower leaves, then quarter it. Peel and quarter the onions. Lightly score a criss-cross into each tomato.

2. Finely grate the lemon zest into a deep 30cm x 40cm roasting tray, then squeeze in the juice. Finely slice and add the coriander stalks, reserving the leaves in a bowl of cold water, then stir in the curry paste. Add the veg and rub the paste mixture all over them, making sure you get into the cuts in the aubergine. Shake into an even layer, spritz with olive oil, season with sea salt and black pepper, and roast for 45 minutes, or until soft and gnarly.

3. Meanwhile, pour the contents of the lime pickle jar into a blender with 150ml of boiling kettle water and blitz until smooth. Refill the jar and stash in the fridge for future meals, decanting the rest into a little bowl.

4. Transfer the tray to a medium-high heat on the hob and pour in the coconut milk. Let it simmer and reduce for 5 minutes, or until you've got a nice saucy consistency, scraping up any sticky goodness from the bottom of the tray. Scatter over the coriander leaves, crush over the nuts and serve drizzled with the lime pickle. Great with wholegrain rice or naans.

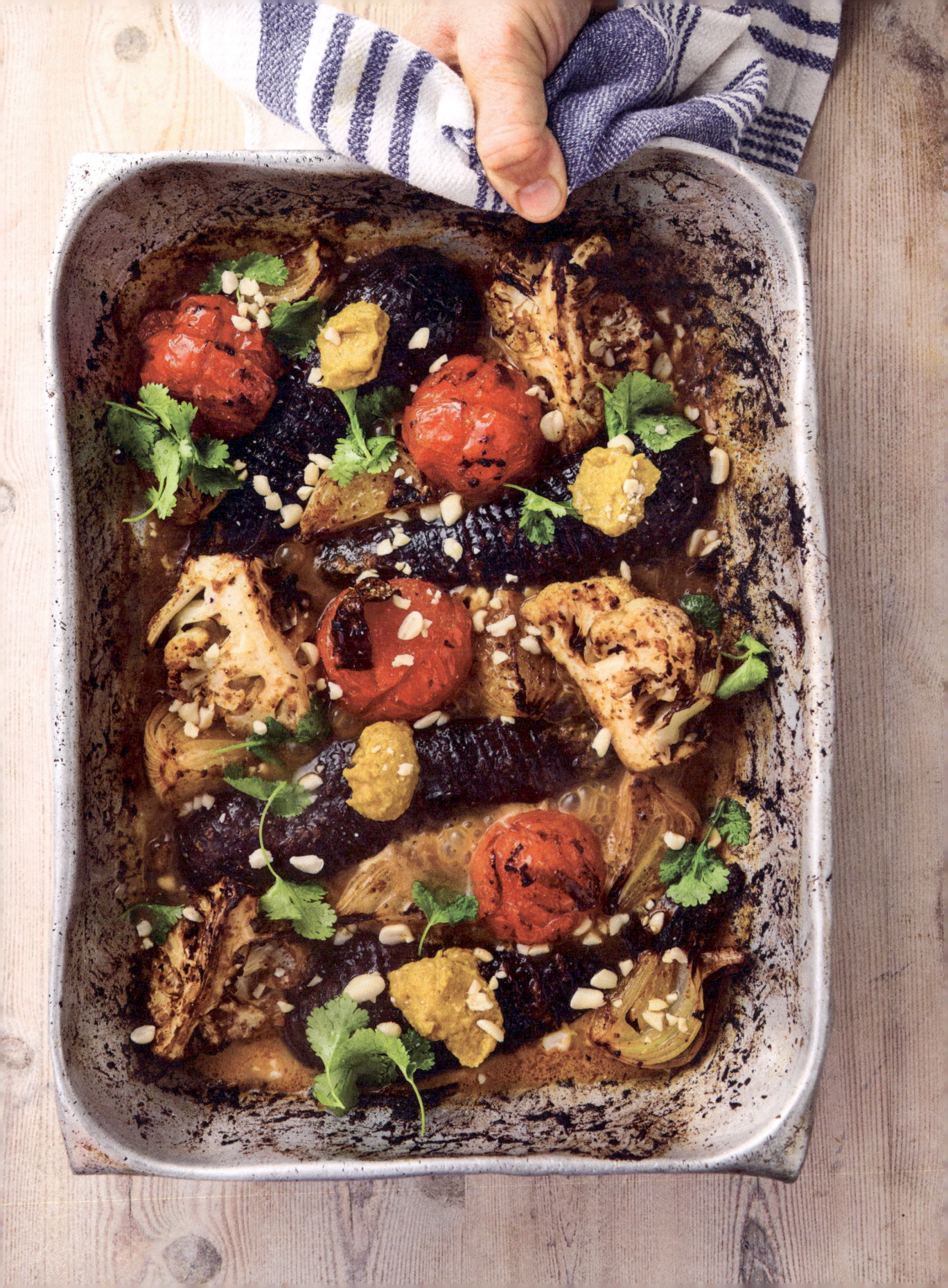

Chicken & mushroom hotpot

Screaming comfort, the shortcuts of tinned soup and gnocchi mean big flavour and convenience

SERVES 4
PREP 10 MINUTES
COOK 1 HOUR

4 large chicken thighs, skin on, bone in

2 onions (320g)

2 large carrots (320g)

½ a bunch of thyme (10g)

320g chestnut mushrooms

1 x 295g tin of condensed mushroom soup

600ml semi-skimmed milk

320g frozen sweetcorn

1 x 570g jar of cannellini beans

2 x 400g bags of potato gnocchi

1 Put a large shallow non-stick casserole pan on a medium-high heat. Pull the skin off the chicken thighs and place it in the pan to render.

2 Season the thighs with a small pinch of sea salt and black pepper, and place in the pan, turning with tongs until golden all over, while you peel the onions and carrots and chop into 3cm chunks, adding as you go. Remove and discard the crispy chicken skin, then strip in the thyme, tear in the mushrooms, and cook for 20 minutes, or until the veg is caramelized, stirring regulary.

3 Now, stir in the soup and milk. Cover with a lid ajar, and simmer gently on a medium heat for 10 minutes. Preheat the oven to 220°C.

4 Stir the sweetcorn and beans, juice and all, into the pan, then gently drop the gnocchi on top. Spritz with a little olive oil, then transfer uncovered to the oven for 30 minutes, or until the chicken pulls easily away from the bone, the gnocchi are golden and the stew is bubbling nicely.

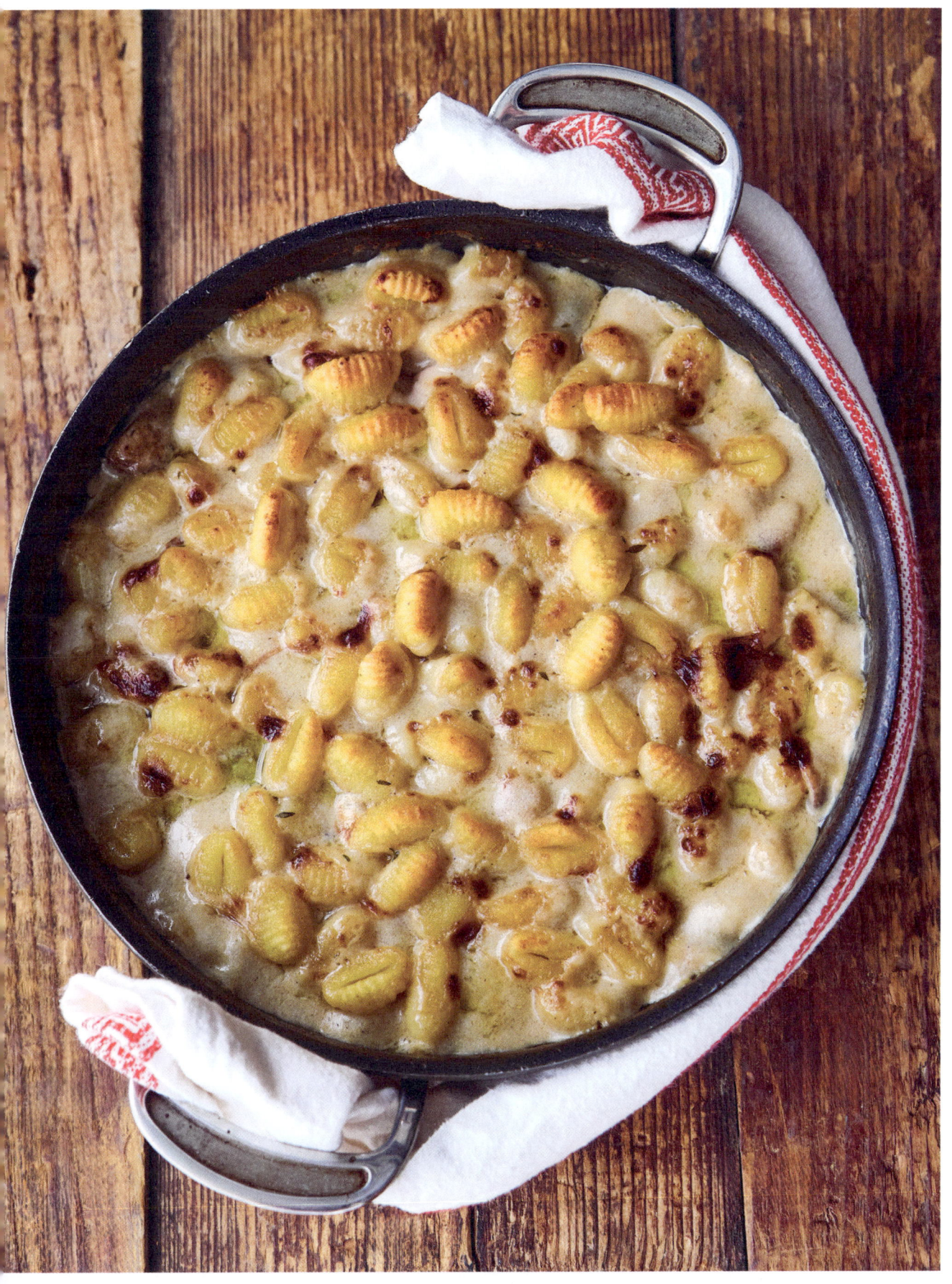

Weekend

3 of your 7 a day

Spring soup & ricotta toasts

A truly spectacular, tasty soup that will get your face smiling and your taste buds singing

SERVES 4
30 MINUTES

2 leeks (320g)

1 x 285g jar of artichoke hearts in oil

320g frozen peas

320g frozen broad beans

1 big bunch of mint (60g)

250g ricotta cheese

20g Parmesan cheese

1 lemon

4 slices of wholemeal sourdough bread

dried red chilli flakes

1 Trim the leeks, then halve lengthways, wash, slice and place in a large deep non-stick pan on a medium heat. Halve and add the artichokes, along with 2 tablespoons of oil from their jar. Cook gently for 15 minutes, or until the leeks are soft and sweet, stirring occasionally. Boil the kettle.

2 Add the peas, broad beans and 1 litre of boiling water, then turn the heat up and bring to the boil while you pick and finely chop the mint leaves. Stir them into the pan, then blend half of the soup, either removing to a blender or in the pan with a stick blender, and stir it back through the rest for a creamier texture. Season to perfection and leave to simmer.

3 In a bowl, beat the ricotta with the finely grated Parmesan and lemon zest, season to perfection and loosen with a little lemon juice, to taste. Toast the bread, then spread 1 heaped tablespoon of the ricotta mixture across each toast, stashing the rest in the fridge for another meal (it will keep for up to 3 days). Add a pinch of chilli flakes to each toast, then portion up the soup and serve with lemon wedges for squeezing over, if you like.

EMBELLISH IT

If you've got one, adding a Parmesan rind with the peas and broad beans will give an incredible depth of flavour. Feel free to add other green veg to the mix, too, such as asparagus, broccoli, green beans or edamame beans.

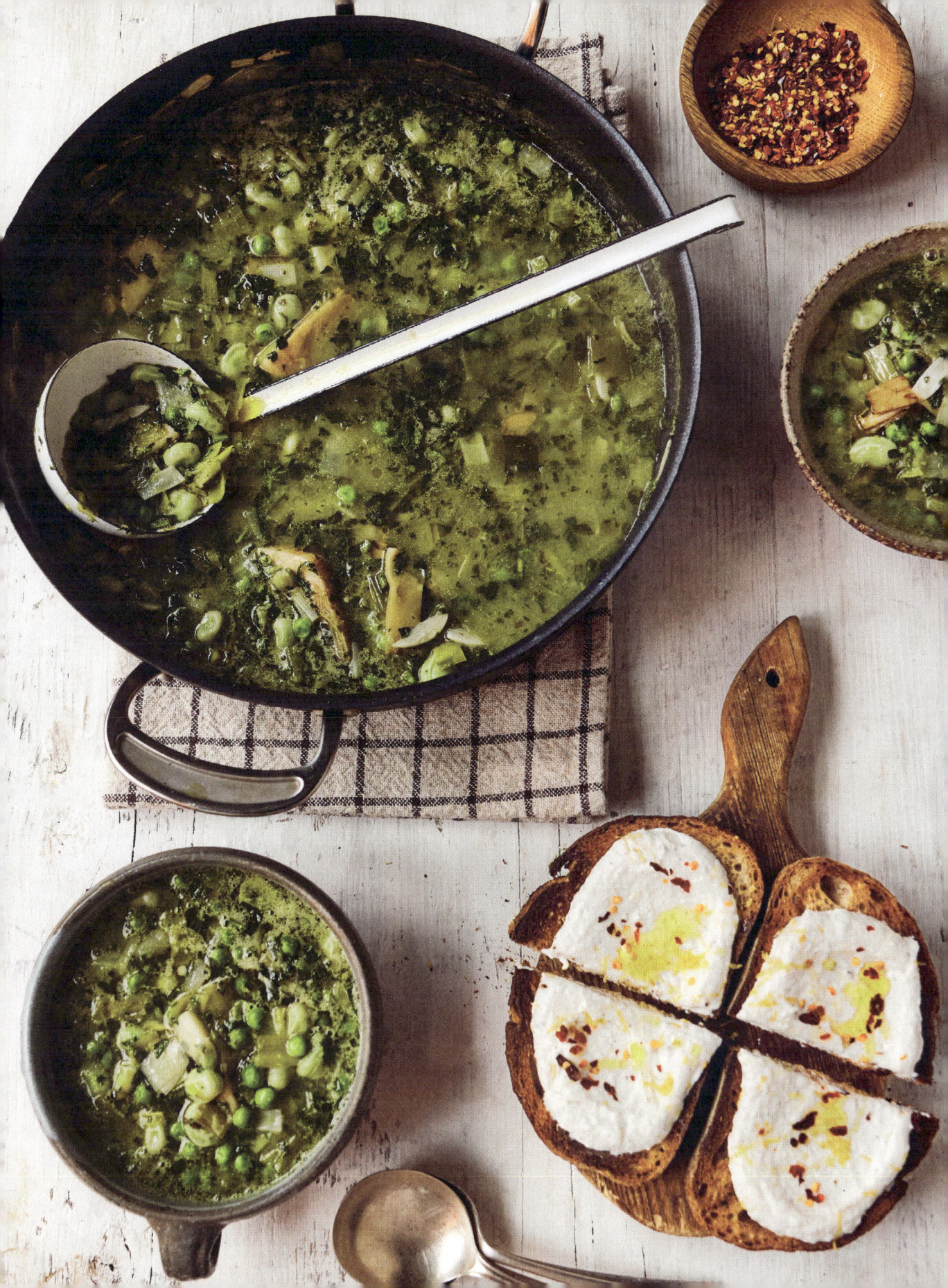

Spiced lamb & lentil soup

This gives me mulligatawny vibes. Think satisfaction and scrumptiousness – like a hug in a mug

SERVES 4
35 MINUTES

250g lamb mince

2 cloves of garlic

2 onions (320g)

2 large carrots (320g)

2 tablespoons curry powder

250g red split lentils

1 jar of lime pickle

1 bunch of coriander (30g)

320g frozen garden peas

10 uncooked poppadoms

1 Put a large shallow casserole pan on a high heat with the mince, breaking it up with a spoon. Dry fry for 10 minutes, or until gnarly, stirring regularly.

2 Peel and finely chop the garlic, onions and carrots. Add to the pan with 1 tablespoon each of olive oil and curry powder, and cook for another 10 minutes, or until starting to caramelize, stirring regularly. Boil the kettle. Stir in the lentils, then pour in 2 litres of boiling water and boil for 10 minutes.

3 Meanwhile, pour the contents of the lime pickle jar into a blender, tear in the coriander stalks, add half a jar of water and blitz until smooth. Refill the jar and stash in the fridge (for up to 1 week), decanting the rest into a bowl.

4 Add the peas to the soup, scrunch in the uncooked poppadoms, and cook for 5 minutes. Stir through the remaining curry powder and the coriander leaves, season to perfection, and serve with the blitzed lime pickle.

VEGGIE LOVE

Swap the lamb mince for 320g of finely chopped or blitzed mushrooms.

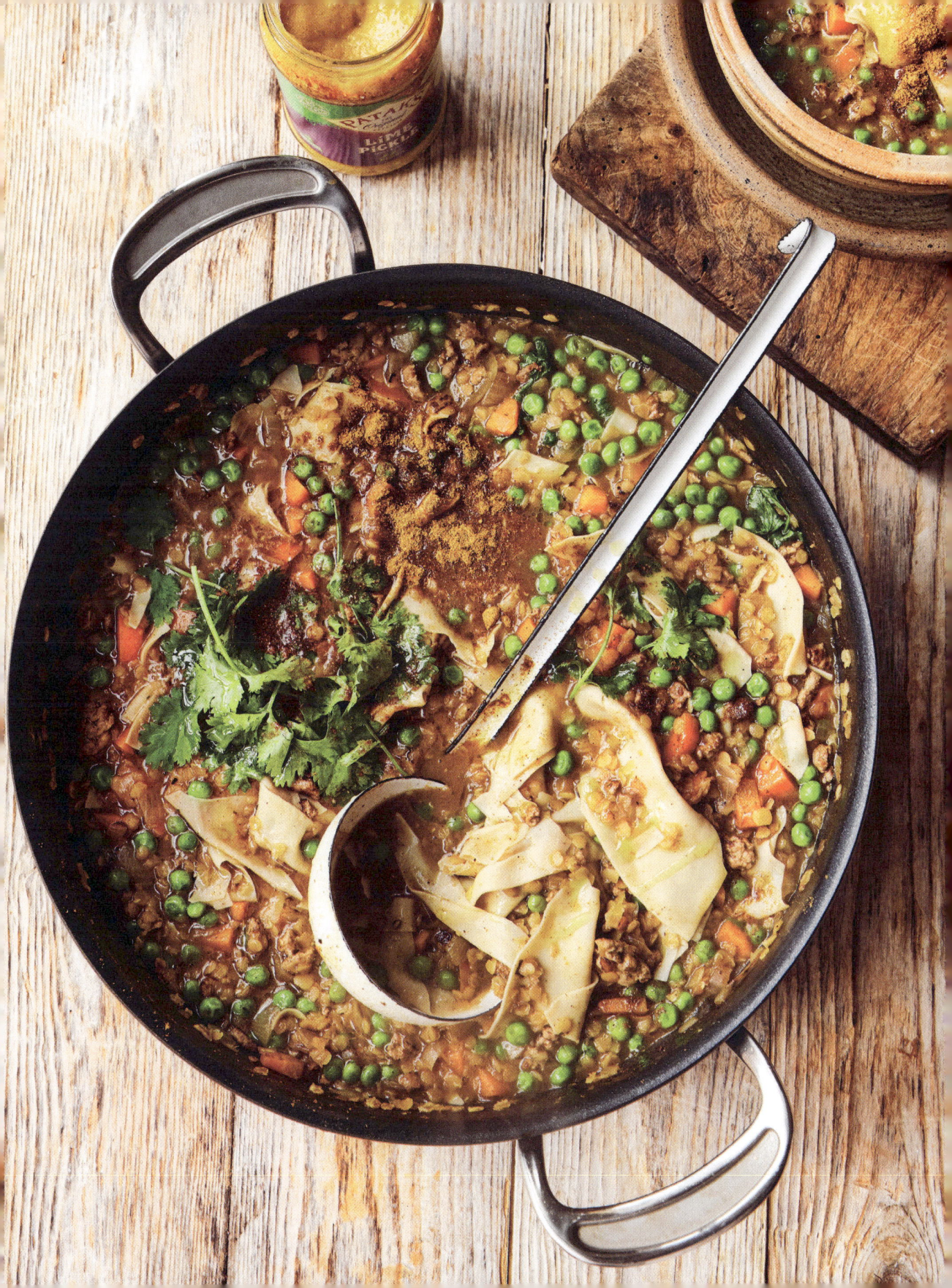

Golden hasselback salmon

Impressive looking yet very easy to prepare, this delicious salmon is the perfect meal to share

SERVES 6
PREP 12 MINUTES
COOK 30 MINUTES

1 x 1kg side of salmon, skin on, scaled, pin-boned

1 lemon

1 bunch of basil (30g)

1 x 50g tin of anchovy fillets in oil

500g ripe tomatoes, on the vine

2 tablespoons harissa paste

300g wholewheat couscous

1 x 700g jar of queen chickpeas

1kg frozen mixed Mediterranean veg

100g natural yoghurt

1 Preheat the oven to 220°C. Use a sharp knife to score through the salmon flesh at 1cm intervals, slicing most of the way through towards the skin.

2 Finely grate the lemon zest on to a board. Pick over most of the basil leaves, reserving some nice ones in a bowl of cold water, and place the stalks in a blender. Add the anchovies to the board with a drizzle of oil from their tin and a pinch of sea salt and black pepper, finely chop together, then rub into all the cuts in the salmon.

3 Add the tomatoes, 1 tablespoon of harissa and 2 tablespoons of red wine vinegar to the blender. Blitz until smooth, season to perfection, then pour into a deep 30cm x 40cm roasting tray and stir in the couscous and chickpeas, juice and all. Sit the prepped salmon on top in the centre, then scatter the frozen veg around it. Cook on the top shelf of the oven for 30 minutes, or until golden and cooked through.

4 Sprinkle over the reserved basil leaves. Use fish slices to move the salmon to a board and portion up, then mix everything left in the tray. Mix the remaining harissa into the yoghurt. Serve with lemon wedges.

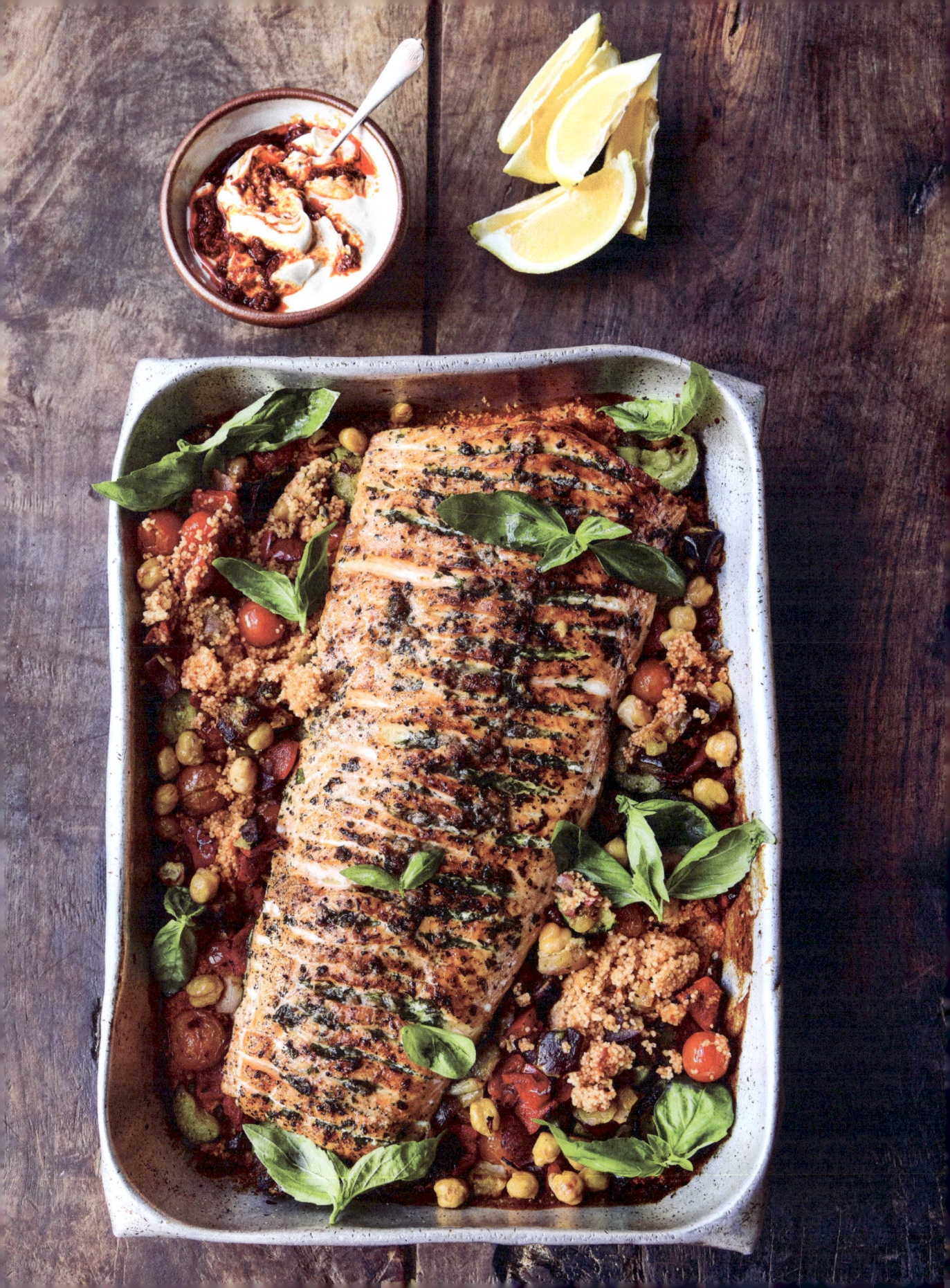

2 of your 7 a day

Healthy fish & chips

Traditional fish and chips just ain't compatible with a health kick, so here's my healthy expression

SERVES 4
45 MINUTES

1kg sweet potatoes

80g panko breadcrumbs

1 egg

4 x 130g white fish fillets, skin off, pin-boned

1 x 400g tin of chickpeas

2 tablespoons tikka masala curry paste

2 lemons

320g frozen peas

½ a bunch of mint (15g)

gherkins, to serve

1 Preheat the oven to 220°C. Wash the sweet potatoes and slice lengthways into thin wedges. In a large roasting tray, toss with 1 tablespoon of olive oil, a pinch of sea salt and lots of black pepper, arrange in a single layer, and roast for 40 minutes, or until golden and cooked through, turning halfway.

2 Put the breadcrumbs on a plate. Beat and season the egg in a shallow bowl. Coat the fish in the egg, then turn in the crumbs, patting them all over. Place on an oil-spritzed tray and roast above the wedges for the last 20 minutes.

3 Pour the chickpeas, juice and all, into a blender and add the curry paste and 200ml of water. Squeeze in the juice of 1 lemon and blitz until smooth. Pour into a small pan on a medium heat and cook for 10 minutes, or until thickened, stirring occasionally, then season to perfection.

4 Cook the peas in a small pan of boiling salted water for 2 minutes, while you pick and finely chop the mint leaves. Drain the peas, toss with the mint and season to perfection. Slice the gherkins (I like to use a crinkle-cut knife).

5 Serve it all together, with lemon wedges and condiments of your choice.

AIR FRYER IT

Cook the chips in the large drawer of an air fryer for 20 minutes at 200°C, or until golden and cooked through, shaking halfway. Cook the fish in the small drawer for 10 minutes at 200°C, or until golden and cooked through.

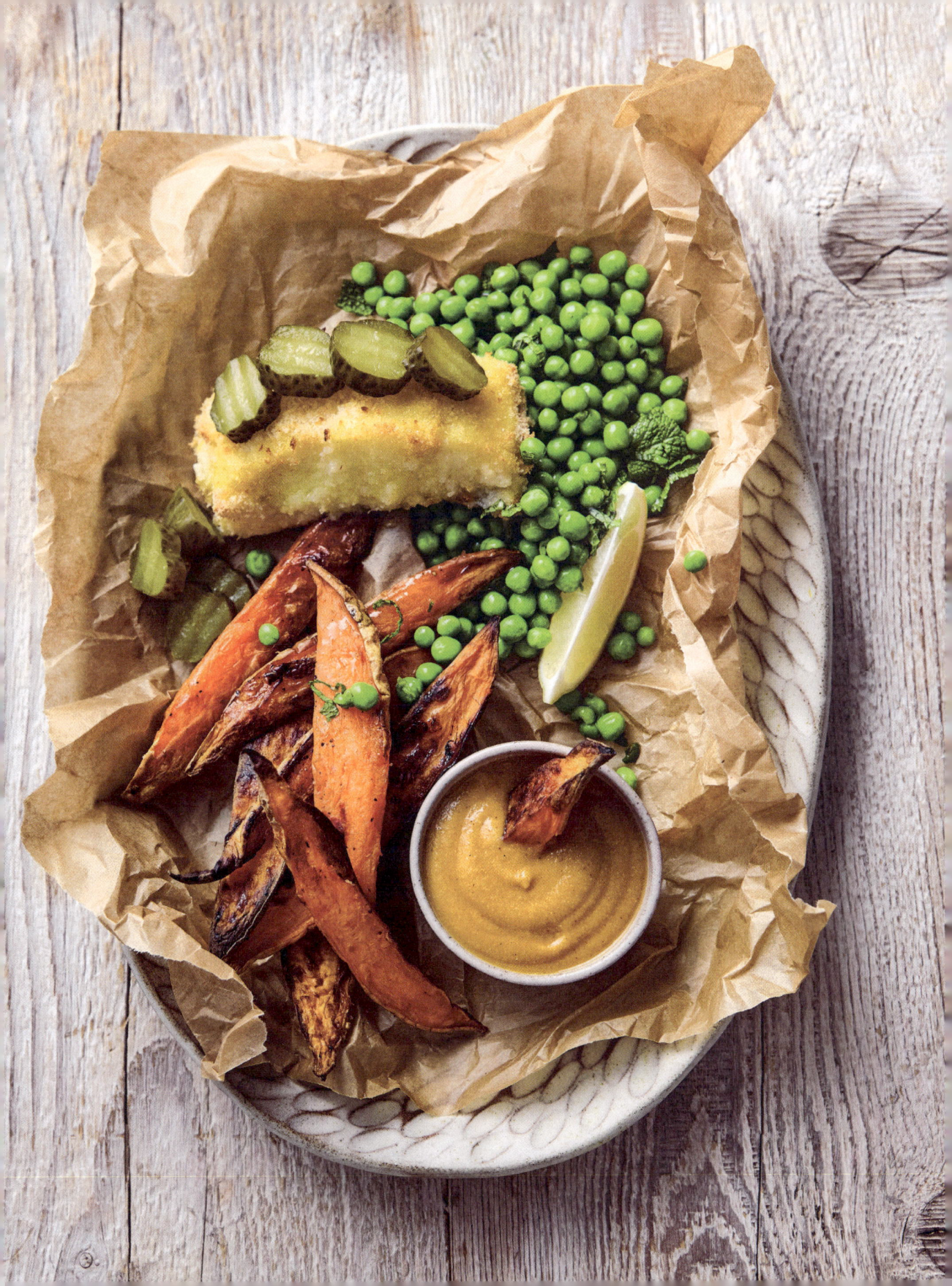

Fish filo parcel & beans

Delicate pastry and fish teamed with spinach and fragrant herbs is a beautiful thing

SERVES 4
45 MINUTES

320g baby spinach

1 bunch of dill (20g)

4 sheets of filo pastry

4 x 130g trout or salmon fillets, skin off, pin-boned

2 cloves of garlic

500g ripe cherry tomatoes

2 x 400g tins of cannellini beans

2 teaspoons Dijon mustard

4 heaped tablespoons natural yoghurt

1 lemon

1 Preheat the oven to 180°C. Put a large shallow casserole pan on a medium-high heat with a spritz of olive oil, the spinach and most of the dill, stalks and all, reserving a few fronds for garnish. Cook for 10 minutes, or until the excess moisture has evaporated, stirring occasionally. Remove to a board, finely chop and season to perfection with sea salt and black pepper.

2 Lay out 2 sheets of overlapping filo on a clean work surface with the short ends facing you. Spritz with olive oil, then put the other 2 sheets on top and spritz again. Sit 2 trout fillets facing each other in the middle at the bottom, so the thinner ends of the fillets overlap, pile the spinach mixture on top in an even layer, then sit the remaining fillets on top. Fold in the sides of the filo, then roll it up into a parcel. Place on an oil-spritzed baking tray, generously spritz with oil and cook for 30 minutes, or until golden and cooked through.

3 Meanwhile, wipe out the pan. Spritz it with oil, then peel, finely chop and add the garlic. Halve and add the tomatoes, and cook on a medium heat for 5 minutes, or until softened. Pour in the beans, juice and all, and simmer for another 5 minutes, or until thickened, then add ½ a tablespoon of red wine vinegar and season to perfection.

4 Stir the Dijon through the yoghurt, and serve it all together, with lemon wedges on the side and the reserved dill scattered over the top.

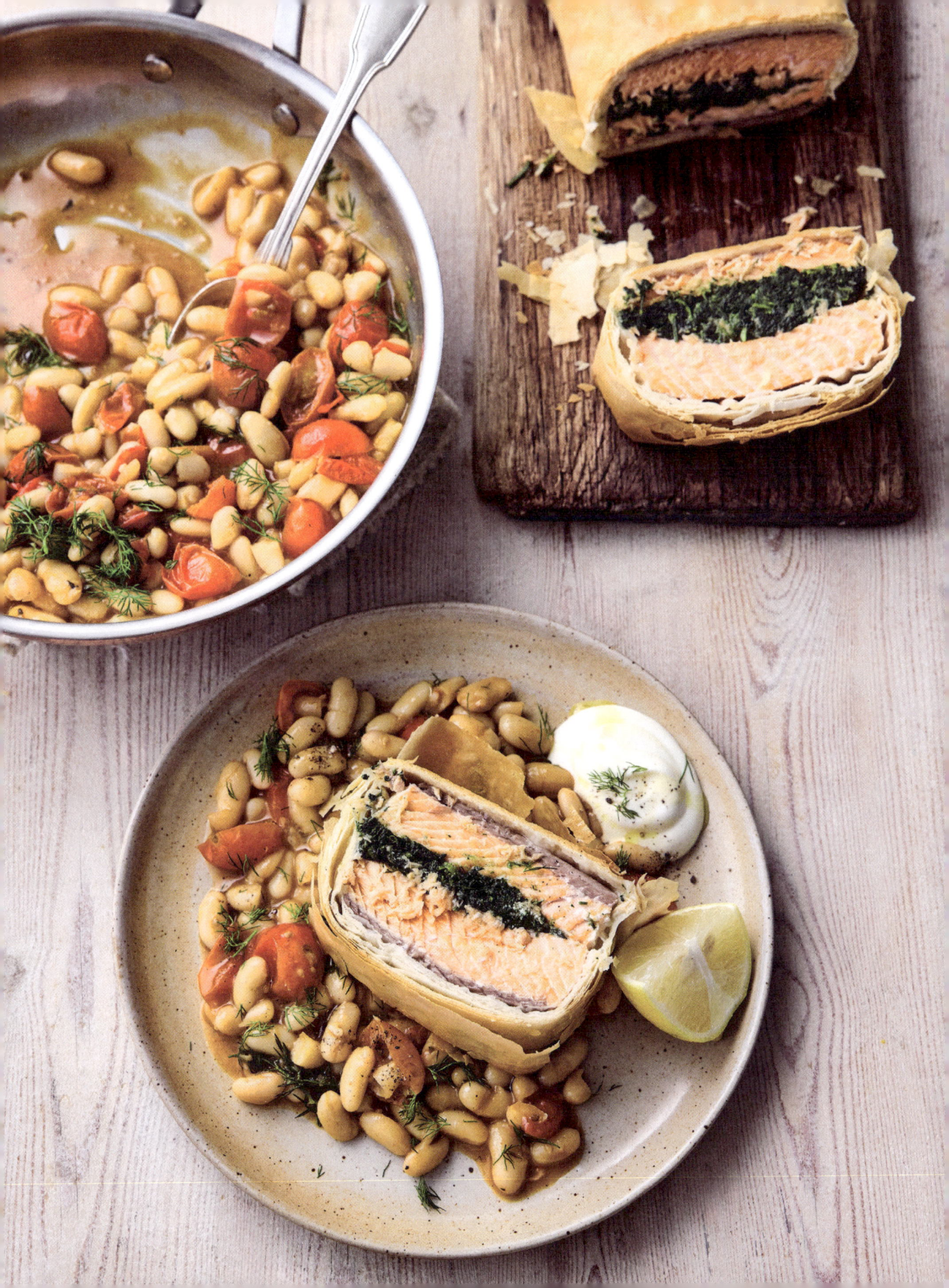

Fish pie soup & eggs on toast

Delicious and satisfying, this is all the elements of a classic fish pie in sumptuous soup form

SERVES 4
46 MINUTES

2 onions (320g)

2 large carrots (320g)

2 leeks (320g)

2 potatoes (320g)

4 teaspoons English mustard, plus extra to taste

2 large eggs

400g mixed frozen fish chunks

½ a bunch of curly parsley (15g)

4 tablespoons soured cream

4 slices of wholemeal sourdough bread

1 Put a large deep non-stick pan on a high heat. Stirring into the pan to dry fry as you go, peel and dice the onions and carrots, trim the leeks, halve lengthways and wash, then chop. Add 2 tablespoons of olive oil and a small pinch of sea salt and black pepper to the pan and cook for 10 minutes, stirring regularly. Boil the kettle.

2 Peel and dice the potatoes, add to the pan with the mustard, pour in 1 litre of boiling kettle water, cover and boil for 10 minutes, adding the eggs to cook for 7 minutes, for soft-boiled. Remove the eggs to cold water.

3 Add the fish to the pan and reduce to a simmer for 10 minutes, or until the fish is cooked through. Finely chop the parsley, stalks and all, and stir half into the soured cream. Toast the bread. Peel and halve or quarter the eggs.

4 Mash some of the soup with a potato masher, creating a creamy consistency. Season to perfection and add extra mustard to taste, then stir through the reserved parsley and drizzle with a little extra virgin olive oil, if you like. Spread the soured cream across the toasts, top with the eggs, and serve.

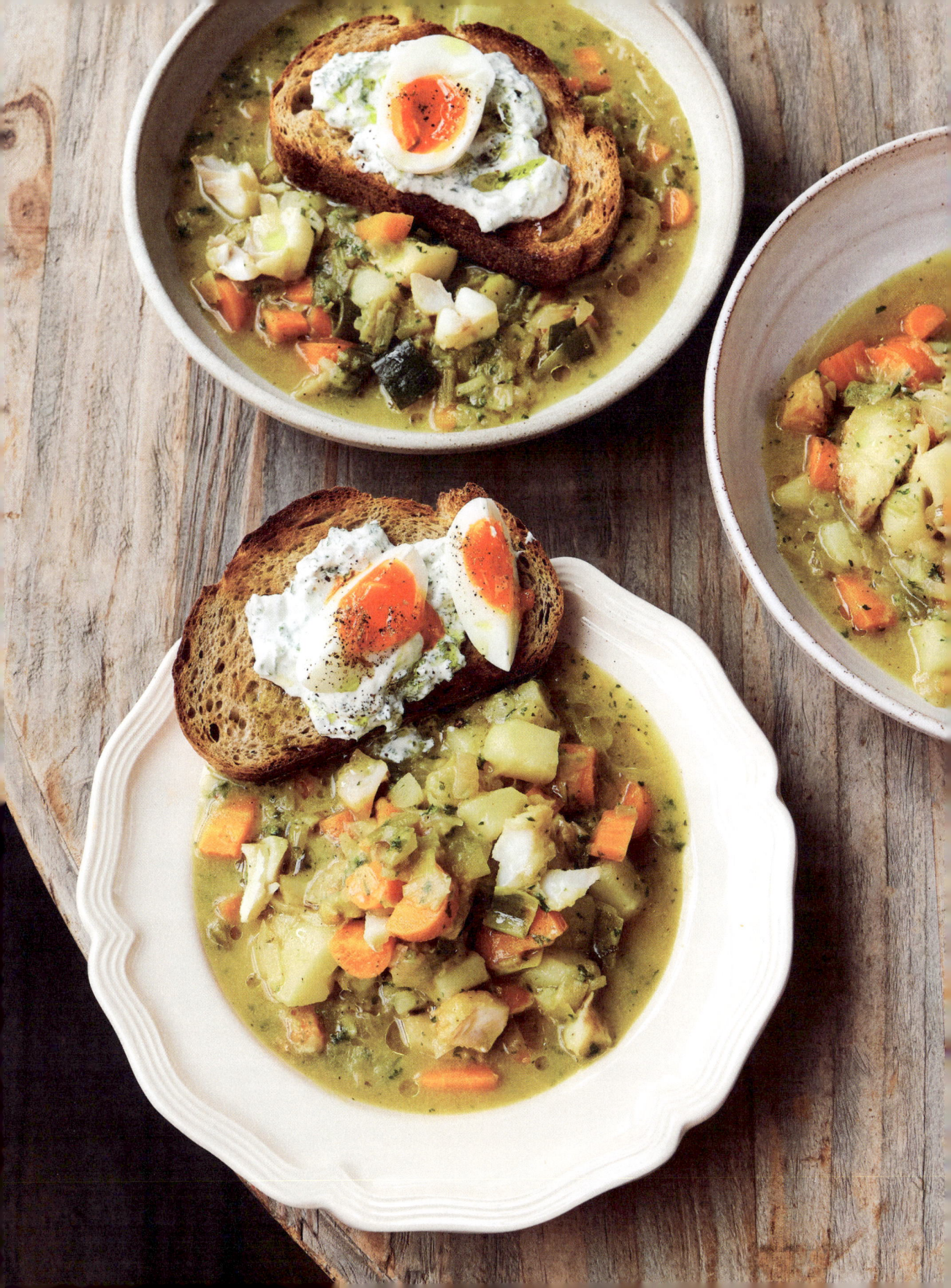

Crispy steamed veggie buns

Buns like these are great for sharing and are a fun way to enjoy different veg

SERVES 4
48 MINUTES

500g self-raising flour, plus extra for dusting

300ml semi-skimmed milk

3 cloves of garlic

3cm piece of ginger

4 spring onions

1 x 225g tin of sliced water chestnuts

500g baby spinach

2 heaped tablespoons hoisin sauce, plus extra to serve

4 carrots (320g)

20g unsalted roasted peanuts or cashew nuts

1 Mix the flour, milk and a pinch of sea salt with a fork, then your clean hands, until you have a dough, knead on a flour-dusted surface, cover and rest.

2 Peel and chop the garlic and ginger with the whites of the spring onions, slicing and reserving the greens. Put it all into a large non-stick frying pan on a high heat with 1 tablespoon of olive oil. Drain and add the water chestnuts, then the spinach, 1 tablespoon of red wine vinegar and the hoisin. Cook down for 10 minutes, stirring regularly until thick and sticky, then tip on to your board, finely chop it all, season to perfection and divide into 8.

3 Roll the dough into a log, cut into 8 equal pieces, then use your thumbs and fingertips to turn and stretch each piece into a 15cm round – you want it slightly thicker in the middle and thinner at the edges. Add a portion of filling to each, then start bringing the opposite edges into the middle, folding and pinching to seal (use a bit of water to help them stick, if needed). Place seal side down in the wiped-out pan with a spritz of oil as you go, and repeat.

4 Place the pan on a medium heat. As soon as you hear a sizzle, pour 250ml of water around the buns and cover the pan. Steam for 12 minutes, while you use a speed-peeler to peel the carrots into ribbons. Toss with 1 tablespoon of red wine vinegar and season to perfection. Crush the nuts.

5 Now, uncover the pan and cook until the buns are crispy and golden on the bottom. Serve with the carrots, sliced green spring onions, crushed nuts and extra hoisin, tearing open the buns and adding the crunchy bits for contrast.

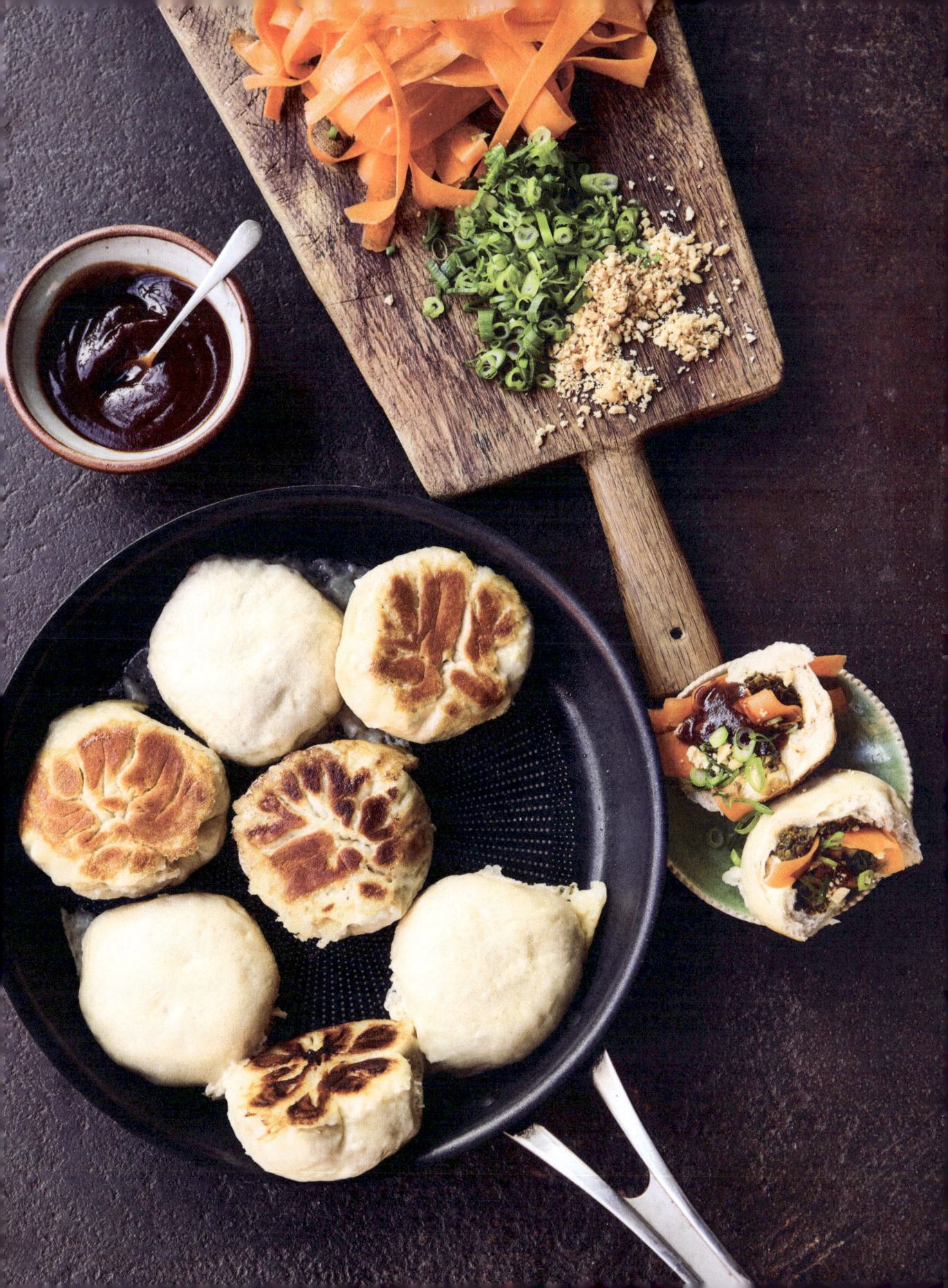

Comforting chickpea soup

Inspired by my love of aloo gobi, this hearty soup will give you a whole heap of comfort

SERVES 4
PREP 15 MINUTES
COOK 25 MINUTES

4cm piece of ginger

4 cloves of garlic

2 onions (320g)

1 small handful of curry leaves

1 head of cauliflower (800g)

500g potatoes

3 tablespoons of your favourite curry paste

60g coconut cream

2 x 400g tins of chickpeas

200g ripe mixed-colour cherry tomatoes

1 Peel and finely chop the ginger, garlic and onions, and place in a large deep non-stick pan on a medium heat with 1 tablespoon of olive oil and the curry leaves. Click off and discard only the tatty outer leaves from the cauliflower, then, adding to the pan as you go, roughly chop the rest, stalk and all. Peel the potatoes, chop into 2cm dice, add to the pan with the curry paste, and cook for 10 minutes, stirring regularly.

2 Stir in the coconut cream, then pour in the chickpeas, juice and all, along with 800ml of boiling kettle water. Cover and boil for 25 minutes, then blend half, either removing to a blender or in the pan with a stick blender, and stir it back through the rest for a creamier texture. Season to perfection.

3 Divide the soup between bowls, then quarter and scatter over the tomatoes. Drizzle with extra virgin olive oil, if you like, and devour.

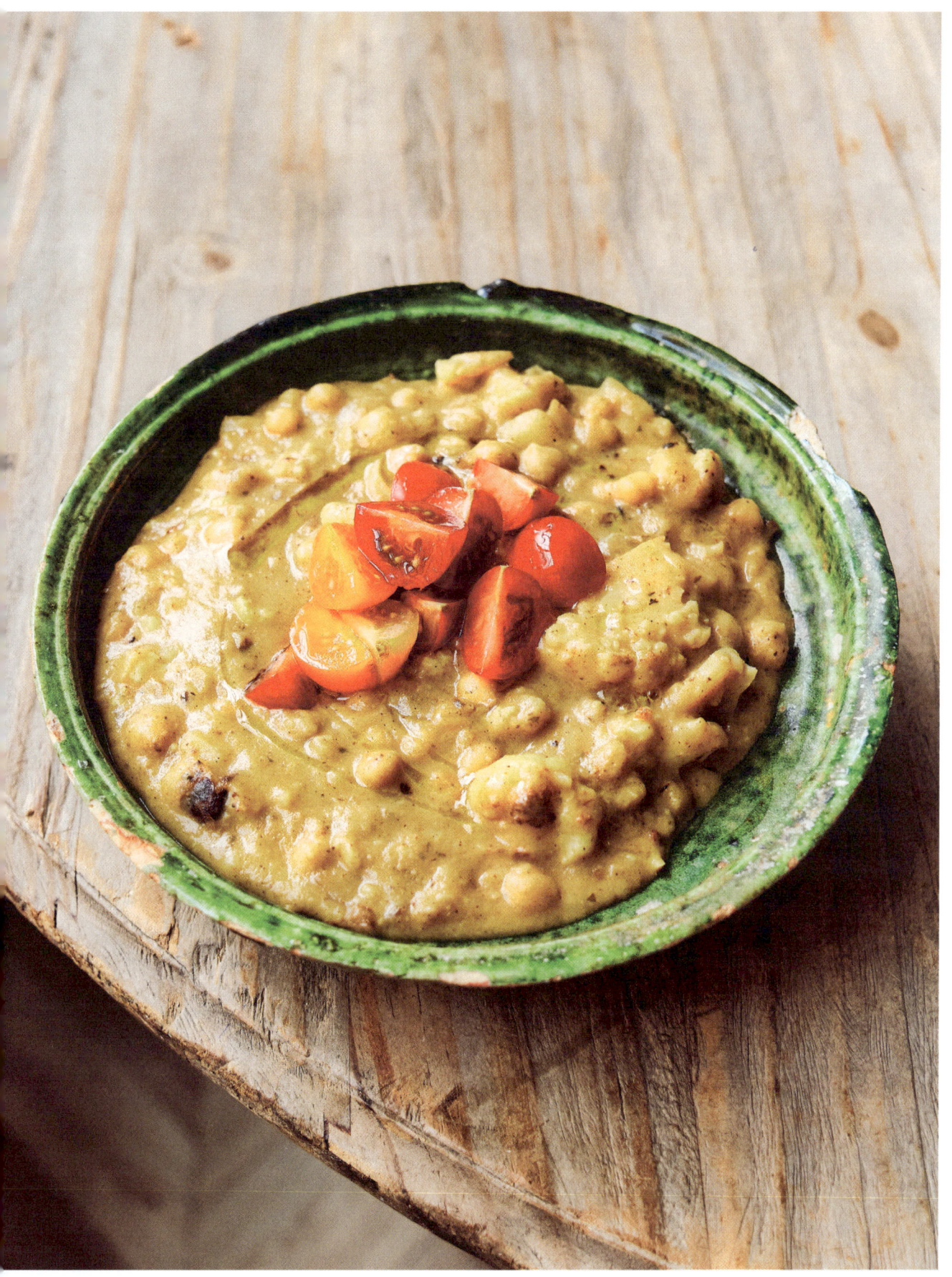

Winter squash & borlotti soup

Embrace the ritual of making soup. You will truly adore the flavour and texture you create here

SERVES 4
50 MINUTES

1 butternut squash (1.2kg)

2 large carrots (320g)

320g celery

1 whole nutmeg, for grating

20g dried porcini mushrooms

1 litre veg or chicken stock

4 sprigs of rosemary

2 x 400g tins of borlotti beans

4 large slices of wholemeal sourdough bread

40g Parmesan cheese

1 Peel and deseed the squash, peel the carrots and celery, then chop it all into 2cm chunks and put into a large shallow non-stick casserole pan on a medium-high heat with 2 tablespoons of olive oil. Add a small pinch of sea salt and plenty of black pepper, finely grate in half the nutmeg, and cook for 30 minutes, or until soft and starting to caramelize, stirring occasionally.

2 Meanwhile, crumble the porcini into a large jug, cover with the hot stock and leave to rehydrate for 20 minutes.

3 Strip the rosemary leaves into the pan, then pour in the beans, juice and all, and add the stock and porcini, discarding the last gritty bit. Simmer for 10 minutes, adding splashes of water to loosen, if needed, then season to perfection and divide between warm bowls.

4 Toast the bread, finely grate over the Parmesan, sit them on top of your soups, and finish with a little drizzle of extra virgin olive oil, if you like.

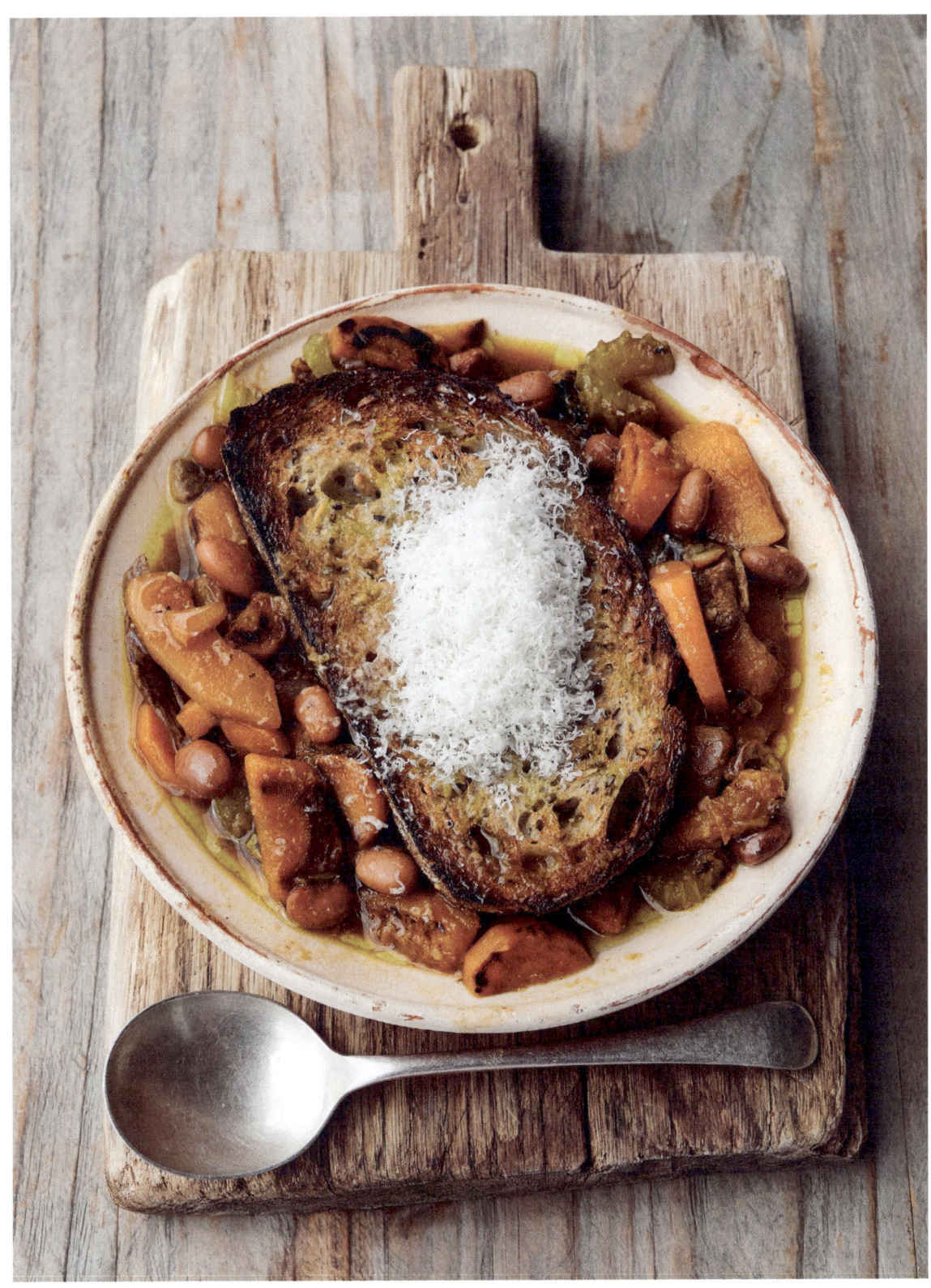

Fragrant veggie filo tart

A really enjoyable celebration of vegetables, interesting textures and contrasting flavours

SERVES 4
58 MINUTES

1 red onion (160g)

1 large bulb of fennel (320g)

1 large aubergine (400g)

2 heaped teaspoons ras el hanout, plus extra to serve

500g ripe tomatoes

120g dried apricots

1 big bunch of mint (60g)

50g wholewheat couscous

125g feta cheese

6 sheets of filo pastry

1. Preheat the oven to 180°C. Put a large shallow non-stick casserole pan on a medium-high heat. Adding as you go, peel the onion, trim the fennel and cut each into eighths, reserving any leafy fennel tops. Slice the aubergines 2cm thick. Dry fry it all for 15 minutes, or until dark and charred, stirring regularly. Boil the kettle.

2. Go into the pan with 2 tablespoons of olive oil and the ras el hanout. Slice and add the tomatoes, along with 1 tablespoon of red wine vinegar, cook for another 15 minutes, stirring occasionally, then turn the heat off.

3. Meanwhile, in a blender, soak the apricots in 220ml of boiling kettle water for a few minutes, blitz until smooth, then decant into a little serving bowl.

4. Roughly chop most of the mint leaves, saving a handful for garnish, stir into the veg, and season to perfection. Arrange it all in a fairly even layer, then sprinkle over the couscous and crumble over 100g of feta. Layer the filo on top, spritzing with oil as you go, and carefully tucking it down the sides of the pan. Transfer to the oven and cook for 20 minutes, or until golden.

5. Carefully and confidently flip the tart out of the pan on to a board, crumble over the rest of the feta and sprinkle over the remaining mint leaves, along with any reserved fennel tops. Serve drizzled with the apricot sauce, and an extra dusting of ras el hanout, if you like. Nice with a simple side salad.

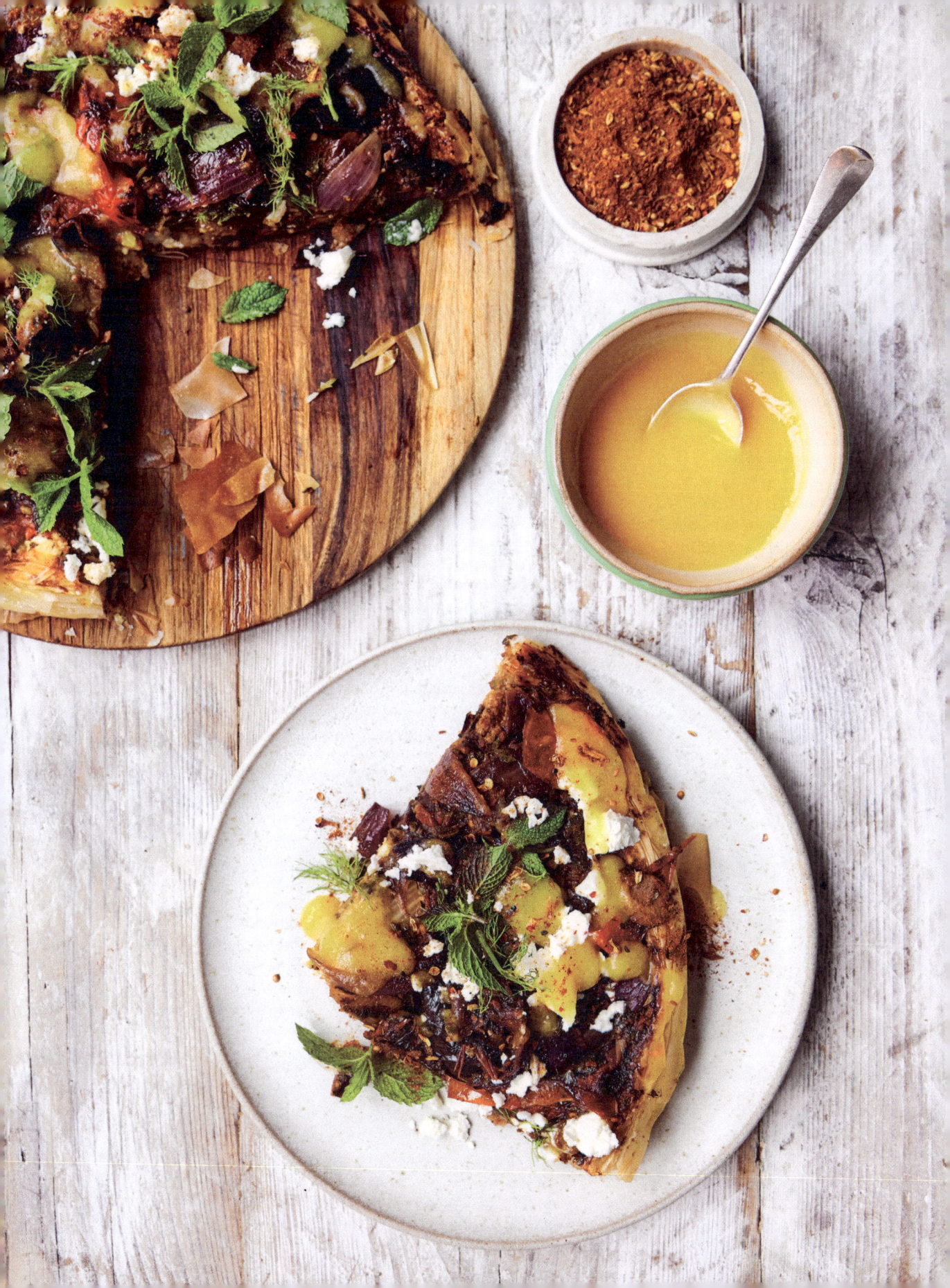

Mushroom riso soup

Adding risotto rice to mushroom soup creates a fun, hearty, comforting bowlful

SERVES 4
1 HOUR

2 onions (320g)

4 carrots (320g)

320g celery

500g chestnut mushrooms

4 cloves of garlic

300g risotto rice

2 litres veg stock

4 sprigs of thyme, flowering if you can get it

1 lemon

50g Parmesan cheese

1 Peel and finely chop the onions, carrots and celery, putting them into a large casserole pan on a medium-high heat with 2 tablespoons of olive oil as you go. Trim, finely slice and add the mushrooms, reserving a few pretty cross-sections for garnish, then peel, finely slice and add the garlic. Cook for 20 minutes, or until softened, stirring regularly.

2 Stir the rice into the pan, then pour in 2 litres of hot stock. Simmer for 20 minutes, or until the rice is cooked, stirring occasionally.

3 Meanwhile, strip the thyme leaves into a pestle and mortar with a small pinch of sea salt, pound into a paste, then loosen with 3 tablespoons of extra virgin olive oil and the lemon juice to make a fragrant oil.

4 You can leave the soup chunky, or blitz some of it, stirring it back through for a creamier texture. Finely grate and stir in most of the Parmesan, then season to perfection and divide between warm bowls. Scatter over the reserved mushroom slices, shave over the remaining Parmesan, finish with a drizzle of thyme oil and pick over some thyme flowers, if you have them.

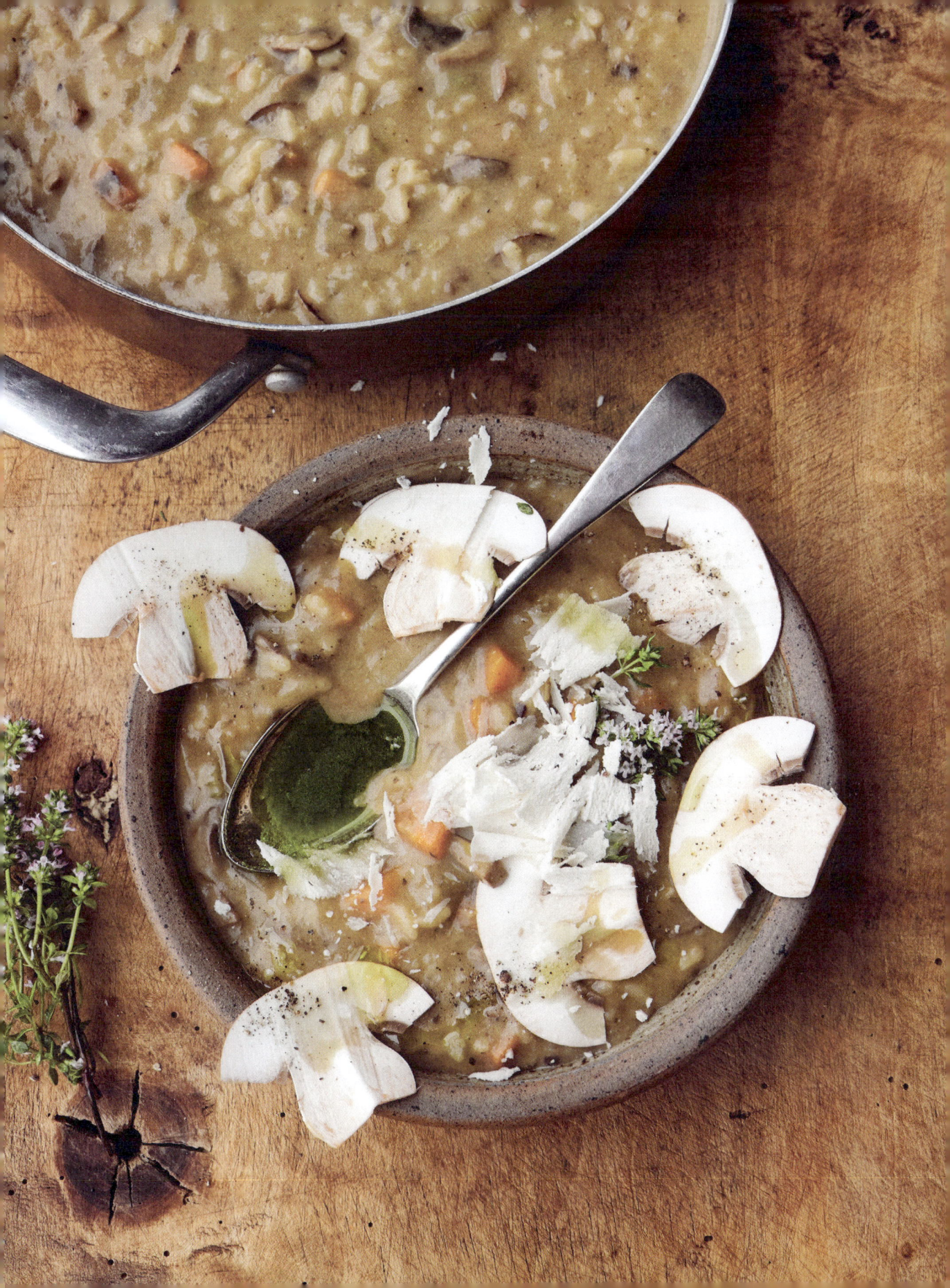

Sumptuous squash risotto

Risotto is one of those magical rituals giving joy in both the making and the eating

SERVES 4

1 HOUR

1 butternut squash (1.2kg)

1 pinch of dried red chilli flakes

2 onions (320g)

320g celery

1.6 litres veg or chicken stock

½ a bunch of rosemary (10g)

300g risotto rice

30g Parmesan cheese, plus extra to serve

180g vac-packed chestnuts

300g cottage cheese

1. Preheat the oven to 180°C. Peel the squash, carefully halve lengthways, then scoop out and discard the seeds. Slice into 3cm-thick moons and toss in a tray with 1 tablespoon of olive oil, the chilli flakes and a pinch of sea salt and black pepper. Roast for 50 minutes, or until soft and starting to caramelize.

2. Peel and finely chop the onions and celery. Put the stock in a pan and leave to simmer on the lowest heat. Put a large high-sided pan on a medium heat with 1 tablespoon of oil, strip in the rosemary leaves, fry until crispy, then use a slotted spoon to remove to a plate, leaving the oil in the pan.

3. Go in with the onion and celery and cook for 10 minutes, stirring regularly. Stir in the rice for 2 minutes, then add a ladleful of stock, stirring constantly until it's been absorbed before adding another. Continue to add ladlefuls of stock until the rice is tender but still holding its shape – around 17 minutes.

4. Mash up three-quarters of the squash and stir into the risotto, finely grate in the Parmesan, then season to perfection. Cover and let it rest while, in a blender, you blitz the chestnuts with the cottage cheese until super-smooth, loosening with splashes of water, if needed, and season to perfection.

5. Divide the risotto between warm bowls. Tear over the remaining squash, spoon over the chestnut cream, sprinkle over the crispy rosemary leaves and serve with an extra grating of Parmesan, if you like.

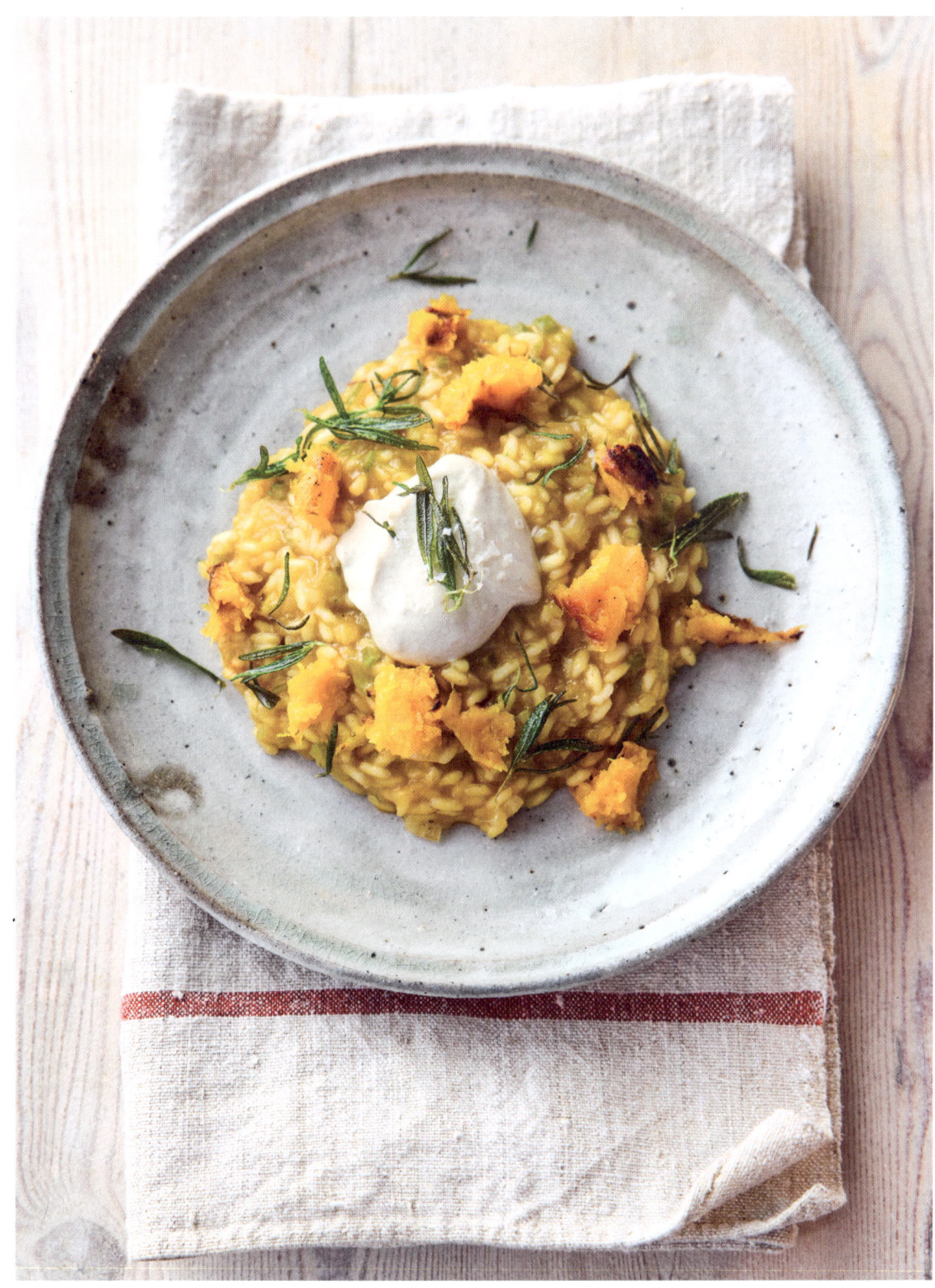

Happy fish pie

Creamy, comforting and ever so delicious, the big question is, are you having eggs, or no eggs?

SERVES 6
PREP 30 MINUTES
COOK 35 MINUTES
PLUS RESTING

1kg potatoes

1 large head of broccoli (480g)

optional: 3 large eggs

3 leeks (480g)

2 heaped tablespoons plain flour

2 teaspoons of your favourite mustard

600ml semi-skimmed milk

800g mixed frozen fish chunks

75g Cheddar cheese

1 bunch of chives (20g)

1 lemon

1 Preheat the oven to 180°C. Peel the potatoes, halving any larger ones, then cook in a pan of boiling salted water for 20 minutes, or until tender. Trim, finely chop and reserve the broccoli stalk. Chop the head into florets and add to the pan with the eggs, if using, for the last 7 minutes. Cool the eggs under cold running water. Drain the potatoes and broccoli, and steam dry.

2 Meanwhile, trim the leeks, halve lengthways, then wash and finely slice. Place in a large shallow casserole pan on a medium heat with 1 tablespoon of olive oil and the chopped broccoli stalk. Cook for 10 minutes, or until soft, stirring regularly. Stir in the flour and mustard, then gradually stir in the milk. Simmer for 5 minutes, stirring occasionally, then season to perfection.

3 Add the fish chunks and simmer for another 5 minutes, then grate in most of the cheese. Finely chop the chives and fold in most of them. Peel, halve and dot in the eggs, if using, and finely grate over the lemon zest.

4 Mash the potato and broccoli – rustic or smooth, the choice is yours. Season to perfection, then spoon over the dish, fork up the top for added texture, grate over the last bit of cheese and spritz with oil. Bake for 35 minutes, or until golden and bubbling. Rest for 5 minutes, sprinkle over the remaining chives, and serve with lemon wedges.

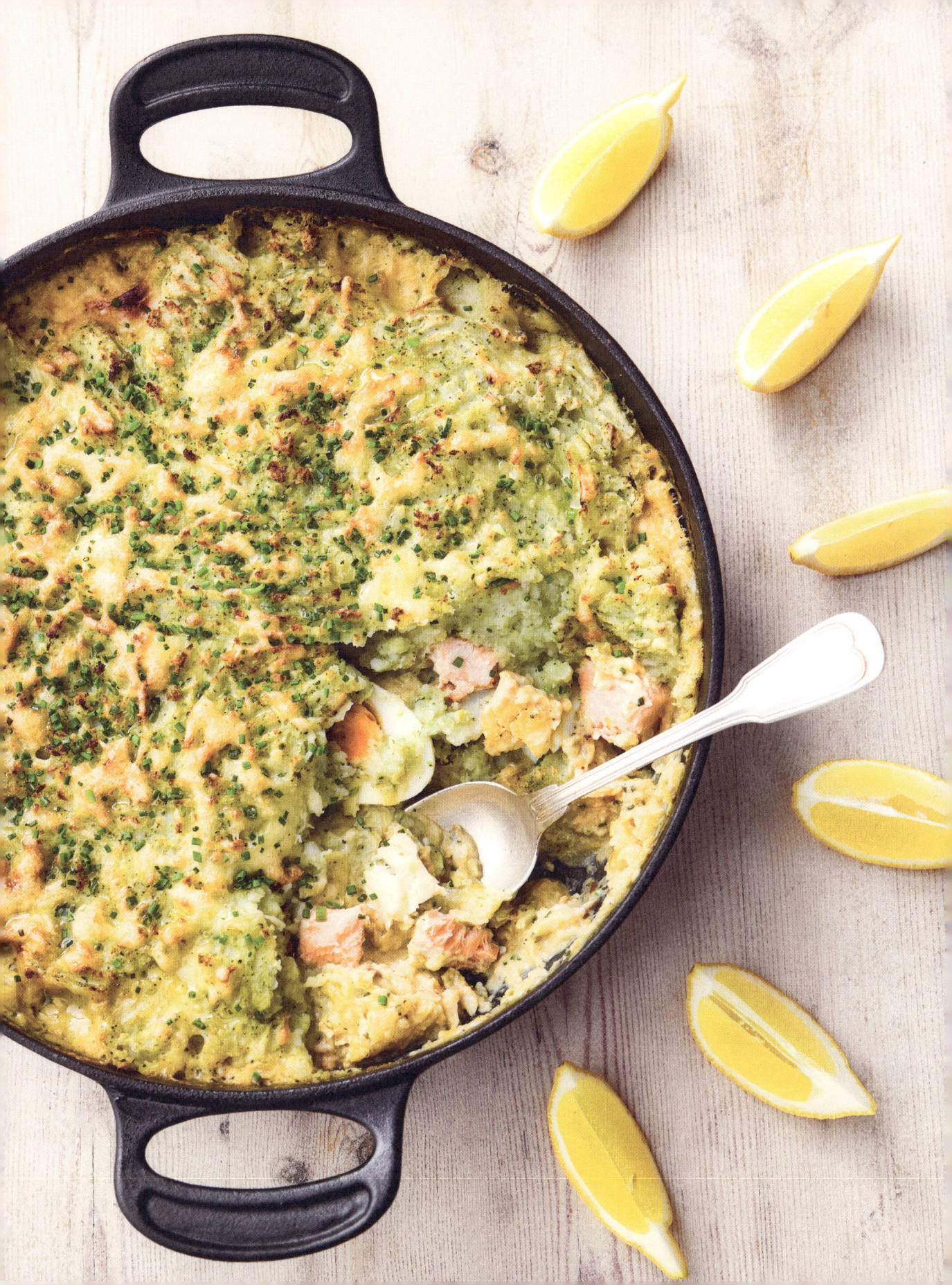

Meatball traybake

Using an old friend like meatballs to get some beans into your life is a tasty, nutritious win

SERVES 4
PREP 10 MINUTES
COOK 1 HOUR

1 large bulb of fennel (320g)

2 red onions (320g)

4 carrots (320g)

1 x 400g tin of cannellini beans

400g beef or pork mince

1 teaspoon dried oregano

2 x 400g tins of plum tomatoes

1 x 460g jar of roasted red peppers

1 lemon

50g feta cheese

1 Preheat the oven to 200°C. Trim the fennel, reserving any leafy tops, peel the onions, then cut it all into wedges and place in a deep 30cm x 40cm roasting tray. Peel, halve and add the carrots. Toss with 1 tablespoon of olive oil, season with sea salt and black pepper, and roast for 40 minutes.

2 Meanwhile, drain the beans and pulse a couple of times in a food processor. Add the mince and oregano, season, and pulse until just combined. With clean wet hands, divide the mixture into 12, roll into balls, then place in a large non-stick frying pan on a medium-high heat with 2 tablespoons of oil and cook until golden all over, turning regularly.

3 Pour the tomatoes and peppers, juice and all, into the processor (there's no need to clean it). Finely grate and reserve the lemon zest, then squeeze the juice into the processor, season and blitz until smooth.

4 Remove the tray from the oven, pour the sauce over the veg, then evenly sit the golden balls around the tray. Return to the oven for a final 20 minutes.

5 To serve, crumble over the feta, sprinkle over the reserved lemon zest and any fennel tops, and drizzle with a little extra virgin olive oil, if you like. Great as it is, or with wholemeal toast, couscous, rice or spaghetti.

VEGGIE LOVE

Veggie mince works very well in place of beef or pork mince.

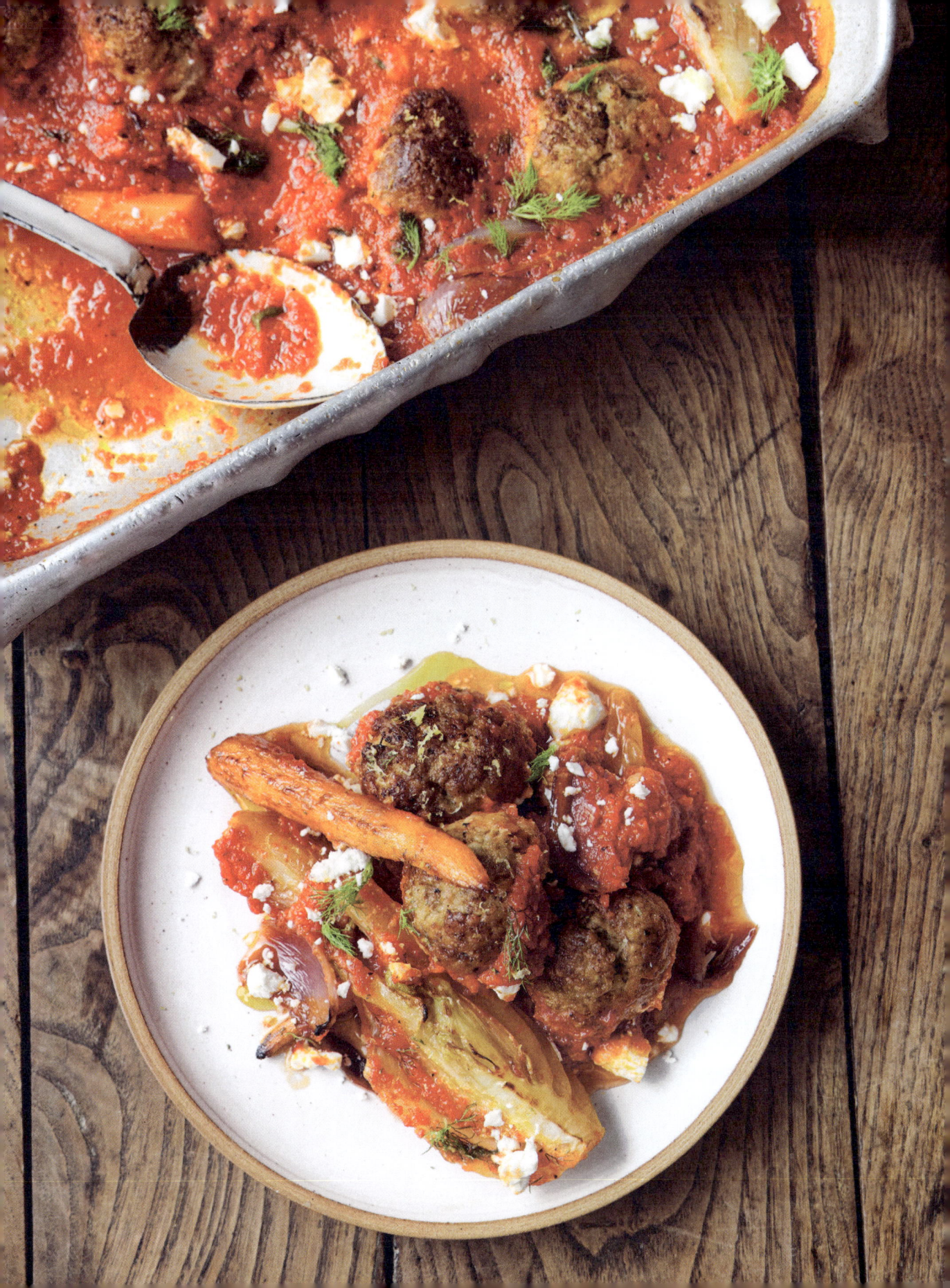

Hearty veg casserole

A real celebration of veggies, this is all about the harmony of fragrance and flavour

SERVES 4
PREP 18 MINUTES
COOK 1 HOUR

2 onions (320g)

½ a butternut squash (600g)

1 large bulb of fennel (320g)

2 courgettes (320g)

320g new potatoes

3 cloves of garlic

120g dried apricots

1 heaped tablespoon ras el hanout

2 x 400g tins of plum tomatoes

50g feta or soft, crumbly vegan cheese

1 Preheat the oven to 200°C. Peel the onions and squash, trim the fennel, then chop it all into 2cm chunks. Put a large shallow casserole pan on a medium heat with 1 tablespoon of olive oil, add the chopped veg, and cook for 15 minutes, or until softened and starting to caramelize, stirring regularly.

2 Meanwhile, very finely slice the courgettes and potatoes into rounds, either by hand with good knife skills, or on a mandolin (use the guard!). Keep aside.

3 Peel and finely slice the garlic. Roughly chop the apricots, then stir both into the pan with the ras el hanout. Cook and stir for 2 minutes, then pour in the tomatoes, breaking them up with your spoon. Mix well, season to perfection, then turn the heat off.

4 Arrange the courgette and potato slices alternately around the edge of the pan on top of the stew, like you see in the picture, gently pressing down to absorb all the flavours. Transfer to the oven and cook for 40 minutes, or until golden, thick, blipping and delicious, crumbling over the feta for the last couple of minutes. Delicious as is, or with a side of rice or couscous.

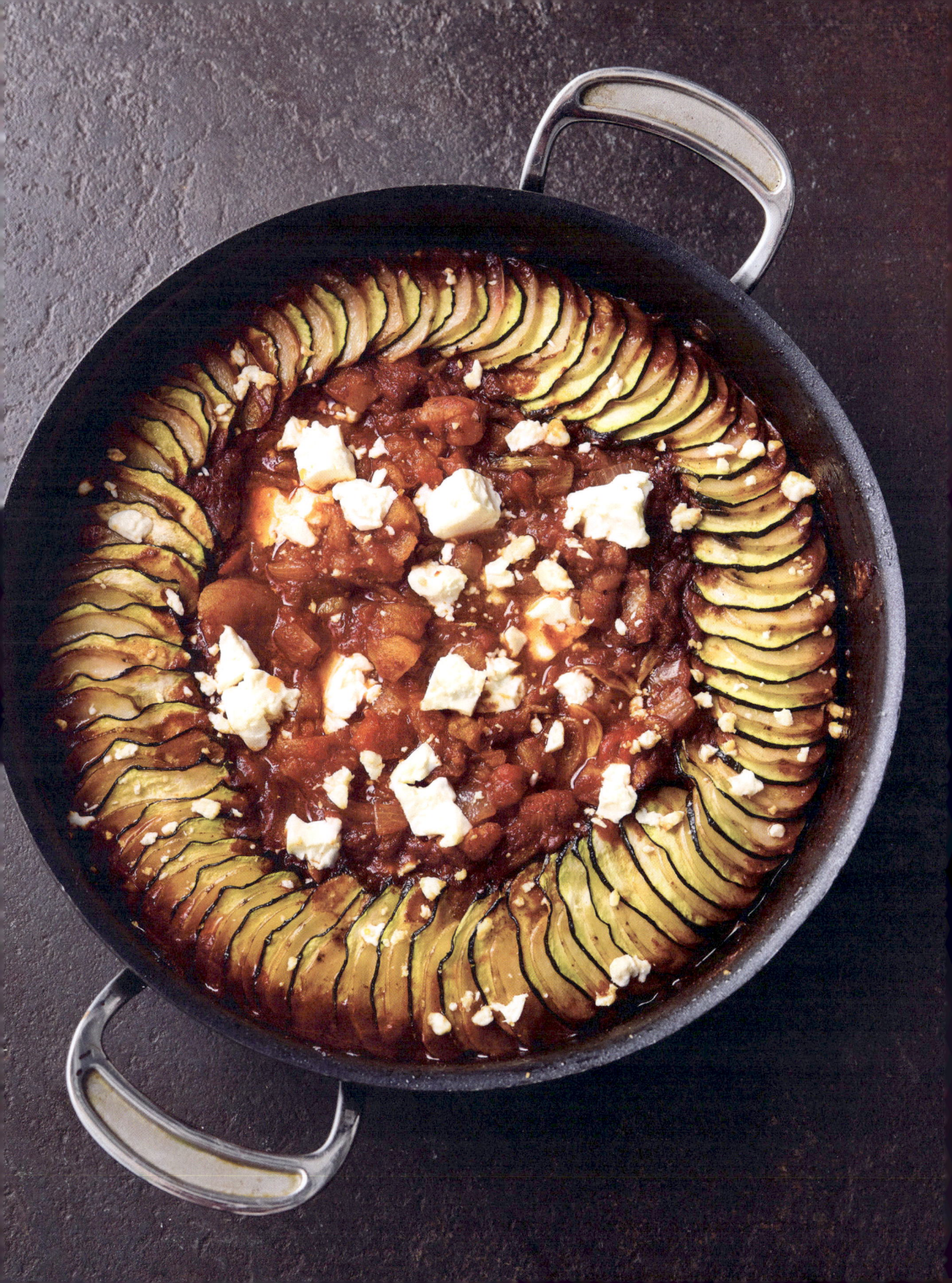

Chipotle chicken & bean soup

With a wonderfully warming level of spice, this hearty veg-packed soup is really almost a stew

SERVES 4
PREP 20 MINUTES
COOK 1 HOUR

4 large chicken thighs, skin on, bone in

320g button mushrooms

2 red onions (320g)

4 carrots (320g)

320g celery

4 teaspoons chipotle chilli paste

2 x 400g tins of butter beans

2 x 400g tins of plum tomatoes

1 small ripe avocado (160g)

1 lime

1 Put a large shallow non-stick casserole pan on a medium-high heat. Pull the skin off the chicken thighs and place it in the pan to render. Once crispy, remove and reserve the skin, leaving the rendered fat in the pan.

2 Lightly season the thighs and place in the pan, turning with tongs until golden all over, while you trim the mushrooms, halving any larger ones, and peel and finely slice the onions, carrots and celery, reserving any nice yellow celery leaves. Remove the chicken to your board, stir the veg into the pan and cook for 10 minutes, stirring regularly.

3 Stir in the chilli paste, put the chicken back in, pour in the beans, juice and all, then add the tomatoes, breaking them up with your spoon, and 1 tin's worth of water. Cover and simmer for 45 minutes, stirring occasionally.

4 Pull out and shred the chicken, discarding the bones, stir it back through the soup and simmer to your desired consistency, then season to perfection.

5 Halve, destone, peel and dice the avo, dress with lime juice, sprinkle over the soup with any reserved celery leaves, and crunch over the chicken skin.

EMBELLISH IT

I like to slice up a couple of corn tortillas and drop them into the soup to heat through before serving for a soft, stodgy result, or you can air-fry, toast or roast them for more of a crunchy crouton vibe. Both ways are delicious.

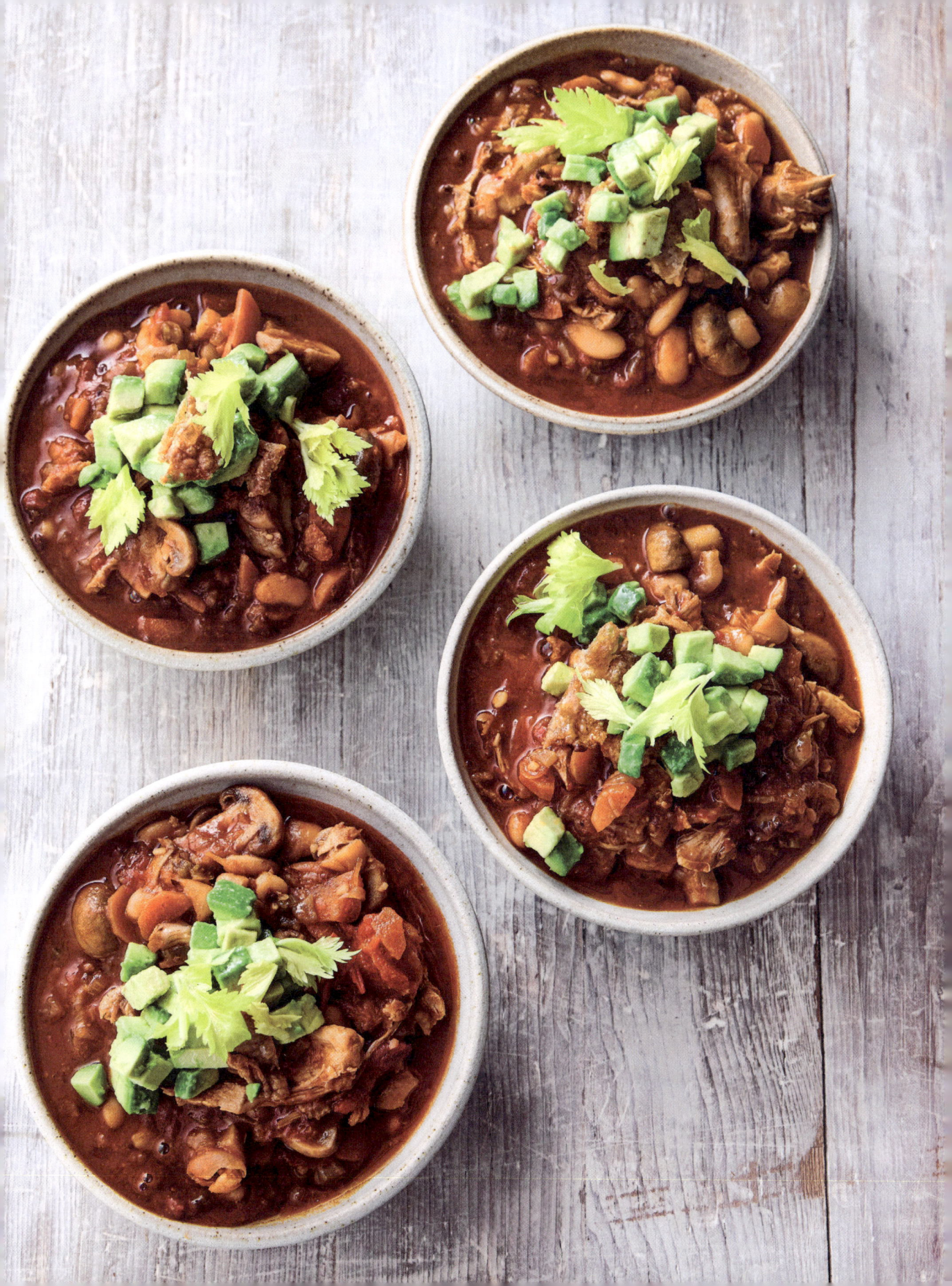

Roast chicken & sticky spuds

Perfect for sharing, this is an epic, fun and delicious roast chicken dish, but not as you know it . . .

SERVES 6
1 HOUR 40 MINUTES

6 onions

10 fresh bay leaves

1 bulb of garlic

1 x 1.5kg whole chicken

480g celeriac

100g natural yoghurt

2 heaped tablespoons wholegrain mustard

1 lemon

1.5kg new potatoes

480g seasonal greens, such as spinach, rainbow chard

1 Preheat the oven to 180°C. Peel and finely slice the onions, toss with 5 bay leaves, the garlic bulb, 2 tablespoons of red wine vinegar and a pinch of black pepper, and scatter into a deep roasting tray. Rub the chicken all over with 1 tablespoon of olive oil and a pinch of seasoning, then place directly on the bars of the oven with the onion tray beneath. Roast for 1 hour 20 minutes, or until golden and cooked through, stirring the onions halfway.

2 Tear the remaining bay leaves into a pestle and mortar, removing the tough stalks, pound with a pinch of salt until you have a paste, then muddle in 1 tablespoon of red wine vinegar and 2 tablespoons of extra virgin olive oil.

3 Peel and coarsely grate or very finely shred the celeriac. Place in a bowl with the yoghurt and mustard, finely grate over the lemon zest, squeeze in the juice, then toss and scrunch together well, and season to perfection.

4 Halving any larger ones, cook the potatoes in a large pan of boiling salted water for 20 minutes, or until tender. Place the greens in a colander, cover, steam above the potatoes until just wilted, then move to a serving bowl. Drain the potatoes and leave to steam dry.

5 Remove the chicken to a board to rest, and get the sticky onions out. Squeeze the soft garlic into the tray, discarding the skins. Break in the potatoes, and toss them through the onions and garlic. Serve with the chicken, slaw and steamed greens, which are delicious tossed in bay oil.

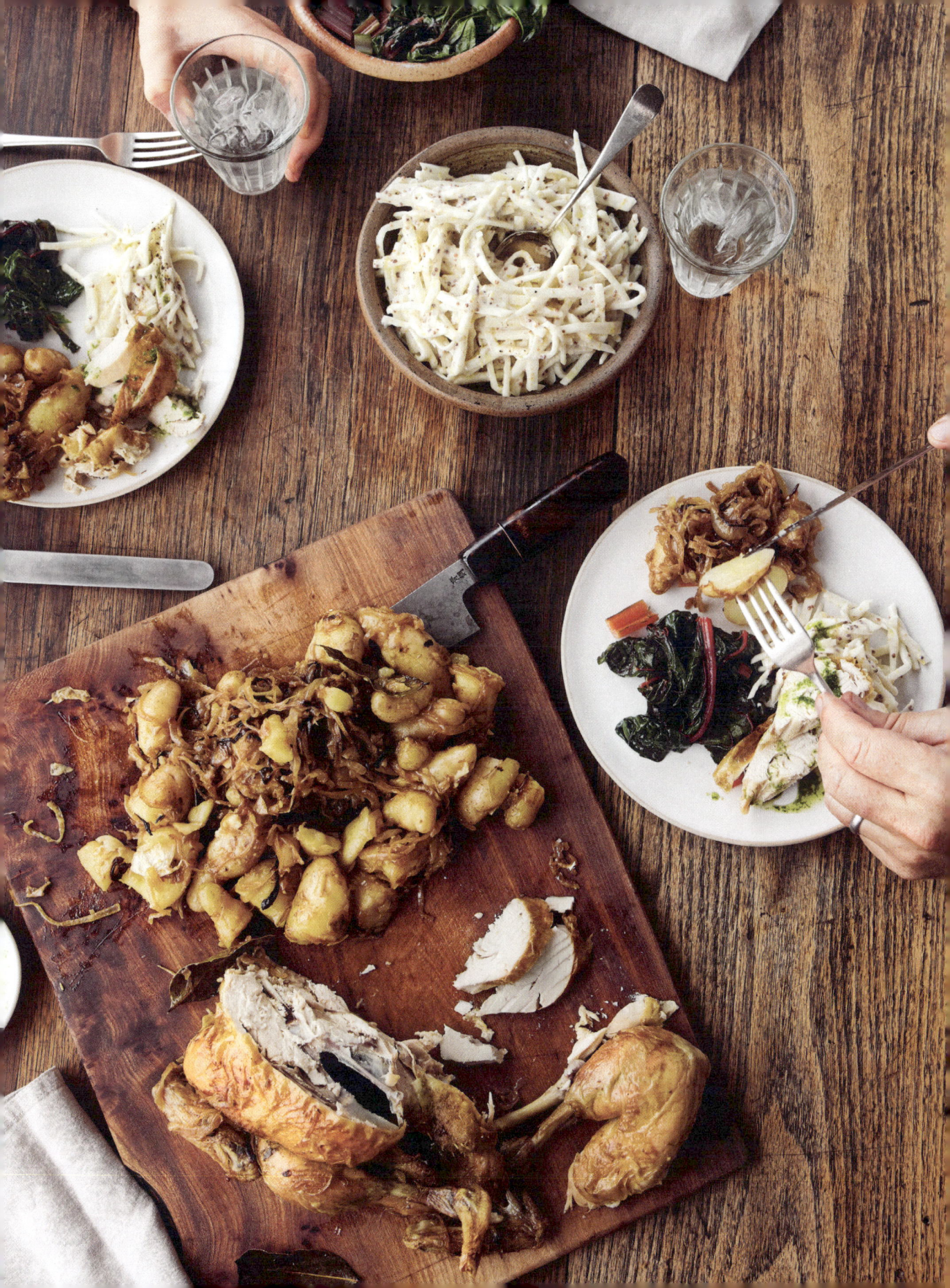

Beef & borlotti bean ragù

Totally scrumptious, think of this as a cousin of the much-loved Bolognese. Eat it, batch it, enjoy it!

SERVES 6
PREP 40 MINUTES
COOK 1 HOUR

500g beef mince

1 good pinch of ground cinnamon

3 red peppers (480g)

3 onions (480g)

3 large carrots (480g)

240g celery

6 cloves of garlic

2 x 400g tins of borlotti beans

1 x 400g tin of plum tomatoes

1 bunch of flat-leaf parsley (30g)

1. Put a large shallow casserole pan on a medium-high heat and go in with 2 tablespoons of olive oil, the mince, cinnamon and a very generous pinch of black pepper. Stir regularly while you deseed and finely chop the peppers, and peel and finely chop the onions, carrots, celery and garlic, adding them to the pan as you go. Cook until softened and golden, stirring regularly.

2. Add 2 tablespoons of red wine vinegar and let it cook away, then pour in the beans, juice and all. Tip in the tomatoes, breaking them up with your spoon, and 1 tin's worth of water, then a good pinch of sea salt. Cover, bring to the boil, then reduce to a simmer for 1 hour, stirring occasionally and uncovering for the last 10 minutes.

3. Use a potato masher to mash up half the ragù, stirring it back through for a better texture, then loosen with a little water, if needed. Taste, then season to perfection with salt, pepper, and a little more red wine vinegar, if you like.

4. Finely chop the parsley, stalks and all, and stir through the ragù. Now, you can serve it as is, with pasta or rice, hunks of bread, or in a jacket potato, or you can turn it into an oven bake, whether straight away or by stashing it in the fridge (up to 3 days), or the freezer (up to 3 months), for a future meal.

VEGGIE LOVE

Simply swap in veggie mince in place of the beef, and cook on a medium heat in step 1.

TURN THE PAGE FOR INSPO!

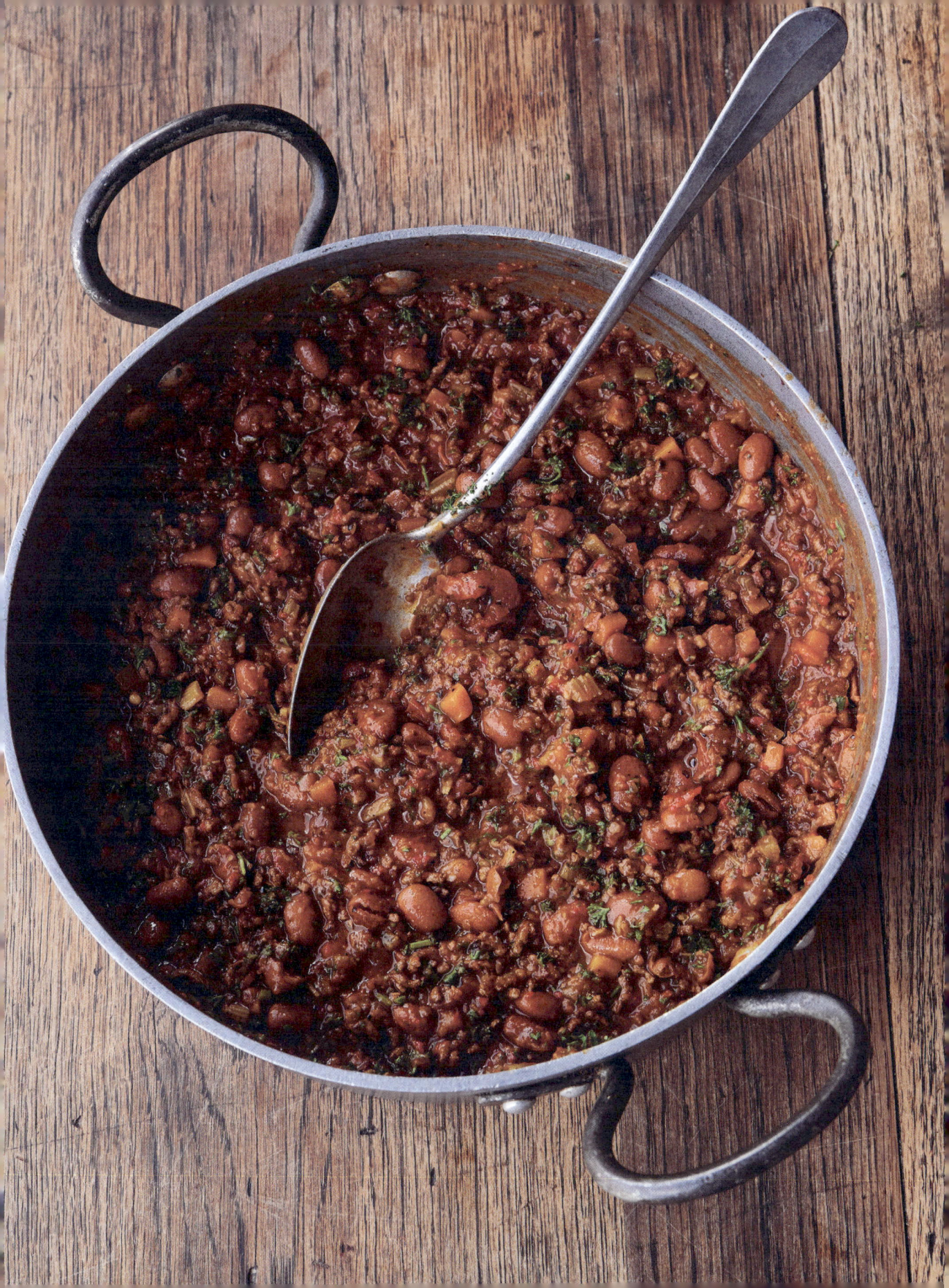

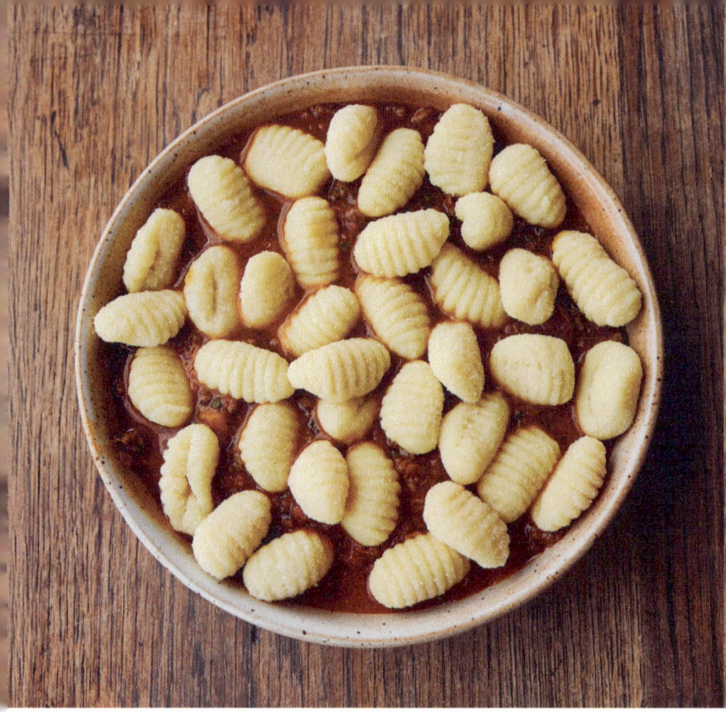

Potato gnocchi

Simply scatter **200g of potato gnocchi** per person over the top, spritz with olive oil, and bake or air-fry at 180°C until piping hot, golden and bubbling.

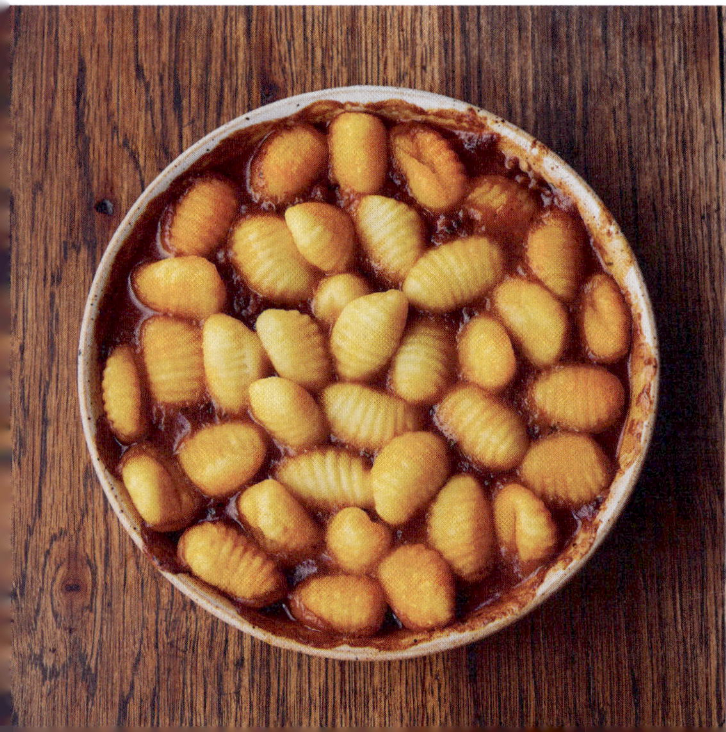

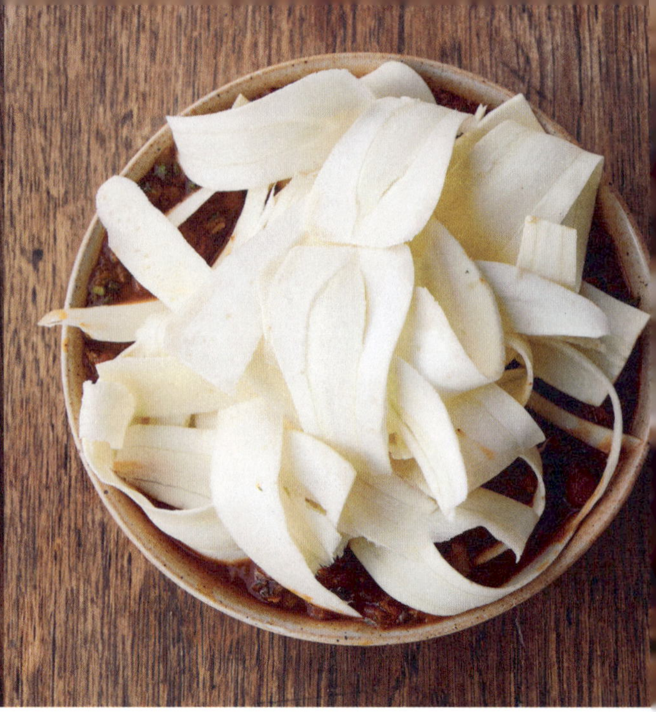

Parsnip ribbons

Speed-peel **parsnips** into ribbons, pile on top of the ragù, spritz with olive oil, season, and bake or air-fry at 180°C until piping hot, golden and bubbling.

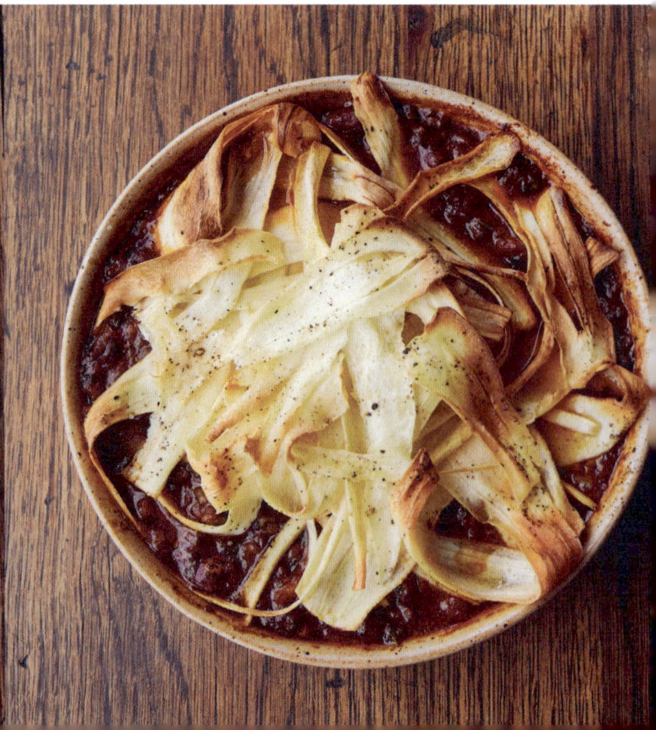

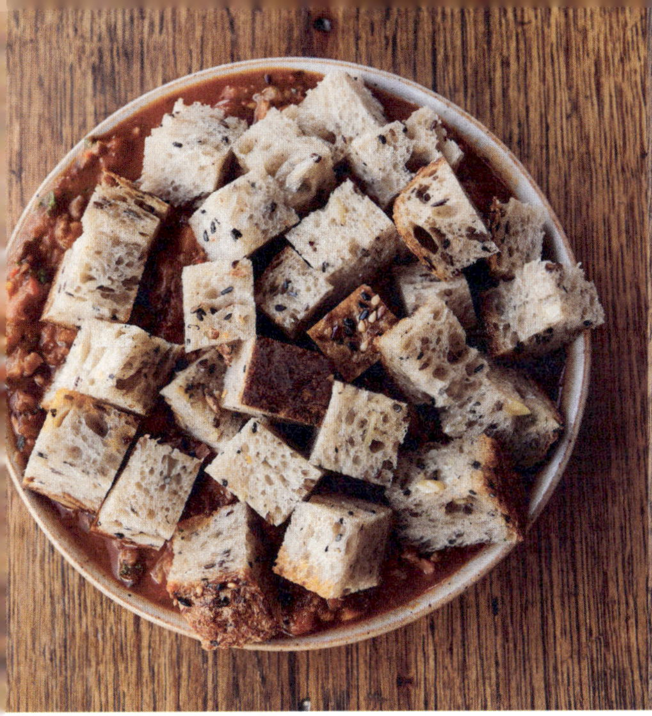

Bread croutons

Slice **seeded sourdough** into chunks, pile on to the ragù, spritz with olive oil, and bake or air-fry at 180°C until piping hot, golden and bubbling.

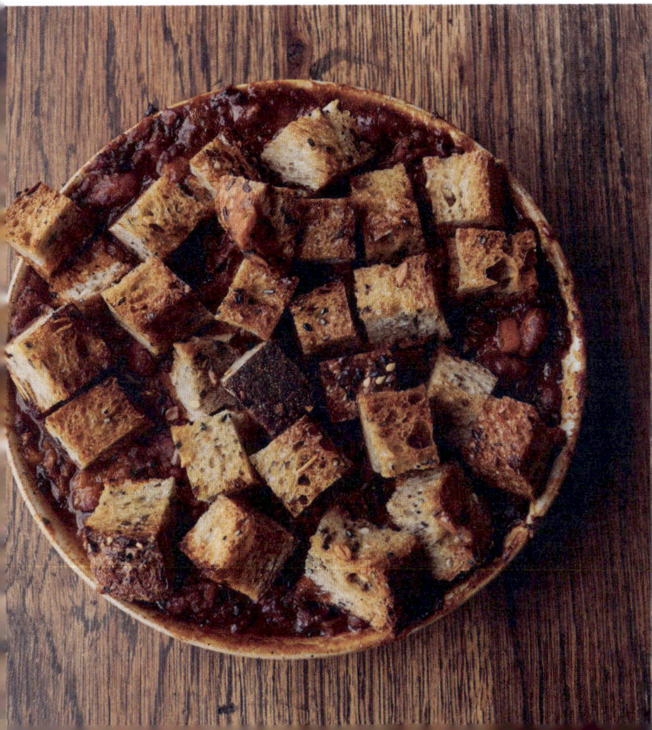

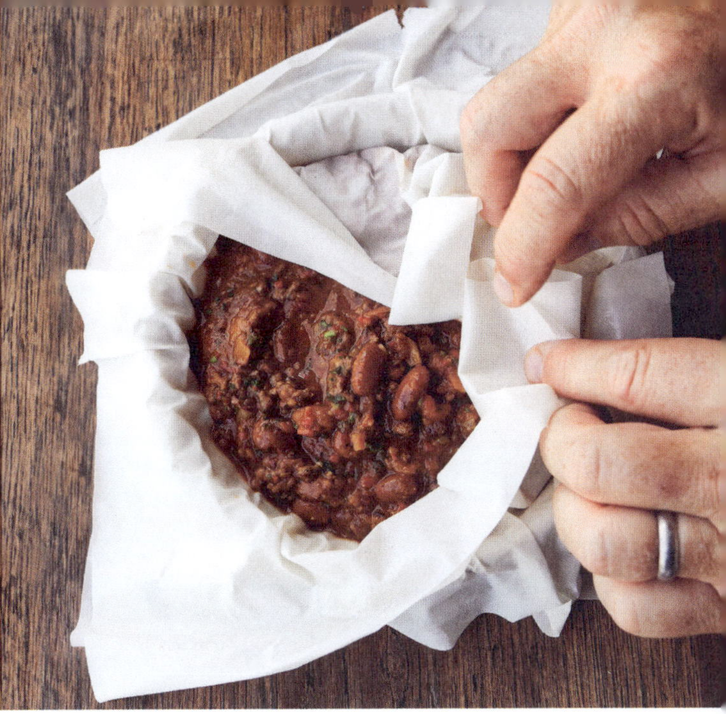

Flaky filo

Line a baking dish with **filo**, add the ragù, then fold in the filo, spritz with olive oil, and bake or air-fry at 180°C until piping hot, golden and bubbling.

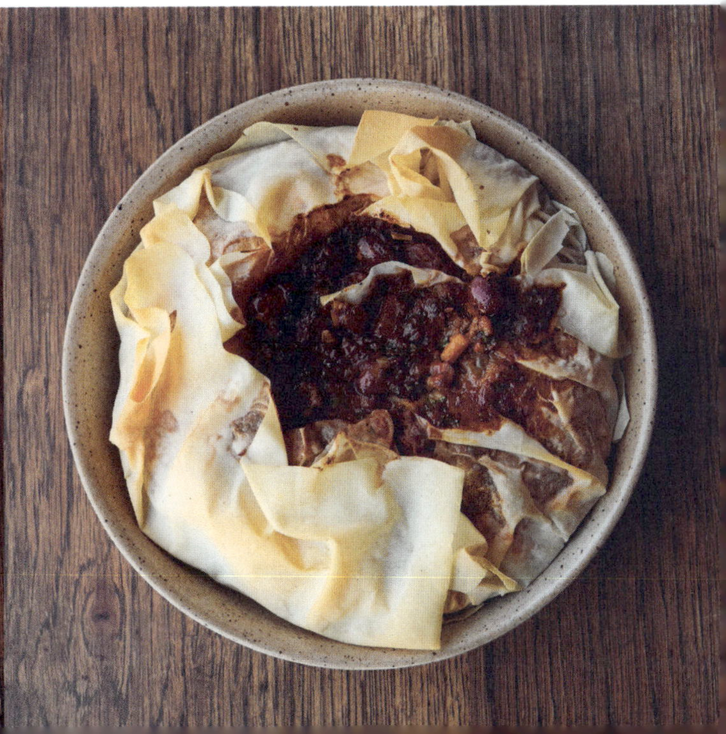

Healthier sweet treats

Cheat's soft-service ice cream

A fun, healthier expression of ice cream, this is both refreshing and delicious

SERVES 1
5 MINUTES

50g ripe banana

80g frozen strawberries

1 heaped tablespoon Greek yoghurt

1 heaped teaspoon tahini or peanut butter

1 teaspoon runny honey

1. Ahead of time, peel, slice and freeze the banana.

2. Once frozen, put the banana into a food processor with the frozen strawberries, yoghurt, tahini or peanut butter and honey. Blitz until smooth.

3. Decant into a chilled bowl, finely grate over an extra frozen strawberry for a fancy finish, if you like, and eat right away.

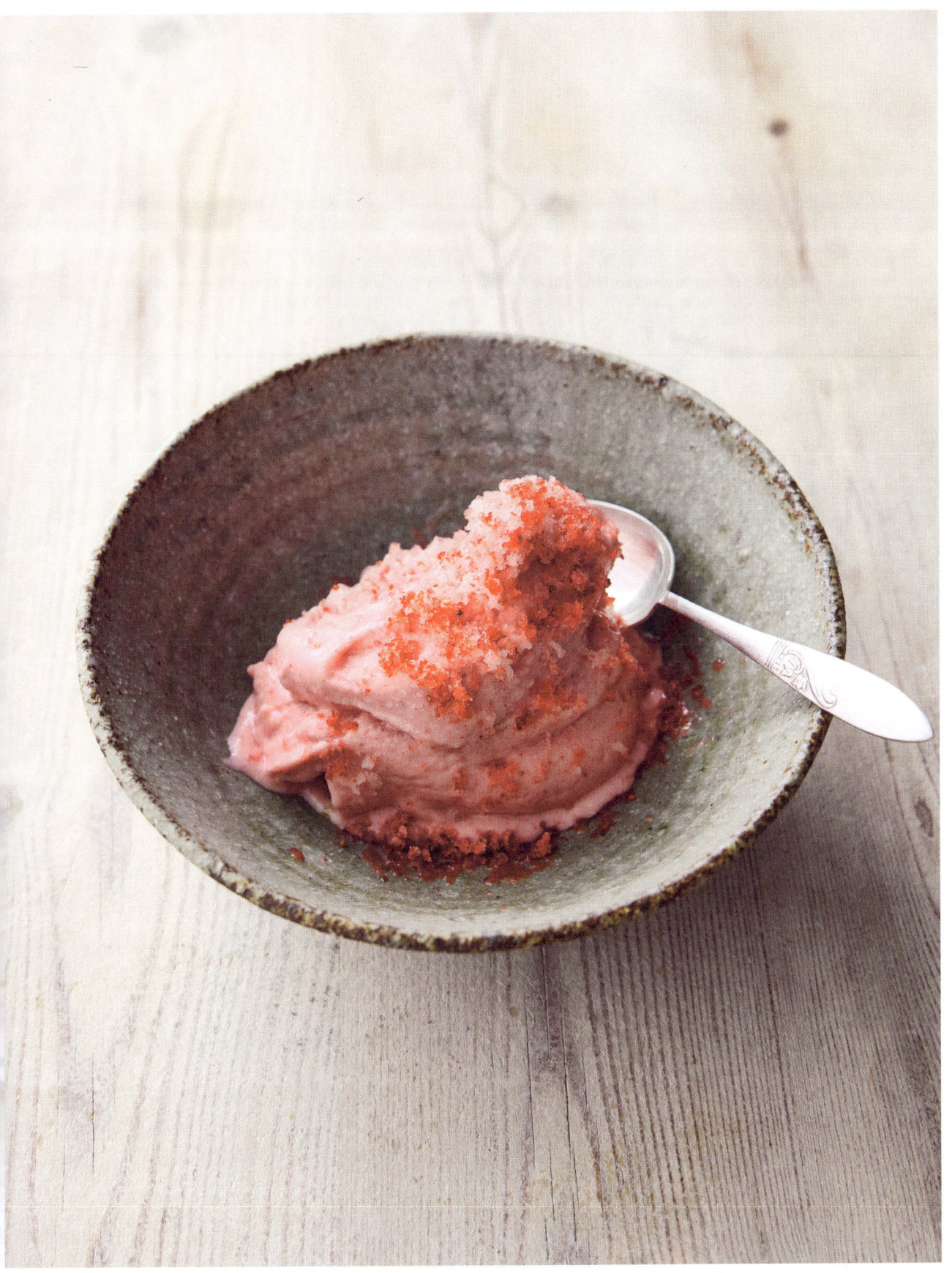

Blackberry smoothie lollies

Smoothies are a big hit in the Oliver household and we love making them into lollies

MAKES 6
8 MINUTES
PLUS FREEZING

1 ripe banana (160g)

150g fresh or frozen blackberries

150g Greek yoghurt

15g milled flaxseed

40g dark chocolate (70%)

optional:
   15g desiccated coconut

1 Peel the banana and place in a blender with the blackberries, yoghurt and flaxseed. Blitz until smooth, then divide between ice lolly moulds and poke in the lollipop sticks. Freeze for at least 6 hours.

2 Snap the chocolate into a heatproof bowl, then melt in the microwave or over a pan of gently simmering water, making sure the water doesn't touch the base of the bowl, stirring occasionally until smooth. Put the coconut into a bowl, if using.

3 Remove the lollies from their moulds and quickly dunk the end of each one into the chocolate, then the coconut, if using. The chocolate should set quickly, so tuck in if you want to, or pop the lollies on a greaseproof-paper-lined tray and return to the freezer for when the mood takes you.

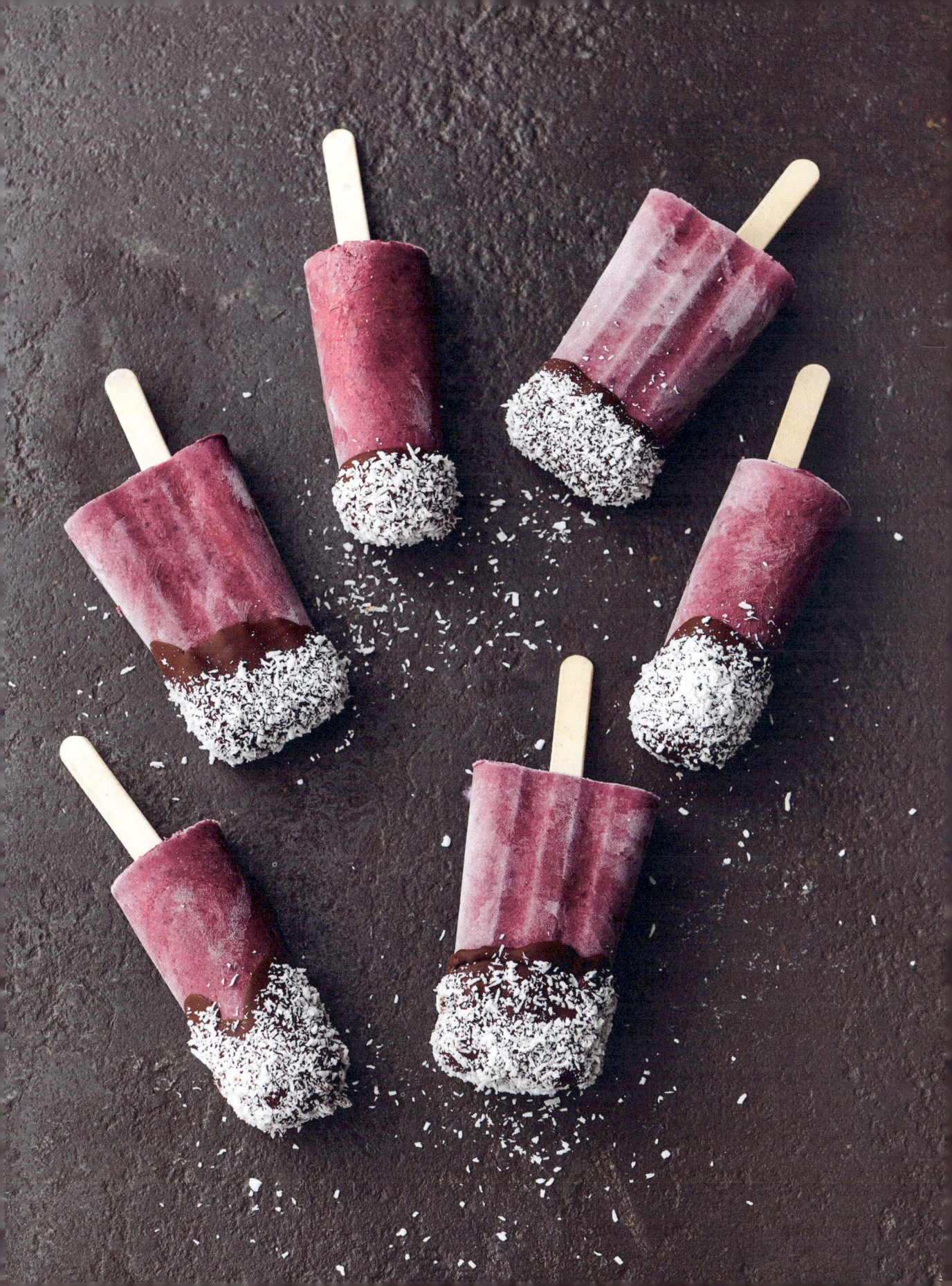

Hot carrot cup cakes

I've reimagined the nostalgic flavours of carrot cake in these tasty and quick microwave cups

SERVES 4
11 MINUTES

100g carrot

1 small ripe banana (80g)

30g dried apricots

1 ball of stem ginger in syrup

30g walnut halves

100g wholemeal self-raising flour

1 teaspoon mixed spice

1 medium egg

80g Greek yoghurt, plus extra to serve

4 oranges

1 Grease four heatproof teacups or shallow mugs with a little olive oil.

2 Wash the carrot and snap into a food processor. Add the peeled banana, apricots, ginger, walnuts, flour, spice, egg and yoghurt. Finely grate in the zest and squeeze in the juice from 1 orange, and pulse until just combined.

3 Divide the mixture between the cups and microwave for 3 minutes on high (800W). Meanwhile, peel and segment or slice the remaining oranges.

4 Leave the cakes to stand for 1 minute, drizzle over a little stem ginger syrup, then turn out and serve with the orange segments, a dollop of yoghurt and an extra drizzle of stem ginger syrup, if you like. Enjoy!

KITCHEN KIT

If you don't have a food processor, finely grate the carrot and zest of 1 orange, mash the banana, and finely chop the apricots, grapes and walnuts, before mixing with the rest of the cake ingredients.

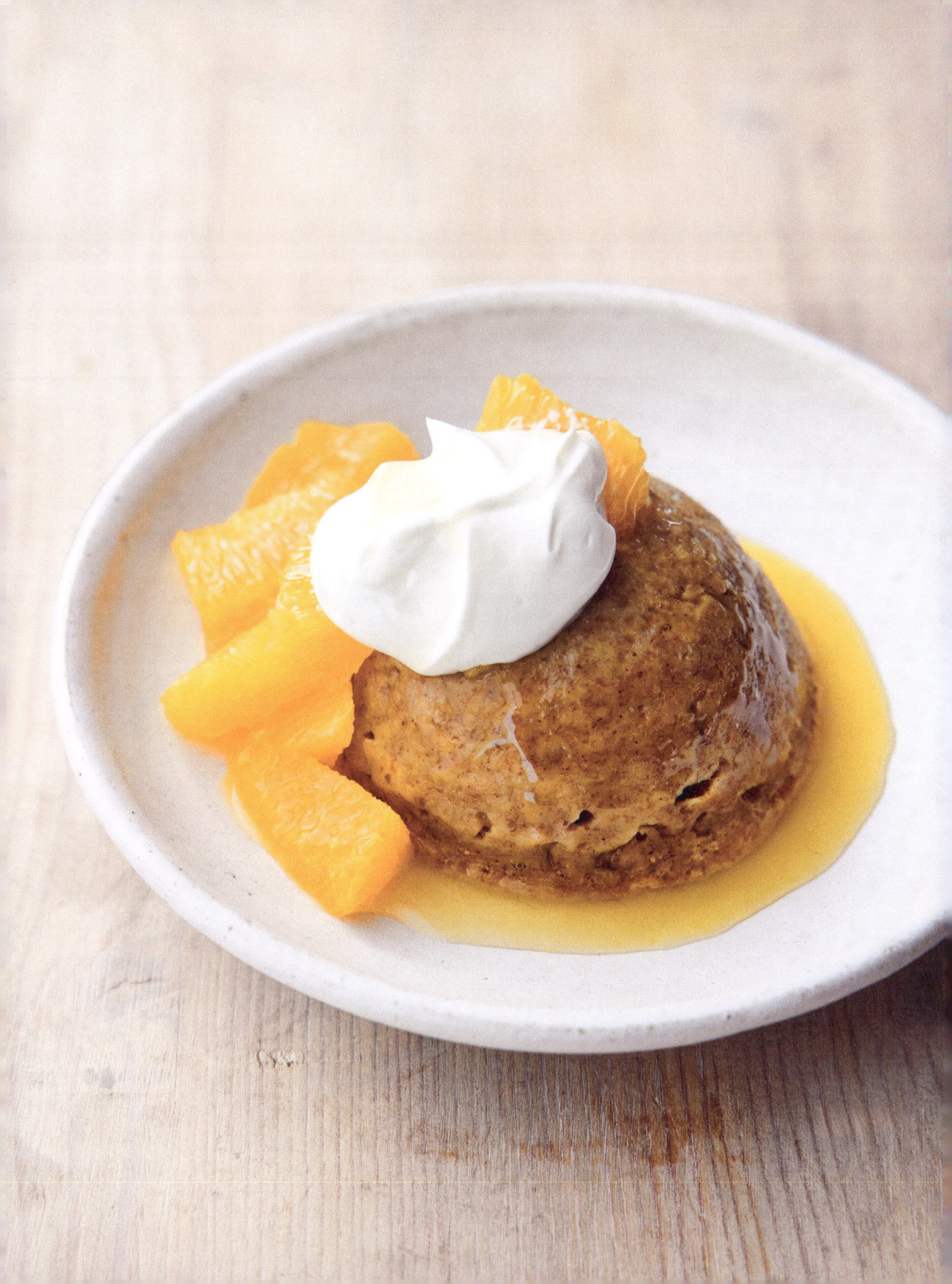

Chocolate orange pots

When only chocolate will do, these pots are sweet, tangy, comforting, silky and utterly delicious

MAKES 6
12 MINUTES

200g pitted Medjool dates

20g blanched hazelnuts

300g silken tofu

4 tablespoons cocoa powder

1 orange

6 heaped tablespoons Greek or plant-based yoghurt

seasonal fruit, such as oranges, cherries, strawberries, raspberries, to serve

1 In a bowl, just cover the dates with boiling kettle water and leave to soak for 5 minutes, then drain. Toast the hazelnuts in a small frying pan until lightly golden, shaking regularly, then crush in a pestle and mortar until fine.

2 Put the dates in a blender with the tofu and cocoa. Finely grate in the orange zest, squeeze in the juice, add 1 ice cube, if you have it, and blitz until super-smooth, stopping to scrape down the sides with a spatula a few times.

3 Decant the mixture between little pots, glasses or cups, and either eat right away, or cover and stash in the fridge until you want them (up to 3 days). Serve each pot with a spoonful of yoghurt, a sprinkling of crushed hazelnuts and some extra fruit, of your choice.

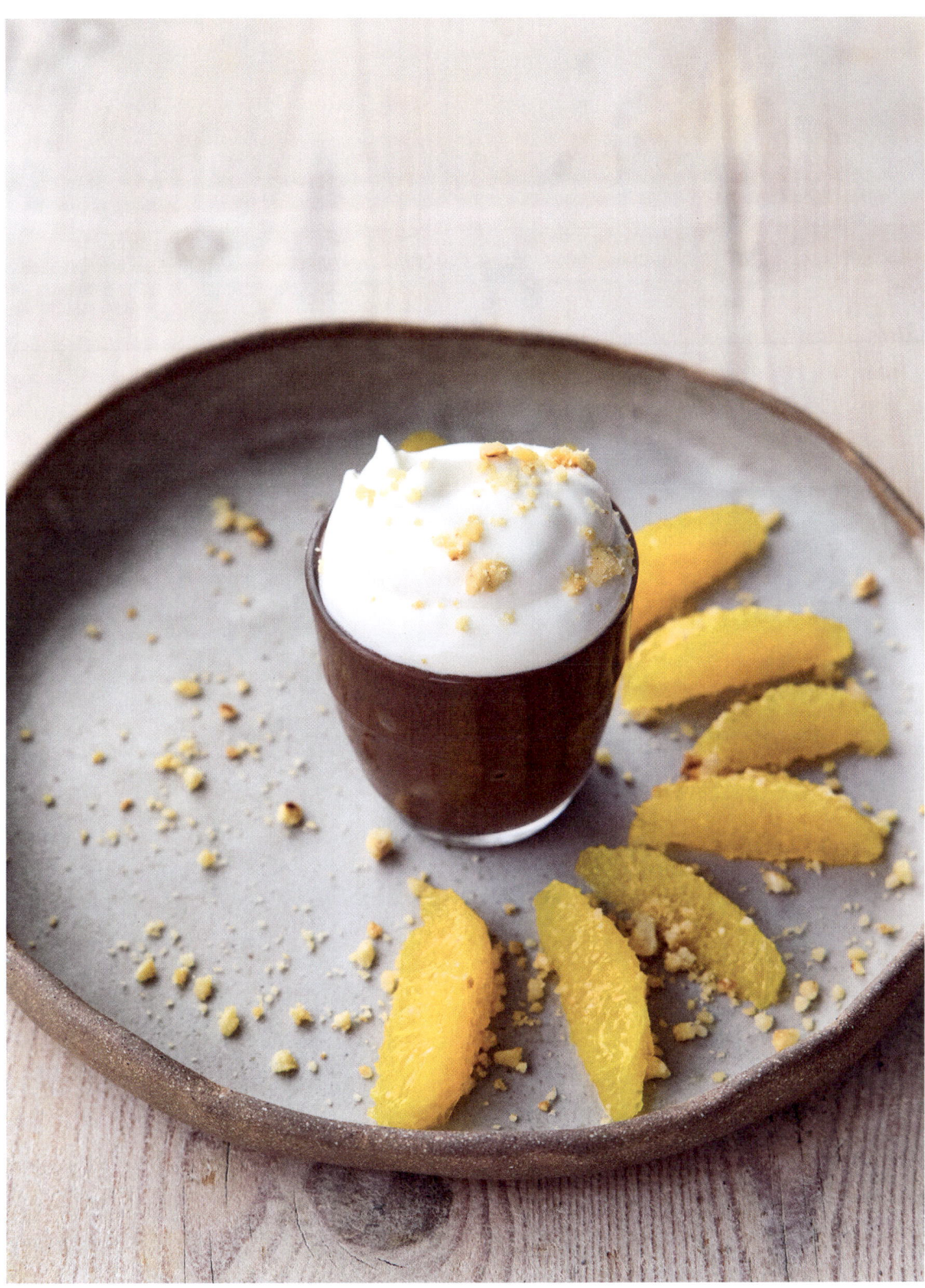

Tahini pretzel yoghurt bark

Using yoghurt as a base for delicious delights is a great way to stretch a sweet treat further

MAKES 10 PORTIONS
12 MINUTES
PLUS FREEZING

50g dark chocolate (70%)

1 teaspoon vanilla bean paste

2 tablespoons runny honey

250g natural yoghurt

2 tablespoons tahini

100g pitted Medjool dates

25g pretzels

1 Line a 25cm x 40cm baking tray with a sheet of greaseproof paper. Snap the chocolate into a heatproof bowl, then melt in the microwave or over a pan of gently simmering water, making sure the water doesn't touch the base of the bowl, stirring occasionally until smooth.

2 Mix the vanilla paste and honey into the yoghurt, then spread it across the lined tray and evenly ripple through the tahini. Finely chop and scatter over the dates, crumble over the pretzels, then erratically drizzle over the melted chocolate to finish. Freeze for at least 2 hours, or until solid.

3 Once frozen, snap into portions and stash in an airtight container, where it will keep happily in the freezer for up to 3 months – if it lasts that long!

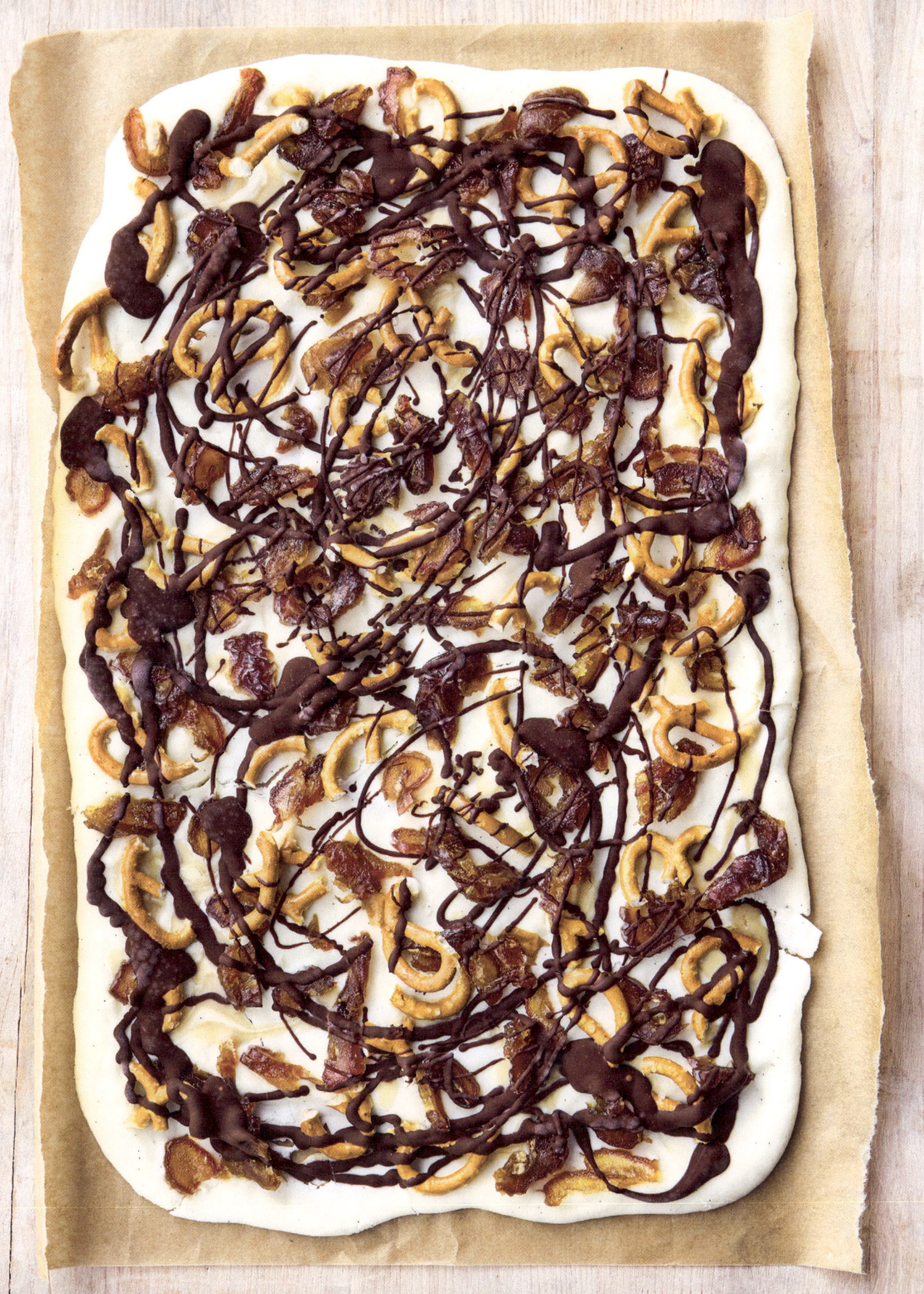

Fizzy berry jellies

Perfect jelly melting on your tongue with the bonus of bubbles that pop as you tuck in

MAKES 6
12 MINUTES
PLUS CHILLING

400ml soda water

500g mixed berries, such as strawberries, blueberries, raspberries

4 leaves of gelatine

4 sprigs of mint

4 tablespoons elderflower cordial

2 ice cubes

18 sponge fingers

3 oranges

6 tablespoons Greek yoghurt

dark chocolate (70%), to serve

1 Pop six cups or glasses (about 200ml each) into the freezer to get super-cold, and chill the soda water and berries in the fridge.

2 In a jug, cover the gelatine with cold water and leave for just 5 minutes, while you hull any strawberries, halving or quartering any large ones. Pick the mint leaves, slicing the bigger leaves, and arrange in the cups or glasses with the rest of the berries.

3 Briefly heat the cordial with 50ml of water in a small pan until it just starts to bubble, then turn the heat off. Remove the gelatine leaves from the jug and whisk into the pan until melted, then chuck in the ice cubes to start to cool the mixture. Pour in the cold soda water, then divide it all between the cups or glasses, gently pressing down to submerge the fruit. Chill in the fridge for at least 6 hours, or until set, hopefully with bubbles suspended.

4 To serve, arrange 3 sponge fingers on each of your serving plates. Zest over the oranges, then squeeze the juice over the sponge fingers, to soften. Carefully dip each jelly mould into a bowl of boiling kettle water for long enough to loosen the jelly, then turn out on to the sponge fingers. Top with yoghurt and scrape or grate over some chocolate, to finish.

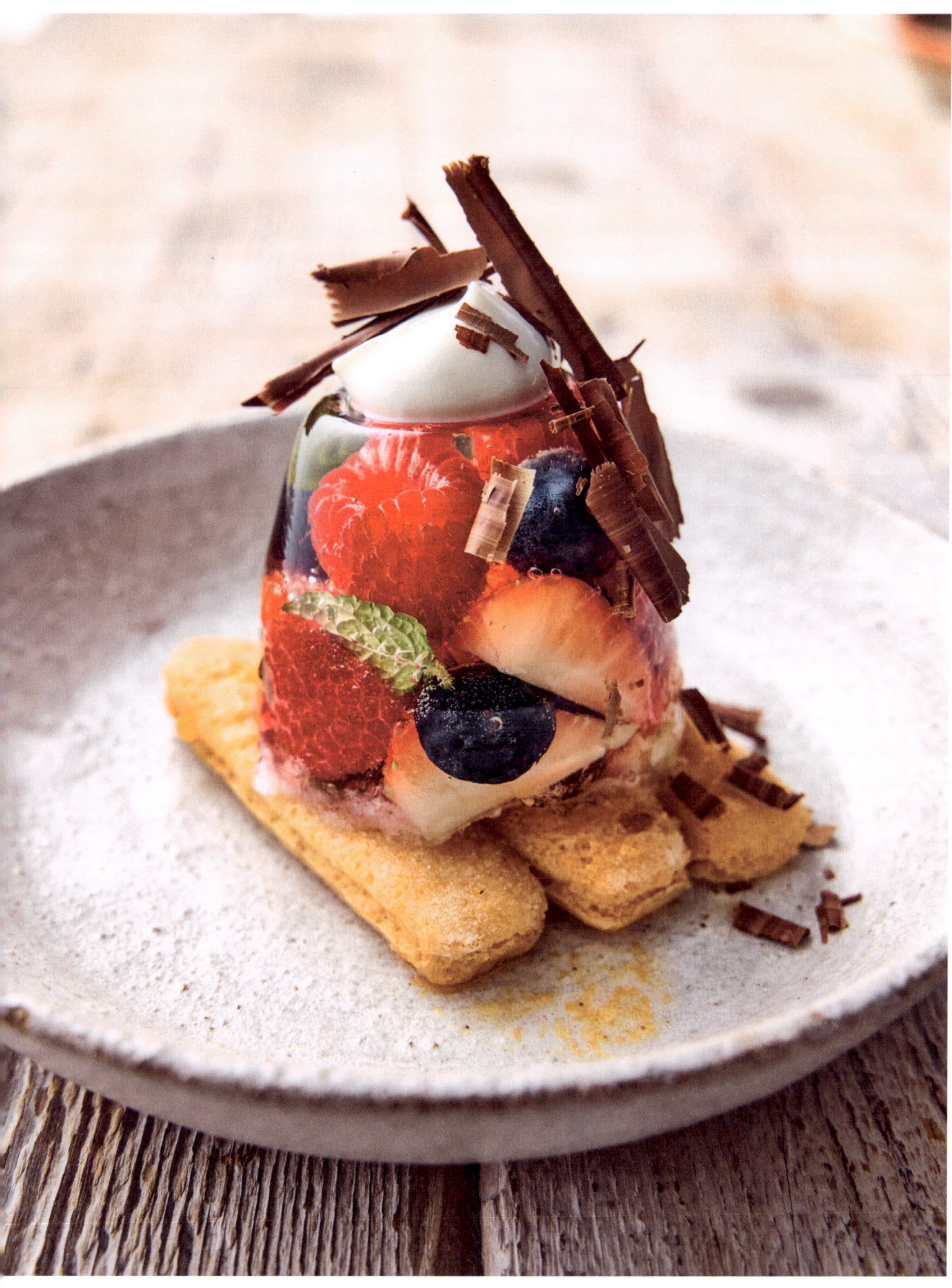

Choccy fro-yo sandwiches

A perfect balance of tang, warmth and comfort, these beauties are a well-worth-it freezer stash

MAKES 16
13 MINUTES
PLUS FREEZING

250g Greek yoghurt

300g fresh or frozen raspberries

4 balls of stem ginger in syrup

20 oatcakes

75g dark chocolate (70%)

1 To make the fro-yo, in a blender, blitz the yoghurt, raspberries, stem ginger balls and 1 tablespoon of their syrup together until smooth.

2 Line a 20cm x 25cm tray with greaseproof paper and arrange 10 oatcakes across the base, snapping to fit, where needed. Pour the fro-yo mixture on top, spreading it out with a spatula to fill the tray. Gently arrange the remaining oatcakes on top, then freeze for at least 3 hours.

3 Snap the chocolate into a heatproof bowl, then melt in the microwave or over a pan of gently simmering water, making sure the water doesn't touch the base of the bowl, stirring occasionally until smooth. Remove the tray from the freezer, erratically drizzle over the chocolate, freeze for a few minutes until set, then use the paper to help you lift the whole thing on to a board and slice into 16 portions. Eat what you will, freezer-stashing the rest.

EASY SWAPS

Swap in any berries you like here for equally delicious results.

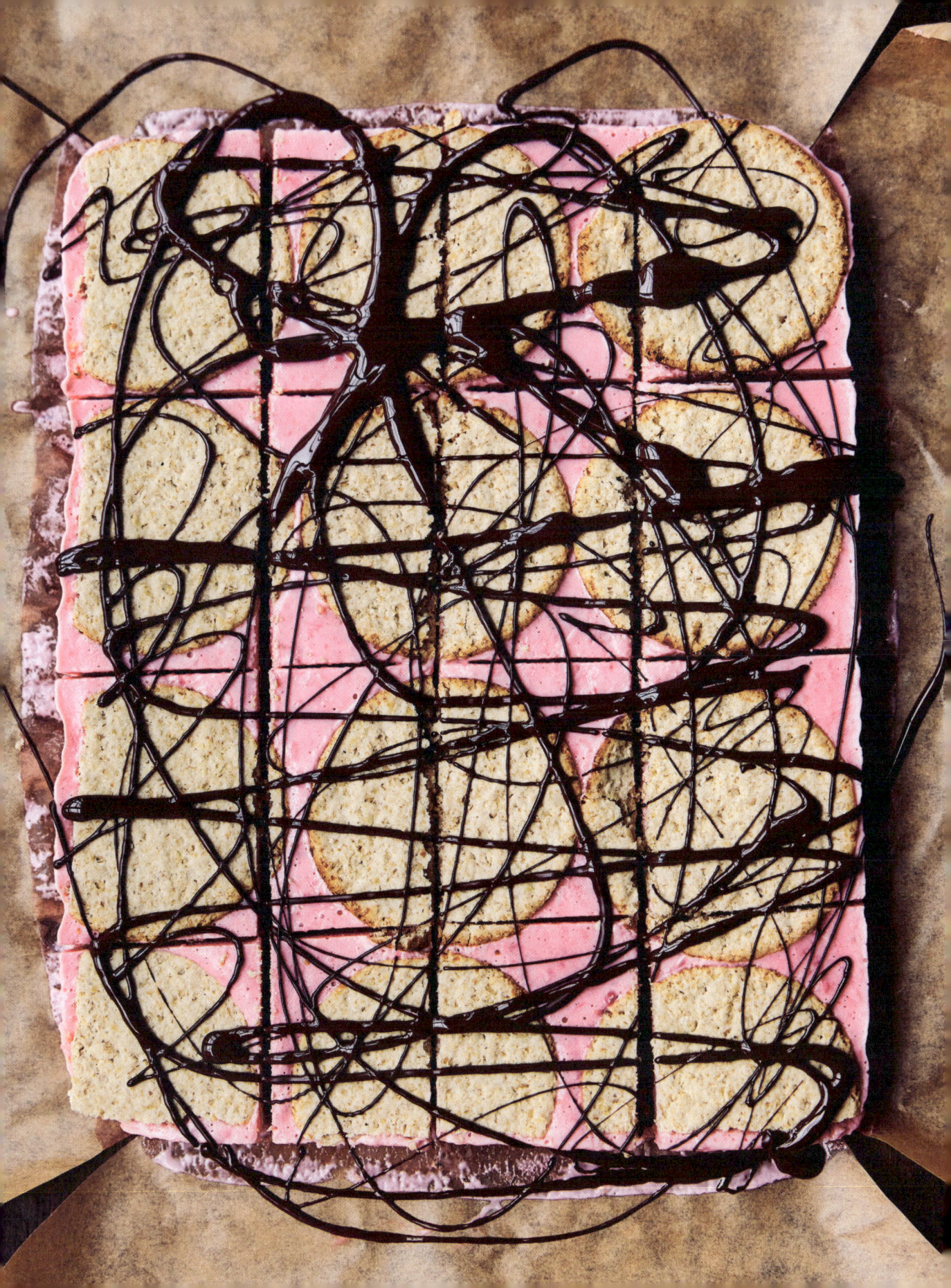

Oaty fridge balls: 2 tasty ways

Having delicious bites like this in stock is a brilliant strategy for keeping healthy eating on track

EACH COMBO MAKES 20 | 13 MINUTES

Almond, apricot & choc

100g dark chocolate (70%)

100g dried apricots

100g toasted flaked almonds

100g porridge oats

100g soft pitted dates

1 tablespoon cocoa powder, for dusting

Snap the chocolate into a food processor, then blitz with everything but the cocoa powder until fine and starting to come together. Divide into 20 and, with clean wet hands, roll into balls. Put the cocoa and balls into a shallow bowl, and gently shake until well coated.

Mango, coconut & vanilla

100g dried mango

100g desiccated coconut, plus extra for dusting

100g porridge oats

100g soft pitted dates

1 tablespoon vanilla bean paste

In a food processor, blitz everything with 1 tablespoon of water until fine and starting to come together. Divide into 20 and, with clean wet hands, roll into balls. Put some extra coconut into a shallow bowl, add the balls and gently shake until well coated.

ALL BALLS

Pop the balls into the fridge or freezer, ready to enjoy as and when you want one! They'll last for up to 1 week in the fridge and 3 months in the freezer.

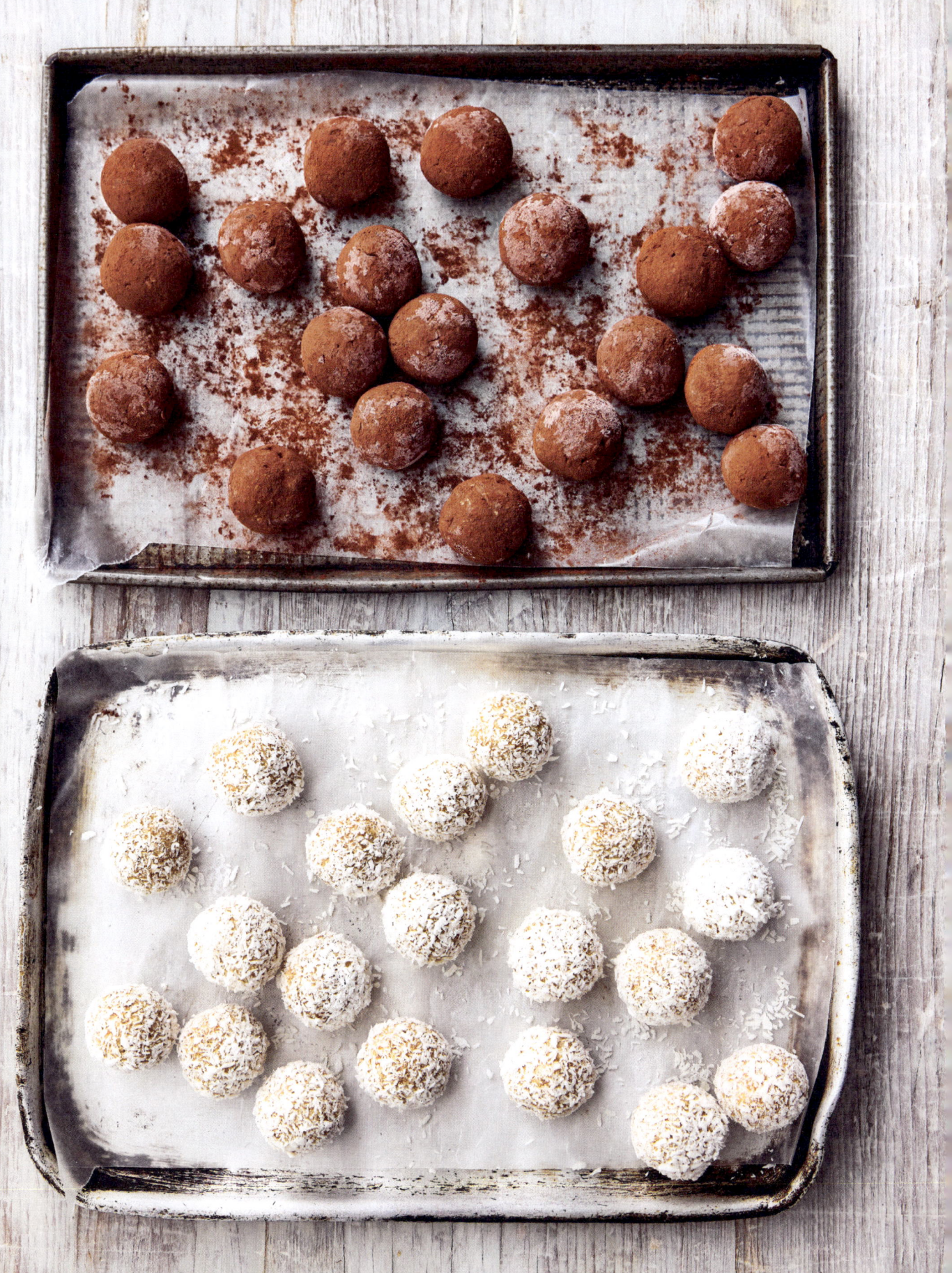

Strawberry filo tarts

Colourfully optimistic, these sweet strawberry tarts are a fun, beautiful pud to share

SERVES 4
22 MINUTES

50g shelled unsalted pistachio nuts

8 sheets of filo pastry

1 orange

ground cinnamon

400g ripe strawberries

1 tablespoon thick balsamic vinegar

1 bay leaf

4 tablespoons natural yoghurt

1 sprig of mint

1 Preheat the oven to 200°C. Lightly crush the pistachios in a pestle and mortar. Spritz one sheet of filo with olive oil. Scatter over some of the pistachios, finely grate over a quarter of the orange zest, add a pinch of cinnamon and a little sprinkle of black pepper (trust me!). Lay over a second sheet of filo, then scruch them up lengthways, concertina style, shape into a loose round, and place on an oil-spritzed baking tray. Repeat with the remaining sheets of filo, then bake for 10 minutes, or until golden and crisp.

2 Meanwhile, hull and quarter the strawberries. Reserving a couple, place in a frying pan on a medium-high heat. Squeeze over the orange juice, add the balsamic, bay and a small pinch of cinnamon, grate in the reserved strawberries, then simmer for 5 minutes, or until thickened.

3 Plate up the filo, divide up the yoghurt, spoon over the syrupy strawberries, sprinkle over the remaining crushed pistachios and pick over the mint.

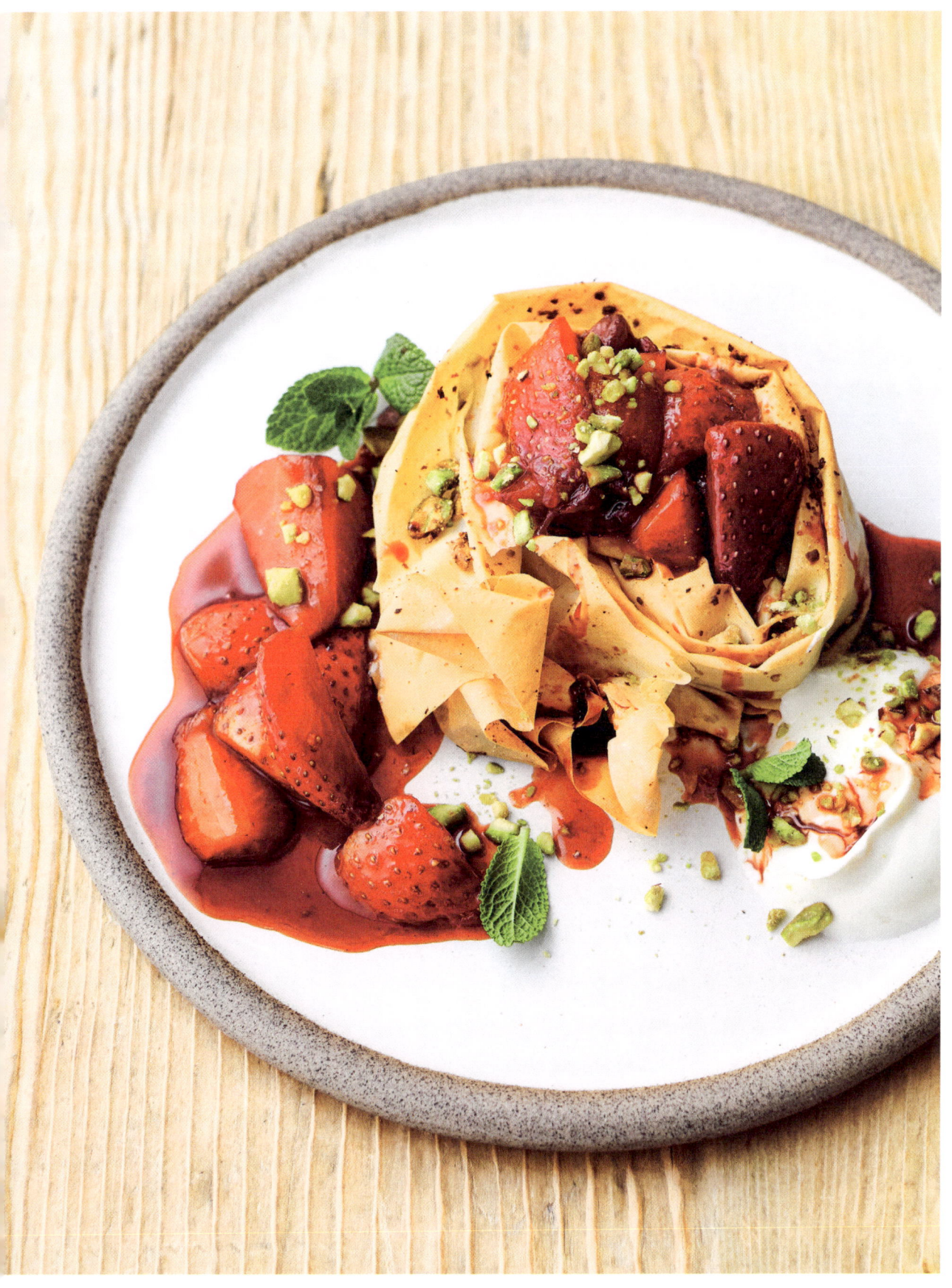

Blueberry muffins

Everyone needs a delicious, fun and happily nutritious blueberry muffin recipe in their lives

MAKES 8
PREP 8 MINUTES
COOK 20 MINUTES

1 ripe banana (160g)

150g self-raising flour

1 teaspoon baking powder

150g natural yoghurt

2 large eggs

2 tablespoons runny honey, plus extra to serve

1 teaspoon vanilla bean paste

50g porridge oats, plus extra for sprinkling

150g blueberries

1 Preheat the oven to 180°C and line a muffin tin with 8 muffin cases.

2 In a food processor, blitz the peeled banana, flour, baking powder, yoghurt, eggs, honey, vanilla, 4 tablespoons of olive oil and a small pinch of sea salt.

3 Fold through the oats and most of the blueberries, then divide between the muffin cases. Poke the remaining berries into the tops, along with an extra sprinkling of oats, and spritz with a little olive oil. Bake for 20 minutes, or until golden and an inserted skewer comes out clean. Cool on a wire rack.

EASY SWAPS

Swap in raspberries or blackberries for equally delicious results.

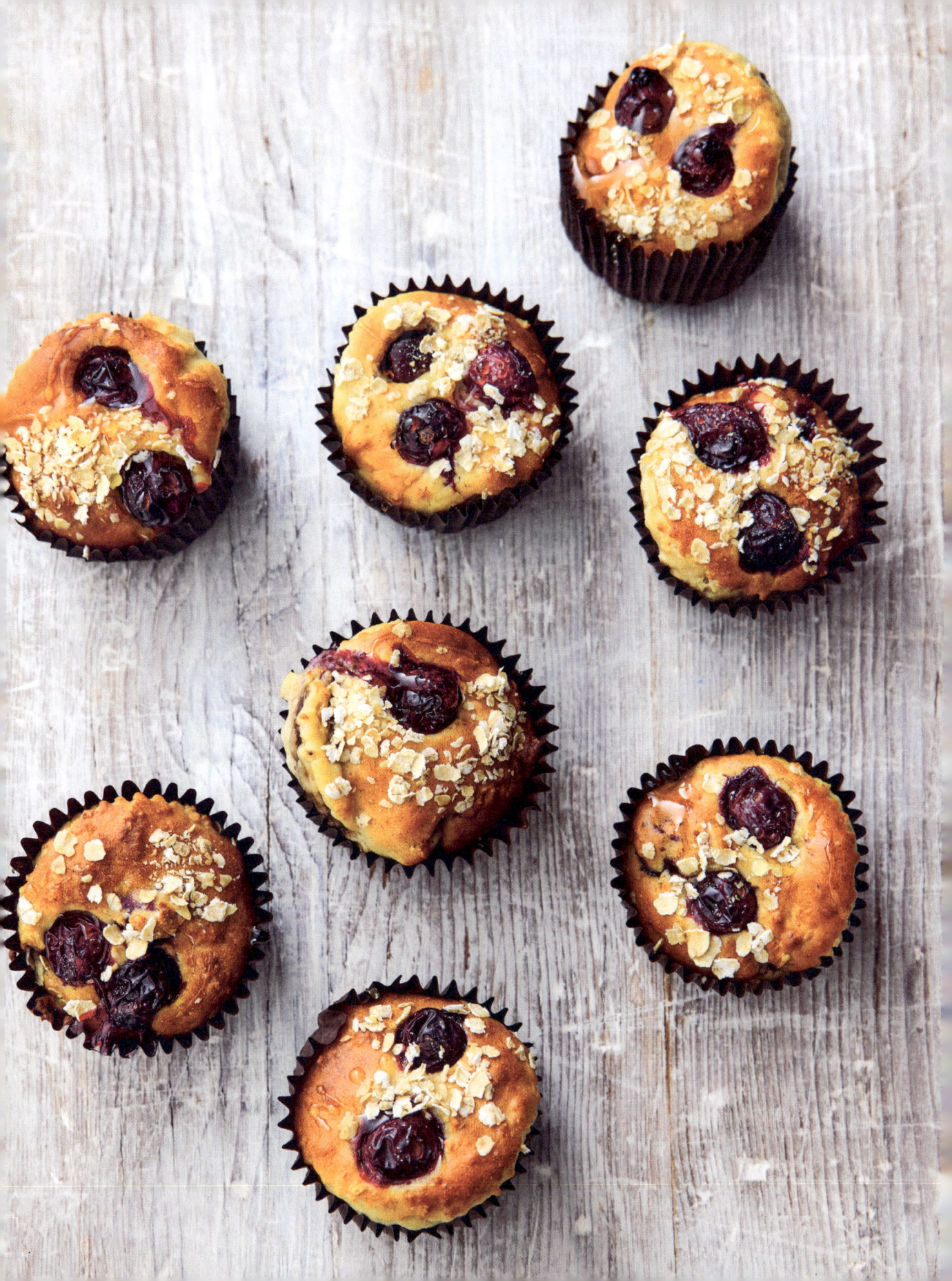

Mini protein bars

If you're protein-bar obsessed, these homemade ones taste good and will save you a bit, too

MAKES 16
PREP 15 MINUTES
COOK 20 MINUTES

2 peeled ripe bananas (320g)

250g porridge oats

150g crunchy peanut butter

3 tablespoons maple syrup

50g chia seeds

1 pinch of ground cinnamon

50g soft pitted dates

50g dark chocolate (70%)

1 Preheat the oven to 180°C. Grease a small deep baking tray or square cake tin (20cm x 20cm) with a little olive oil and line with greaseproof paper.

2 In a bowl, peel and mash the bananas. Add the oats, peanut butter, maple syrup, chia and cinnamon. Finely chop and add the dates, then mix well.

3 Transfer to the lined tin, squash down into an even layer and lightly score into 16 equal-sized bars. Bake for 20 minutes, or until golden.

4 Snap the chocolate into a heatproof bowl, then melt in the microwave or over a pan of gently simmering water, making sure the water doesn't touch the base of the bowl, stirring occasionally until smooth, then drizzle over the bars. Leave to cool before slicing. Store in an airtight container for up to 1 week, or freeze for up to 3 months.

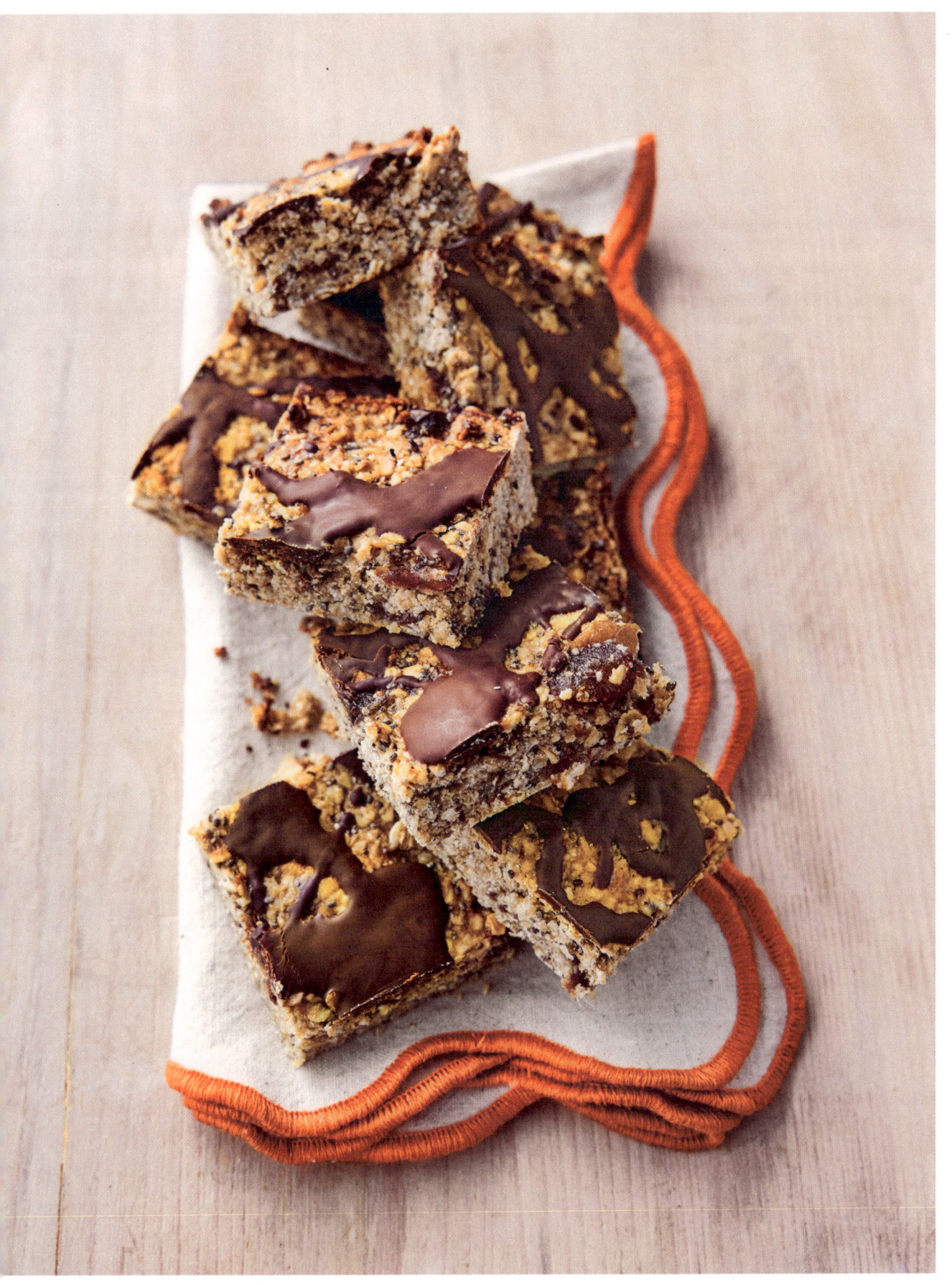

Banana & almond cake

Brilliant bananas and almonds take centre stage in this deliciously moreish chuck-it-all-in cake

SERVES 12
PREP 11 MINUTES
COOK 45 MINUTES

500g peeled ripe bananas

2 large eggs

250g ground almonds

1 tablespoon baking powder

1 teaspoon ground cinnamon

100g natural yoghurt, plus extra to serve

100ml maple syrup, plus extra for brushing

2 teaspoons vanilla bean paste

1 Preheat the oven to 170°C. Grease a deep 23cm springform cake tin with olive oil and line the base with greaseproof paper.

2 Put 350g of the peeled bananas into a food processor, crack in the eggs, and add all of the remaining ingredients. Go in with 50ml of olive oil, add a small pinch of sea salt, then blitz until smooth. Tip the mixture into the cake tin and spread out evenly. Slice the remaining bananas and arrange on top, then bake for 45 minutes, or until an inserted skewer comes out clean.

3 Remove from the oven, brush with a little maple syrup, and leave to cool for 10 minutes. Run a palette knife around the edge of the tin, then release the cake and transfer to a wire rack to cool, or serve warm.

LEFTOVER LOVE

Slice the cake, wrap each portion, and stash in the freezer for another day (up to 3 months). Simply defrost when you want a slice, and enjoy!

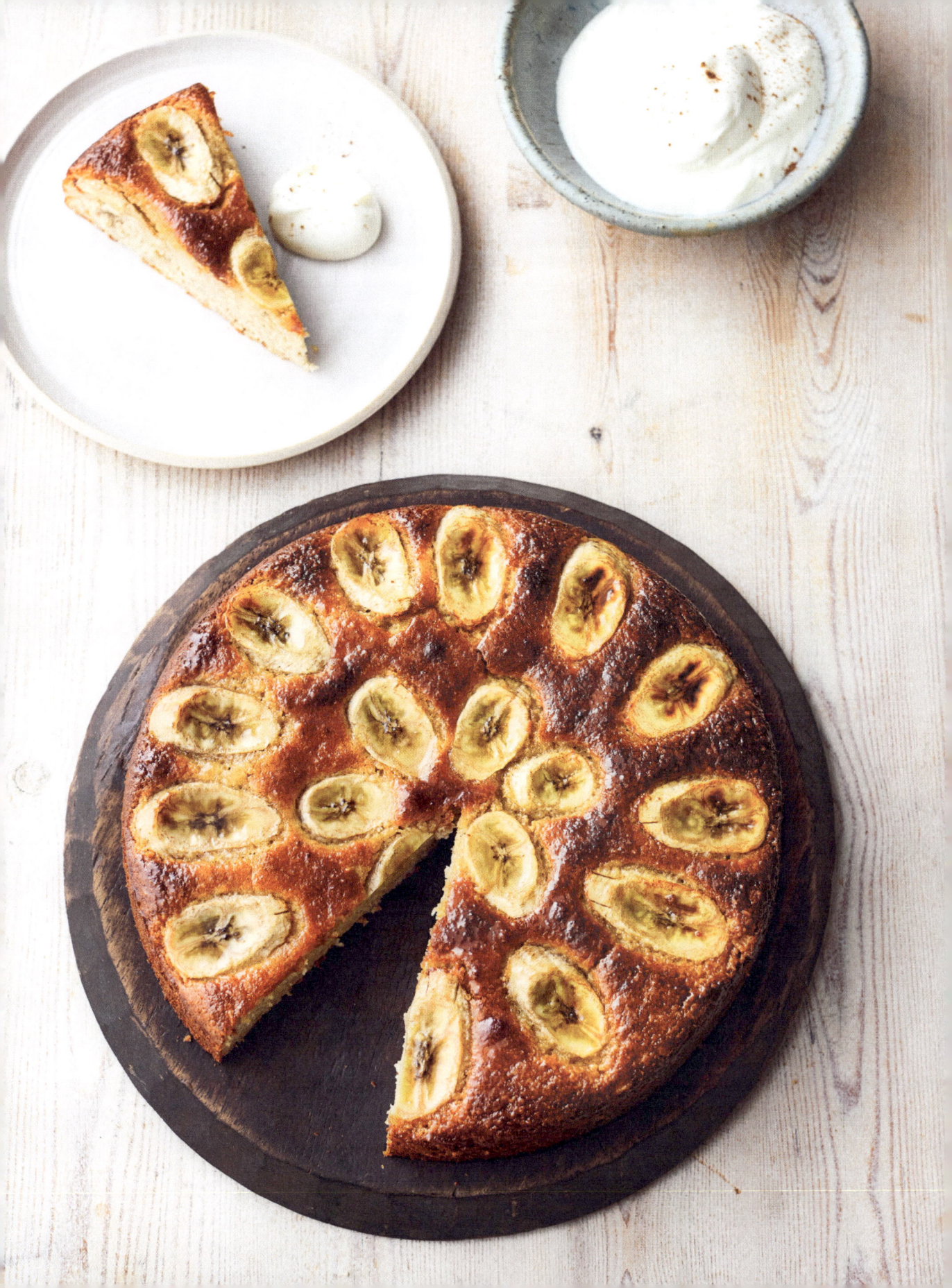

Drinks

Fresh infused waters

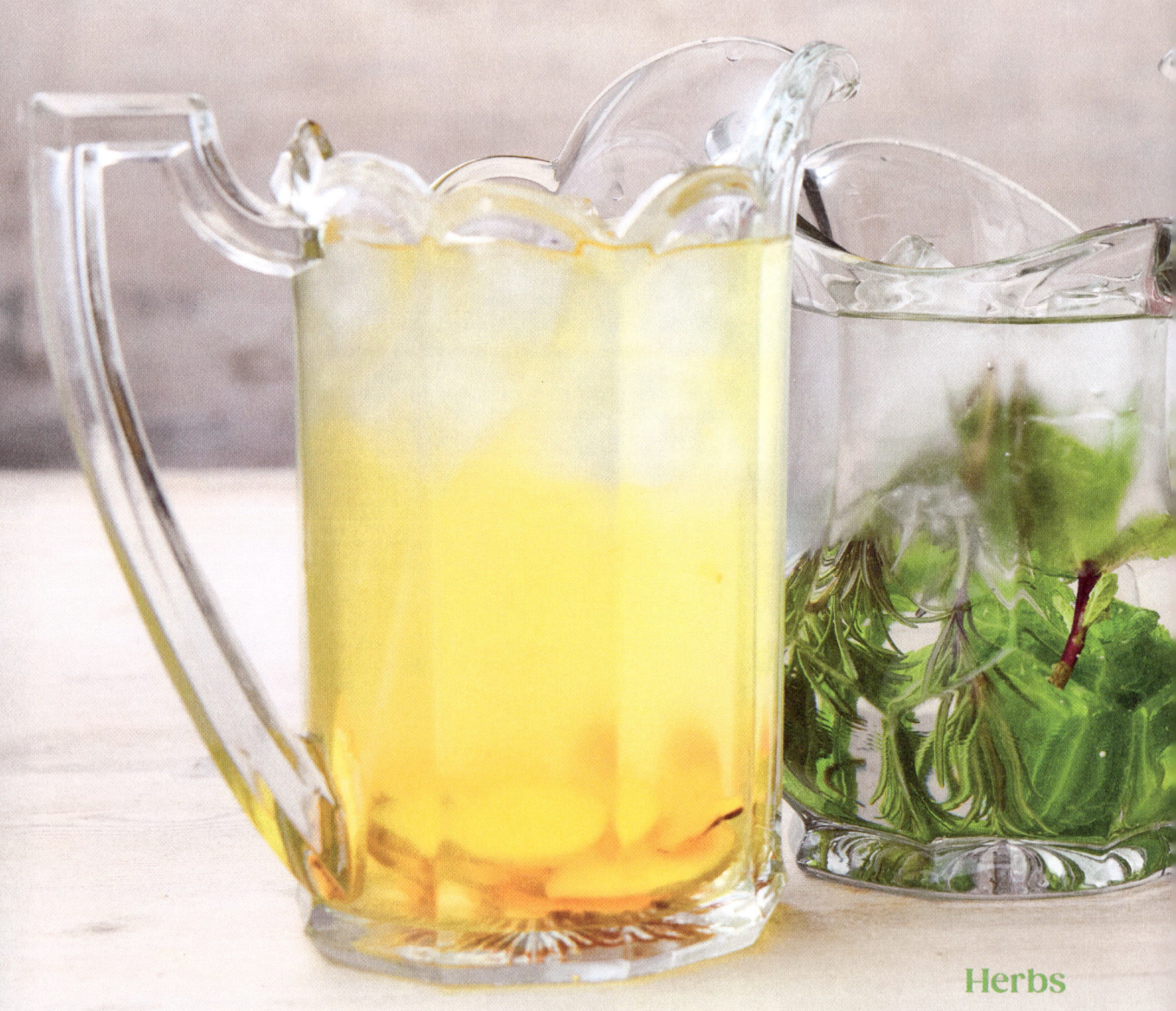

Roots
such as ginger & turmeric

Herbs
such as mint & rosemary

In order to thrive, we need water, and I'm here to help you hydrate in style! Here's some inspo to help you have fun with different colourful infusions.

In a jug, simply steep your chosen combo in a little boiled water for 5 minutes, then top up the jug with cold water and a handful of ice cubes, and enjoy!

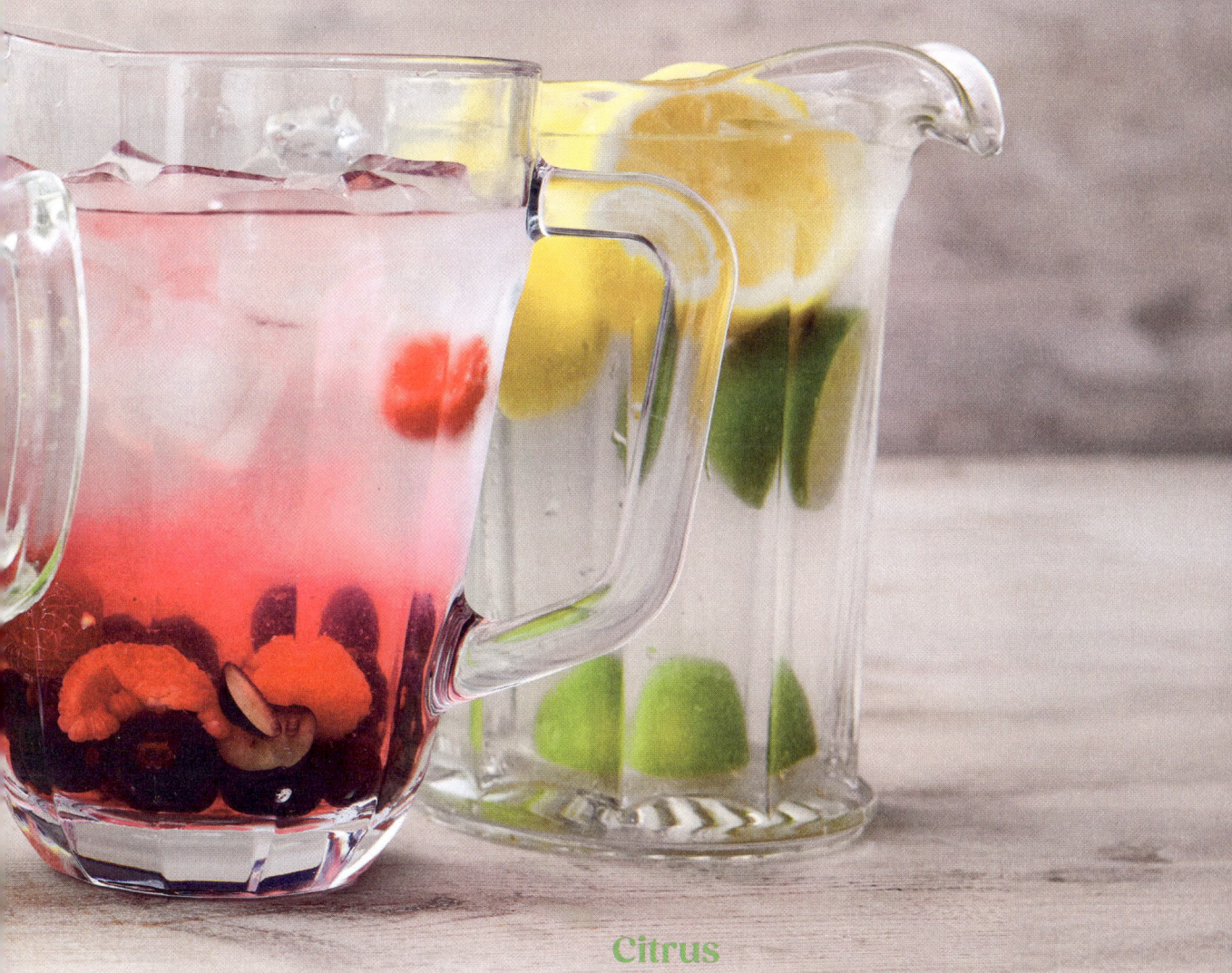

Berries
such as blueberries & raspberries

Citrus
such as lemon & lime

Morning kickstarter

Surprise and invigorate your senses with this punchy kickstarter, which turns good old water into a megamix of flavour and goodness. Nutritious ingredients like cayenne, turmeric and cinnamon are all super-high in iron for metabolic function, red blood cell formation and oxygen transportation, as well as helping to prevent tiredness and fatigue – it's a powerful combo!

MAKES 6 SERVINGS
7 MINUTES
PLUS FREEZING

2 sprigs of mint

12cm piece of ginger

1 teaspoon cayenne pepper

1 teaspoon ground turmeric

1 teaspoon ground cinnamon

4 tablespoons cider vinegar

1 lemon

optional: runny honey

1 Pick the mint leaves into an ice cube tray. Peel and finely grate the ginger into a bowl, add all the spices and the vinegar, squeeze in the lemon juice, mix, then divide into the tray. Top up with water and freeze until needed.

2 To enjoy, simply pop 1 large or 3 regular frozen kickstarter cubes (depending on the size of your ice cube tray) into a mug, and pour over boiling kettle water. Sweeten to taste with a little honey, if you like, and enjoy.

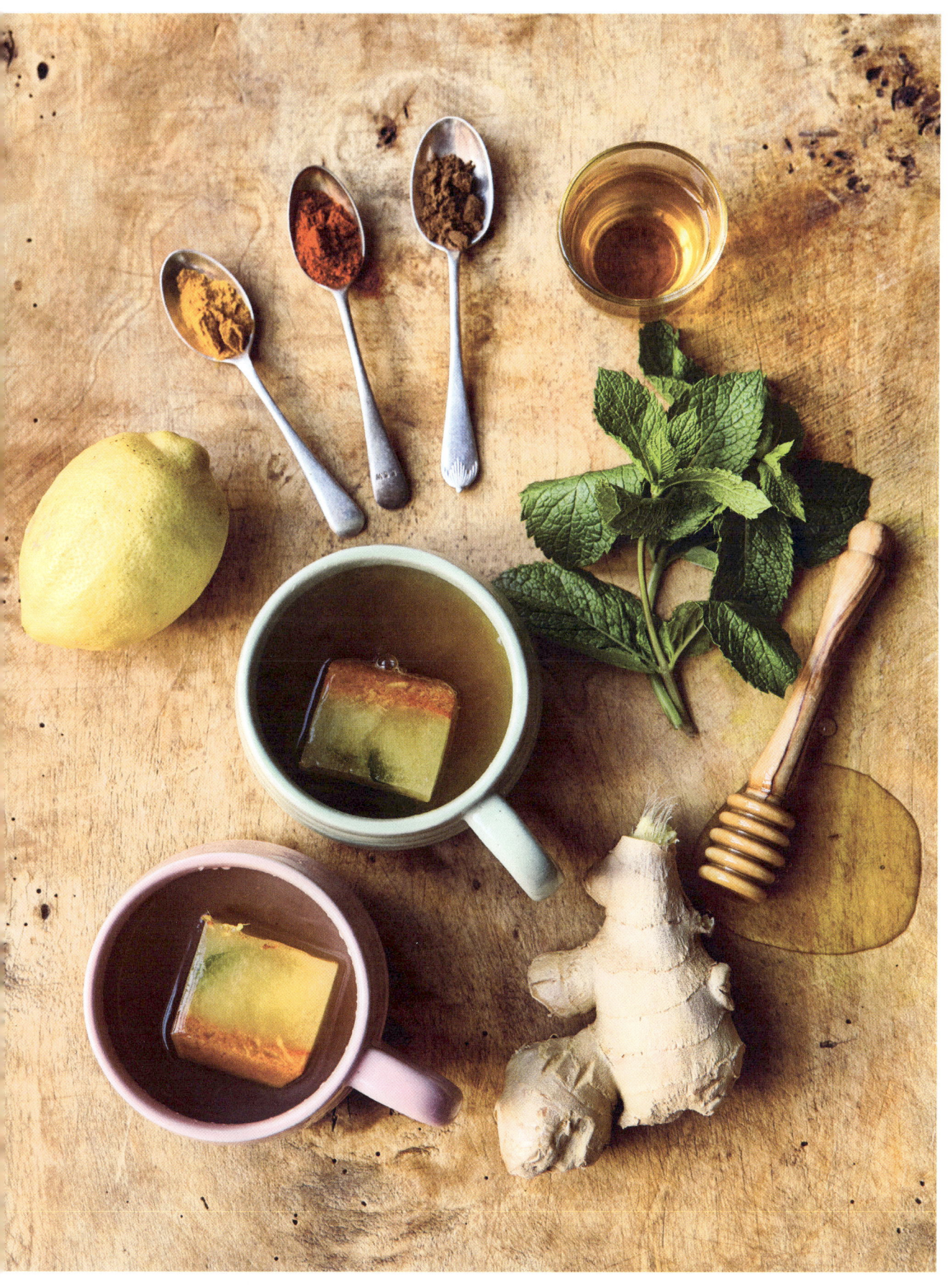

Green goddess smoothie

SERVES 1 | **4 MINUTES**

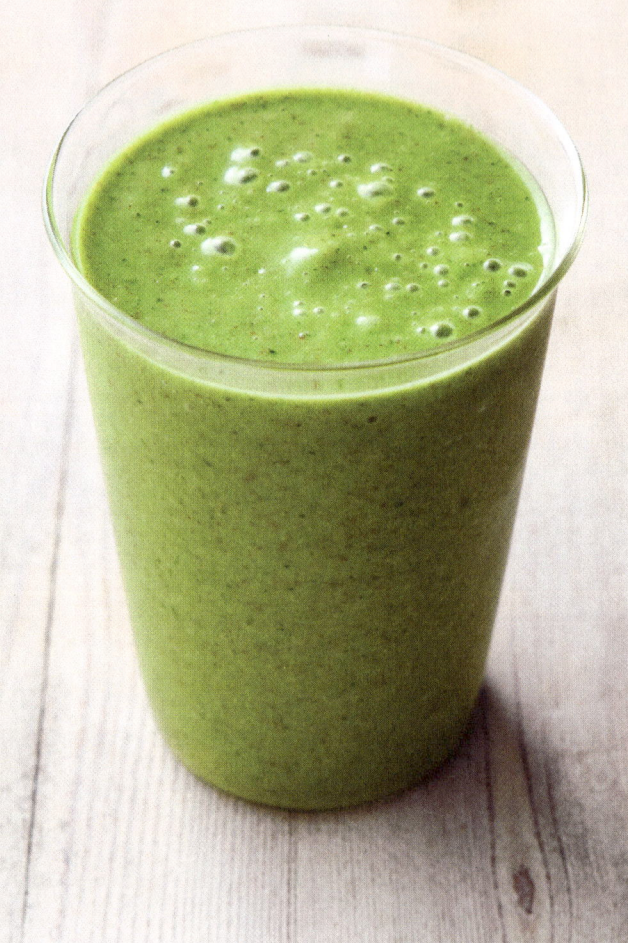

Finely grate the zest of **1 lime** into a blender and squeeze in the juice. Pick in the leaves from **4 sprigs of mint**, add **½ a small peeled banana (40g)**, **40g of peeled ripe avocado**, **40g of baby spinach**, **1 heaped teaspoon of cashew or your favourite nut butter** and **100ml of coconut water**. Chuck in **1 handful of ice cubes** and blitz until smooth, loosening with splashes of water until you get the perfect drinkable consistency. Pour into a glass or decant into a bottle, and enjoy.

Merry berry smoothie

SERVES 1 | 4 MINUTES

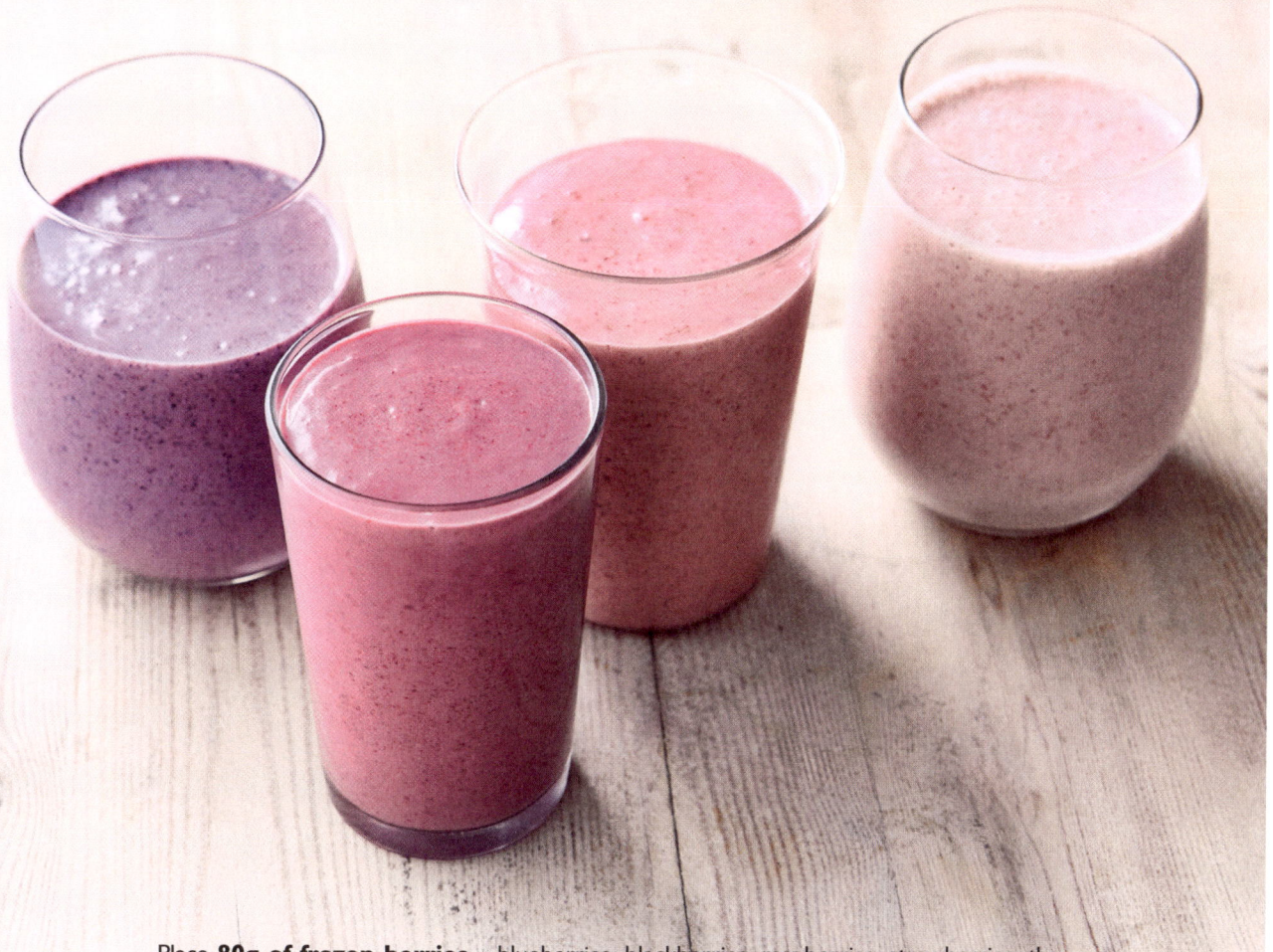

Place **80g of frozen berries** – blueberries, blackberries, raspberries, strawberries, the choice is yours – in a blender with **25g of dried cranberries, 10g of chia seeds, 30g of porridge oats, 1 teaspoon of almond butter and 150ml of semi-skimmed milk or your favourite fortified plant-based milk**. Chuck in **1 handful of ice cubes** and blitz until smooth, loosening with splashes of water until you get the perfect drinkable consistency. Pour into a glass or decant into a bottle, and enjoy.

Post-workout protein smoothie

SERVES 1 | 5 MINUTES

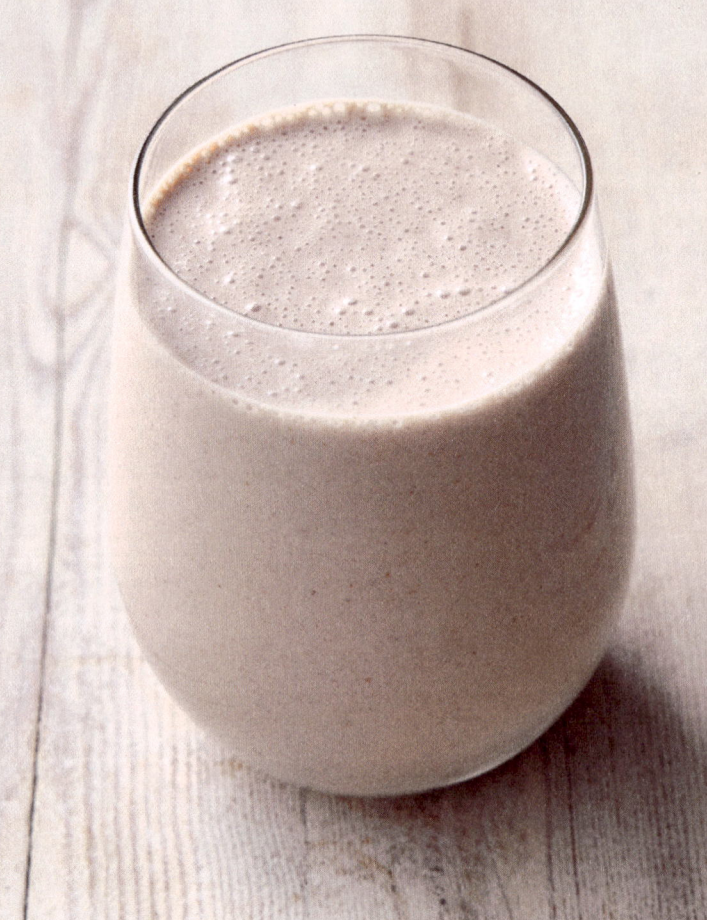

Peel **1 small ripe banana (80g)** and place in a blender with **150g of cottage cheese, 30g of porridge oats, 2 soft pitted dates (25g), 1 pinch of cocoa powder** and **150ml of semi-skimmed milk**. Chuck in **1 handful of ice cubes** and blitz until smooth, loosening with splashes of water until you get the perfect drinkable consistency. Pour into a glass or decant into a bottle, and enjoy.

Matcha & kefir smoothie

SERVES 1 | **5 MINUTES**

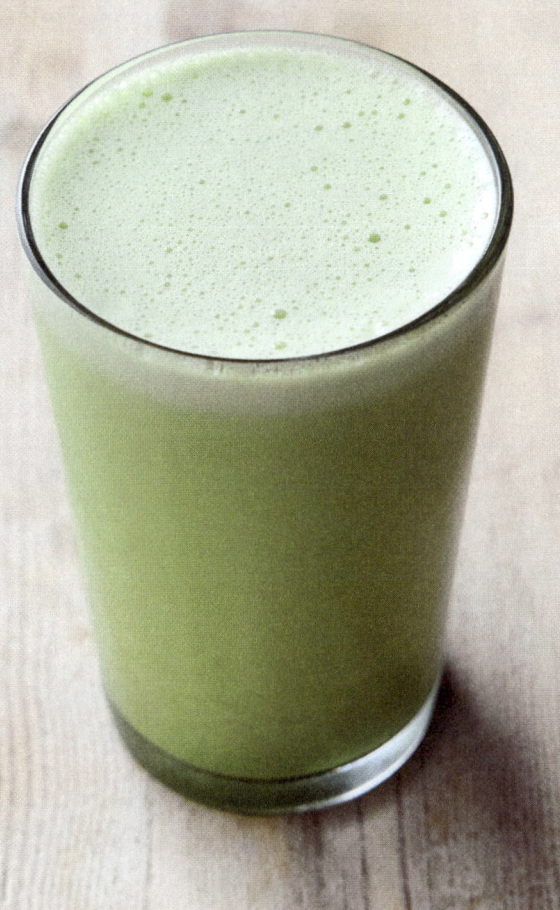

Put **1 teaspoon of good-quality matcha powder** into a blender with 65ml of hot water (not boiling). Add **½ a teaspoon of vanilla bean paste** and **175ml of kefir or unsweetened fortified almond plant milk**. Chuck in **1 handful of ice cubes** and blitz until smooth and foamy, loosening with splashes of water until you get the perfect drinkable consistency. Pour into a glass or decant into a bottle, and enjoy.

Whipped coffee

SERVES 2 | **2 MINUTES**

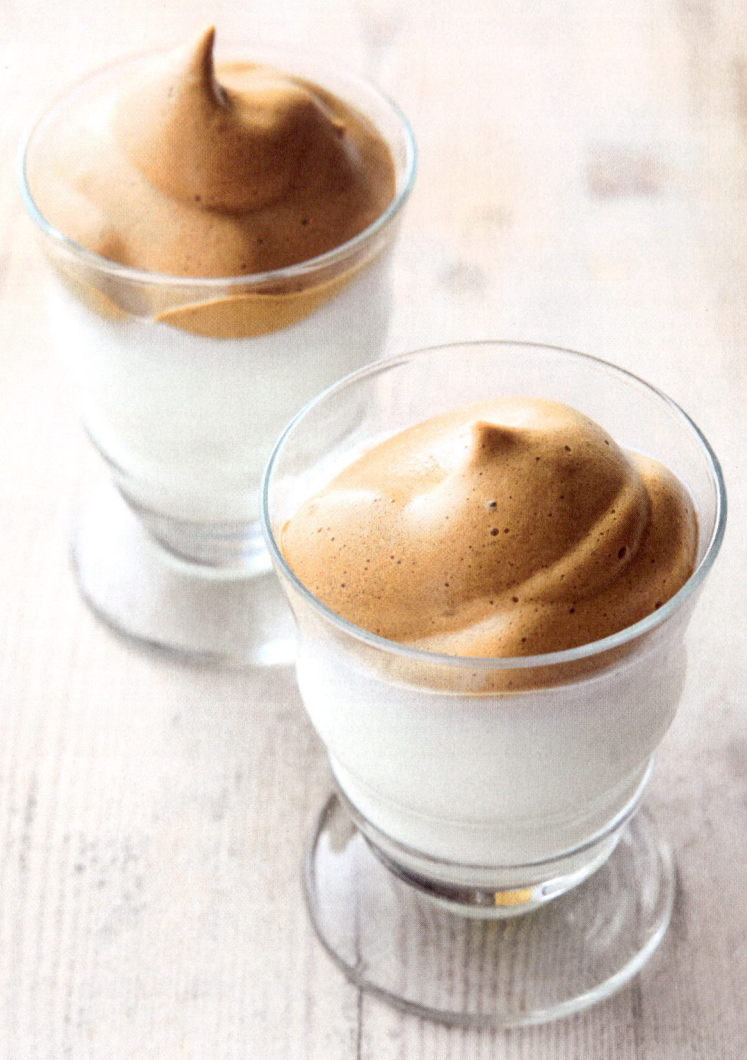

In an electric milk frother or in a jug using a handheld milk frother or balloon whisk, whip **1 tablespoon of instant coffee** with 1 tablespoon of boiling kettle water and **1 teaspoon of runny honey**, until it forms stiff peaks. Divide up to **400ml of kefir or your favourite milk or fortified plant-based milk** between two glasses, and spoon the coffee foam on top. Swirl together, and enjoy.

Gennaro's coffee

SERVES 2 | 1 MINUTE, PLUS BREWING

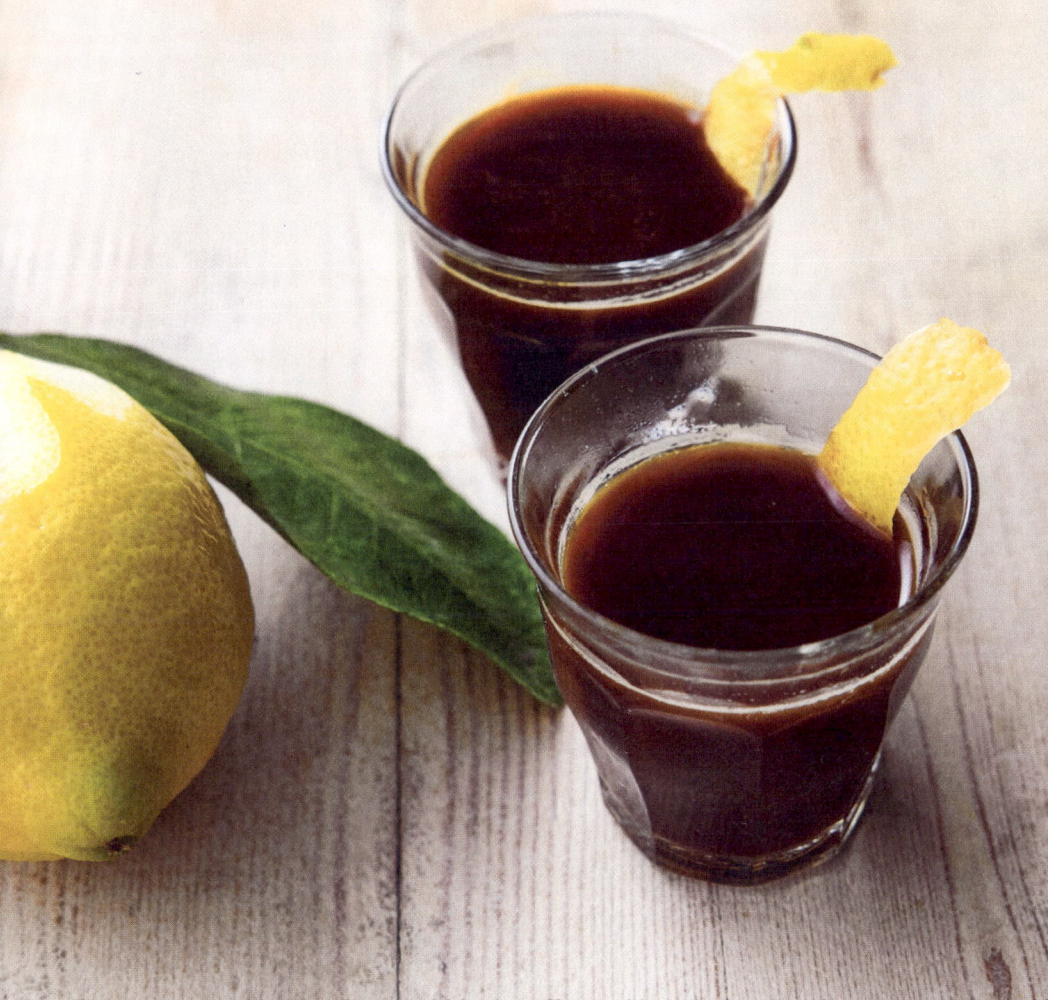

Make a small cafetière of **black coffee** and let it brew, or make **two espressos**. Use a speed-peeler to strip off a couple of chunky pieces of **lemon or orange peel** and roll them up to stimulate the natural oils. Divide the coffee between two small glasses or cups, and add a piece of citrus peel to each to infuse with flavour. Sweeten to taste with **runny honey, if desired**, and enjoy.

Cooking sustainably & kitchen notes

Celebrate quality & seasonality

As is often the case in cooking, using quality ingredients really does make a difference to the success of the recipes. I've tried to keep the number of ingredients under control, so I'm hoping that will give you the excuse to trade up where you can, buying the best veggies, fish or meat you can find. Also, remember that shopping in season always allows your food to be more delicious and more affordable. When it comes to veg and fruit, remember to give everything a nice wash before you start cooking, especially if you're using stuff raw. Ingredients that are noticeably more delicious when you choose the best quality are: sourdough, tinned tomatoes, cheese, beans and chickpeas, jarred and tinned fish, crunchy peanut & sesame chilli oil, peanut butter, sea salt, honey, dark chocolate, cocoa powder and coffee.

Focusing on fish & seafood

Fish and seafood are an incredibly delicious source of protein, but literally the minute they're caught they start to deteriorate in freshness, so you want to buy them as close to the day of your meal as you can – I wouldn't endorse them being stored in the fridge for days, you're better off with frozen if that's the case (see page 173). I recommend planning your fish and seafood dinners around your shopping days. Make sure you choose responsibly sourced fish and seafood – look for the MSC logo, or talk to your fishmonger and take their advice. Try to mix up your choices, choosing seasonal, sustainable options as they're available. If you can only find farmed fish, make sure you look for the RSPCA Assured or ASC logo to ensure your fish is responsibly sourced. Jarred and tinned fish are great options, too, particularly when it comes to oily fish.

Meat & eggs

When it comes to meat, of course I'm going to endorse higher-welfare farming practices, like organic or free-range. Animals should be raised well, free to roam, display natural behaviours and live a stress-free healthy life. Like most things, you pay more for quality. I'm always a believer that if you take a couple of minutes to plan your weekly menus you can be clever about using cheaper cuts of meat, or you could try cooking some of my meat-reduced and meat-free dishes, which should give you the opportunity to trade up to quality proteins when you do choose them. Butchers can be very helpful – they can order stuff in especially for you and can ensure you have the exact weights you need. Unless essential to a recipe, I try not to specify egg sizes. Hens naturally lay a variety of sizes of egg, so look for mixed-size boxes when shopping to support the best possible welfare standards. When it comes to eggs and anything containing egg, such as pasta or mayo – always choose free-range or organic.

Dial up your dairy

With staple dairy products, like milk, yoghurt, cottage cheese and butter, please trade up to organic if you can. Unlike meat, it is only slightly more expensive and I couldn't recommend it enough, if it's available to you. Every time you buy organic, you vote for a better food system that supports the highest standards of animal welfare, where both cows and land are well looked after.

Maximizing flavour

In this book I use a lot of what I like to call 'flavour bombs' or 'shortcuts': widely available ingredients that allow you to add big bonus flavour, fast, often bolstering the taste of a dish in one super-charged ingredient. Much-loved pastes include harissa, miso, gochujang, pesto, tahini and many curry pastes, and pickles. Useful things in brine include jarred roasted red peppers, jarred sliced jalapeños, pickled ginger, olives and capers. Helpful things in oil: anchovies and artichokes. I love spices and blends like dukkah, curry powder, dried red chilli flakes, smoked paprika and ground cinnamon, to name a few, as well as nuts, seeds and dried fruit, and crunchy things like Bombay mix, poppadoms and crispbreads to add texture; cracking condiments, such as mustards, chilli oils and sauces, mango chutney and lime pickle, as well as super sauces like hoisin, soy, black bean and sweet chilli dipping sauce. These items guarantee flavour and consistency, educate your palate and save hours of time in preparation. Most are non-perishable, which means you're not under pressure to use them up super-quickly.

Bigging up fresh herbs

Fresh herbs are a gift to any cook. Instead of buying them, why not grow them yourself in the garden or in a pot on your windowsill? Herbs allow you to add single-minded flavour to a dish, without the need to over-season, which is good for everyone. They're also packed with all sorts of incredible qualities on the nutritional front – we like that. And don't forget dried herbs; they're non-perishable and super-convenient to have ready and raring to go in the cupboard.

Fridge organization

When juggling space in the fridge, remember that raw meat and fish should be well wrapped and placed on the bottom shelf to avoid cross-contamination. Any food that is ready to eat, whether it's cooked or it doesn't need to be cooked, should be stored on a higher shelf.

The freezer is your friend

For busy people, without doubt your freezer, if stocked correctly, is your closest ally. There are just a few basic rules when it comes to really utilizing it well. If you're batch cooking, remember to let food cool thoroughly before freezing – break it down into portions so it cools quicker, and get it into the freezer within 2 hours. Make sure everything is well wrapped, and labelled for future reference. Thaw in the fridge before use, and use within 48 hours. If you've frozen cooked food, don't freeze it again after reheating or defrosting it. Nutritionally speaking, freezing veg and fruit quickly after harvesting retains the nutritional value very efficiently, often trumping fresh equivalents that have been stuck in the supply chain for a while. You will see me using frozen veg and fruit (which I love!) in these recipes – it's super-convenient and widely available.

Oven & air fryer lovin'

Recipes are tested in fan ovens – find conversions for conventional, °F and gas online. Recipes that use an air fryer are tested in a single (4.2 litre) or dual (8.3 litre) air fryer – all air fryers are different, so results may vary.

A note from Jamie's nutrition team

Our job is to make sure that Jamie can be super-creative, while also ensuring that all recipes meet our guidelines. Every book has a different brief, and Eat Yourself Healthy is about recipes you can cook any day of the week, being confident that you're making a good choice as 100% of the recipes fit into our everyday food guidelines. For clarity and so that you can make informed choices, we've presented easy-to-read nutrition info for each dish on pages 298 to 303 (displayed per serving). We also want to inspire a more sustainable way of eating, so 88% of the recipes are either meat-free or meat-reduced (meaning they contain at least 30% less meat than a regular portion size). Food is fun, joyful and creative – it gives us energy and plays a crucial role in keeping our bodies healthy. Remember, a nutritious, varied and balanced diet and regular exercise are the keys to a healthier lifestyle. We don't label foods as 'good' or 'bad' – there's a place for everything. We encourage an understanding of the difference between nutritious foods for everyday consumption and those to be enjoyed occasionally. For more info about our guidelines and how we analyse recipes, please visit jamieoliver.com/nutrition.

Rozzie Batchelar – Senior Nutritionist, RNutr (food)

A bit about balance

Balance is key when it comes to eating well. Balance your plate right and keep your portion control in check, and you can be confident that you're giving yourself a great start on the path to good health. It's important to consume a variety of foods to ensure we get the nutrients our bodies need to stay healthy. You don't have to be spot-on every day – just try to get your balance right across the week. If you eat meat and fish, as a general guide for main meals you want at least two portions of fish a week, one of which should be oily. Split the rest of the week's main meals between brilliant plant-based meals, some poultry and a little red meat. An all-vegetarian diet can be perfectly healthy, too.

What's the balance?

The UK government's Eatwell Guide shows us what a healthy balance of food looks like. The figures below indicate the proportion of each food group that's recommended across the day.

THE FIVE FOOD GROUPS (UK)	PROPORTION
Vegetables & fruit	40%
Starchy carbohydrates (bread, rice, potatoes, pasta)	38%
Protein (lean meat, fish, eggs, beans, other non-dairy sources)	12%
Dairy foods, milk & dairy alternatives	8%
Unsaturated fats (such as oils)	1%
AND DON'T FORGET TO DRINK PLENTY OF WATER, TOO	

Try to only consume foods and drinks high in fat, salt or sugar occasionally.

Vegetables & fruit

To live a good, healthy life, vegetables and fruit should sit right at the heart of your diet. Veg and fruit come in all kinds of colours, shapes, sizes, flavours and textures, and contain different vitamins and minerals, which each play a part in keeping our bodies healthy and optimal, so variety is key. Eat the rainbow, mixing up your choices as much as you can and embracing the seasons so you're getting produce at its best and its most nutritious. As an absolute minimum, aim for at least 5 portions of fresh, frozen or tinned veg and fruit every day of the week, enjoying more wherever possible. 80g (or a large handful) counts as one portion. You can also count one 30g portion of dried fruit, one 80g portion of cooked beans or pulses, and 150ml of unsweetened veg or fruit juice per day.

Starchy carbohydrates

Carbs provide us with a large proportion of the energy needed to make our bodies move, and to ensure our organs have the fuel they need to function. When you can, choose fibre-rich wholegrain and wholewheat varieties. 260g is the recommended daily amount of carbohydrates for the average adult, with up to 90g coming from total sugars, which includes natural sugars found in whole fruit, milk and milk products, and no more than 30g of free sugars. Free sugars are those added to food and drink, including sugar found in honey, syrups, fruit juice and smoothies. Fibre is classified as a carbohydrate and is mainly found in plant-based foods such as wholegrains, veg and fruit. It helps to keep our digestive systems healthy, control our blood-sugar levels and maintain healthy cholesterol levels. Adults should be aiming for at least 30g of fibre each day.

Protein

Think of protein as the building blocks of our bodies – it's used for everything that's important to how we grow and repair. Try to vary your proteins to include more beans and pulses, and two sources of sustainably sourced fish per week (one of which is oily), and reduce red and processed meat if your diet is high in these. Choose lean cuts of animal-based protein where you can. Beans, peas and lentils are great alternatives to meat because they're naturally low in fat and, as well as protein, they contain fibre and some vitamins and minerals. Other nutritious protein sources include tofu, eggs, nuts and seeds. Variety is key! The requirement for an average woman aged 19 to 50 is 45g per day, with 55g for men in the same age bracket.

Dairy foods, milk & dairy alternatives

This food group offers an amazing array of nutrients when eaten in the right amounts. Favour organic dairy milk and yoghurt, and small amounts of cheese, in this category; the lower-fat varieties (with no added sugar) are equally brilliant and worth embracing. If opting for plant-based versions, I think it's great that we have choice, but it's really important to look for unsweetened fortified options that have added calcium, iodine and vitamin B12 in the ingredients list, to avoid missing out on the key nutrients provided by dairy milk.

Unsaturated fats

While we only need small amounts, we do require healthier fats. Choose unsaturated sources where you can, such as olive and liquid vegetable oils, nuts, seeds, avocado and omega-3 rich oily fish. Generally speaking, it's recommended that the average woman has no more than 70g of fat per day, with less than 20g of that from saturated fat, and the average man no more than 90g, with less than 30g from saturated fat.

Drink plenty of water

To be the best you can be, stay hydrated. Water is essential to life, and to every function of the human body! In general, women aged 14 and over need at least 2 litres per day, and men in the same age bracket need at least 2.5 litres per day.

Energy & nutrition info

The average woman needs 2,000 calories per day, while the average man needs roughly 2,500. These figures are a rough guide, and what we eat needs to be considered in relation to factors like your age, build, lifestyle and activity levels.

Nutrition

Pink Shredded Wheat — PAGE 34

ENERGY	FAT	SAT FAT	PROTEIN	CARBS	SUGARS	SALT	FIBRE
362kcal	17.8g	1.5g	13g	42.2g	5.1g	0.2g	9.1g

Cheat's bircher muesli — PAGE 34

ENERGY	FAT	SAT FAT	PROTEIN	CARBS	SUGARS	SALT	FIBRE
286kcal	6.9g	2.2g	11.6g	46.6g	22.4g	0.4g	9.7g

Nutty banana oats — PAGE 34

ENERGY	FAT	SAT FAT	PROTEIN	CARBS	SUGARS	SALT	FIBRE
319kcal	9.8g	1.9g	10.5g	47g	23.4g	0.3g	4.1g

Piña colada muesli — PAGE 34

ENERGY	FAT	SAT FAT	PROTEIN	CARBS	SUGARS	SALT	FIBRE
294kcal	6.5g	3.2g	6.9g	91.2g	16.1g	0.3g	6g

5-minute tasty toppers (option A) — PAGE 36

ENERGY	FAT	SAT FAT	PROTEIN	CARBS	SUGARS	SALT	FIBRE
326kcal	18g	1.6g	12.2g	26.4g	11.4g	0.4g	8.1g

Box grater fruit salad — PAGE 38

ENERGY	FAT	SAT FAT	PROTEIN	CARBS	SUGARS	SALT	FIBRE
344kcal	9.2g	3.9g	7.6g	61.9g	57.9g	0.1g	6.9g

Frosty porridge — PAGE 40

ENERGY	FAT	SAT FAT	PROTEIN	CARBS	SUGARS	SALT	FIBRE
400kcal	12.5g	3g	12.4g	63.3g	25.6g	0g	4.3g

Smoked salmon & rye omelette — PAGE 42

ENERGY	FAT	SAT FAT	PROTEIN	CARBS	SUGARS	SALT	FIBRE
380kcal	18.4g	5.3g	33.5g	20.5g	3.7g	1.8g	4.3g

Speedy stuffed apple — PAGE 44

ENERGY	FAT	SAT FAT	PROTEIN	CARBS	SUGARS	SALT	FIBRE
264kcal	14.7g	4g	6.4g	28.6g	26.7g	0g	2.1g

Mothership overnight oats — PAGE 46

ENERGY	FAT	SAT FAT	PROTEIN	CARBS	SUGARS	SALT	FIBRE
311kcal	6.1g	1.9g	10.2g	57.5g	21g	0.1g	5.4g

Spicy tofu & sweet pepper eggs — PAGE 50

ENERGY	FAT	SAT FAT	PROTEIN	CARBS	SUGARS	SALT	FIBRE
274kcal	18g	3.9g	23.6g	5.1g	4g	1g	2.1g

Golden cheese & jammy berries — PAGE 52

ENERGY	FAT	SAT FAT	PROTEIN	CARBS	SUGARS	SALT	FIBRE
330kcal	15.1g	6g	11.7g	37.1g	20.9g	0.8g	3g

Dukkah poached eggs — PAGE 54

ENERGY	FAT	SAT FAT	PROTEIN	CARBS	SUGARS	SALT	FIBRE
398kcal	18.8g	4g	18.3g	39.2g	11.1g	1.4g	9g

Extraordinary brekkie smush-in — PAGE 56

ENERGY	FAT	SAT FAT	PROTEIN	CARBS	SUGARS	SALT	FIBRE
389kcal	13.8g	4g	13.8g	53.1g	30.7g	0.7g	5.5g

One-cup pancakes (sweet version) — PAGE 58

ENERGY	FAT	SAT FAT	PROTEIN	CARBS	SUGARS	SALT	FIBRE
174kcal	3.5g	1.1g	9.5g	25.1g	3.9g	0.1g	3.4g

Cheesy beans on toast — PAGE 62

ENERGY	FAT	SAT FAT	PROTEIN	CARBS	SUGARS	SALT	FIBRE
400kcal	13.9g	6g	20.9g	48.4g	16.1g	0.8g	10.1g

Easy egg & bean filo twists — PAGE 64

ENERGY	FAT	SAT FAT	PROTEIN	CARBS	SUGARS	SALT	FIBRE
400kcal	17.1g	4.8g	22.5g	42.3g	11.3g	1.6g	11.3g

Granola fruit cups — PAGE 66

ENERGY	FAT	SAT FAT	PROTEIN	CARBS	SUGARS	SALT	FIBRE
245kcal	11g	1.7g	6.1g	33.1g	17.9g	0.1g	3.6g

Batch-it-up protein rolls — PAGE 68

ENERGY	FAT	SAT FAT	PROTEIN	CARBS	SUGARS	SALT	FIBRE
358kcal	11.9g	2.9g	17.4g	48.5g	3.3g	0.5g	6.6g

Prawn cocktail for one — PAGE 72

ENERGY	FAT	SAT FAT	PROTEIN	CARBS	SUGARS	SALT	FIBRE
334kcal	7g	3.4g	36g	36g	24.7g	1.8g	4.6g

Speedy kedgeree — PAGE 74
ENERGY	FAT	SAT FAT	PROTEIN	CARBS	SUGARS	SALT	FIBRE
598kcal	26.2g	5.1g	41.6g	50.2g	8.7g	1.6g	12.2g

Creamy walnut coleslaw — PAGE 76
ENERGY	FAT	SAT FAT	PROTEIN	CARBS	SUGARS	SALT	FIBRE
438kcal	23.8g	4.3g	7.4g	48.6g	42.6g	1.2g	14.1g

Warm lentil salad — PAGE 78
ENERGY	FAT	SAT FAT	PROTEIN	CARBS	SUGARS	SALT	FIBRE
344kcal	18.1g	4.7g	13.1g	32.7g	15.7g	0.6g	10.2g

Harissa tuna platter — PAGE 80
ENERGY	FAT	SAT FAT	PROTEIN	CARBS	SUGARS	SALT	FIBRE
427kcal	17.7g	6g	20.7g	49.4g	11.3g	1.8g	10g

Curried fried eggs & grain salad — PAGE 82
ENERGY	FAT	SAT FAT	PROTEIN	CARBS	SUGARS	SALT	FIBRE
499kcal	21.5g	4.8g	22g	54.2g	14.5g	1.8g	8.1g

Speedy silky omelette — PAGE 84
ENERGY	FAT	SAT FAT	PROTEIN	CARBS	SUGARS	SALT	FIBRE
462kcal	18.4g	6g	37.1g	30.3g	5g	0.9g	18.1g

Prawn & noodle salad — PAGE 86
ENERGY	FAT	SAT FAT	PROTEIN	CARBS	SUGARS	SALT	FIBRE
358kcal	2.9g	0.4g	23.1g	61g	21.4g	1.2g	4.3g

Crispy sardine & avo wrap — PAGE 88
ENERGY	FAT	SAT FAT	PROTEIN	CARBS	SUGARS	SALT	FIBRE
500kcal	26.9g	5.6g	25.8g	37.2g	10.1g	1.6g	7.6g

Chopped rainbow salad — PAGE 90
ENERGY	FAT	SAT FAT	PROTEIN	CARBS	SUGARS	SALT	FIBRE
539kcal	26.2g	4.4g	12.2g	66.6g	45.6g	1.2g	11.8g

Salmon, beet & potato salad — PAGE 92
ENERGY	FAT	SAT FAT	PROTEIN	CARBS	SUGARS	SALT	FIBRE
546kcal	24.1g	4.2g	30.2g	51.7g	17.4g	1.6g	8.3g

Sardines on toast & tomato salad — PAGE 94
ENERGY	FAT	SAT FAT	PROTEIN	CARBS	SUGARS	SALT	FIBRE
491kcal	20g	3.5g	24.1g	49.3g	18.4g	1.5g	14.3g

Sesame miso shred salad — PAGE 96
ENERGY	FAT	SAT FAT	PROTEIN	CARBS	SUGARS	SALT	FIBRE
290kcal	18.6g	2.7g	9g	23.8g	16.8g	0.5g	9.4g

Black bean houmous salad wrap — PAGE 98
ENERGY	FAT	SAT FAT	PROTEIN	CARBS	SUGARS	SALT	FIBRE
463kcal	20.7g	6g	19.2g	41.8g	6.2g	1g	18.6g

Fluffy spring veg omelette — PAGE 102
ENERGY	FAT	SAT FAT	PROTEIN	CARBS	SUGARS	SALT	FIBRE
430kcal	18.2g	5.1g	29.2g	37.2g	5.8g	1.5g	9.3g

Carrot gazpacho — PAGE 104
ENERGY	FAT	SAT FAT	PROTEIN	CARBS	SUGARS	SALT	FIBRE
413kcal	14.9g	3.7g	14.6g	56.8g	26g	1.6g	8.9g

Pea & feta egg warm salad — PAGE 106
ENERGY	FAT	SAT FAT	PROTEIN	CARBS	SUGARS	SALT	FIBRE
474kcal	17.1g	5.9g	26.7g	58.4g	8.4g	1.6g	7.4g

Soy eggs & crispy mackerel rice — PAGE 108
ENERGY	FAT	SAT FAT	PROTEIN	CARBS	SUGARS	SALT	FIBRE
508kcal	23.4g	5.5g	32.9g	41.8g	5.1g	1.8g	12.2g

Chickpea arrabbiata — PAGE 110
ENERGY	FAT	SAT FAT	PROTEIN	CARBS	SUGARS	SALT	FIBRE
411kcal	15.7g	5.5g	18.4g	46.9g	10.4g	0.6g	4.4g

Crispy bean & anchovy eggs — PAGE 112
ENERGY	FAT	SAT FAT	PROTEIN	CARBS	SUGARS	SALT	FIBRE
375kcal	21.1g	5.6g	25.1g	23.5g	6.4g	1g	8.8g

Smashed salad — PAGE 114
ENERGY	FAT	SAT FAT	PROTEIN	CARBS	SUGARS	SALT	FIBRE
335kcal	19.9g	4.5g	9.4g	31.2g	25.1g	0.8g	9.2g

Herby chickpea & feta salad — PAGE 116
ENERGY	FAT	SAT FAT	PROTEIN	CARBS	SUGARS	SALT	FIBRE
554kcal	15.2g	4.5g	24.1g	84.5g	7.7g	0.9g	16.1g

Curried egg & rice pots — PAGE 118
ENERGY	FAT	SAT FAT	PROTEIN	CARBS	SUGARS	SALT	FIBRE
599kcal	23.2g	5.8g	32.7g	66.5g	10.2g	1.2g	14.1g

Tuna & broccoli pasta — PAGE 120

ENERGY	FAT	SAT FAT	PROTEIN	CARBS	SUGARS	SALT	FIBRE
464kcal	19.7g	2.9g	23.1g	47g	6.8g	1.7g	7.9g

Avo & black bean omelette — PAGE 122

ENERGY	FAT	SAT FAT	PROTEIN	CARBS	SUGARS	SALT	FIBRE
448kcal	22.3g	6g	27.8g	28.5g	5.6g	1.1g	16.5g

Carrot & sweet potato fritters — PAGE 124

ENERGY	FAT	SAT FAT	PROTEIN	CARBS	SUGARS	SALT	FIBRE
600kcal	18.6g	5.1g	30g	84g	9.2g	1.7g	14.3g

Crispy mackerel buns — PAGE 126

ENERGY	FAT	SAT FAT	PROTEIN	CARBS	SUGARS	SALT	FIBRE
466kcal	21.3g	5.5g	25.4g	42.1g	18.6g	1.7g	7.8g

Smashed flatbread burger — PAGE 130

ENERGY	FAT	SAT FAT	PROTEIN	CARBS	SUGARS	SALT	FIBRE
553kcal	20.8g	5.9g	35g	55.4g	5.5g	1.6g	7.6g

Super-green stir-fry — PAGE 132

ENERGY	FAT	SAT FAT	PROTEIN	CARBS	SUGARS	SALT	FIBRE
358kcal	9.1g	2g	23.6g	53.1g	26.9g	0.6g	14.3g

Easy prawn curry — PAGE 134

ENERGY	FAT	SAT FAT	PROTEIN	CARBS	SUGARS	SALT	FIBRE
600kcal	17.8g	6g	30.9g	79.5g	27.7g	1.2g	14.4g

Creamy peanut chicken — PAGE 136

ENERGY	FAT	SAT FAT	PROTEIN	CARBS	SUGARS	SALT	FIBRE
542kcal	19.8g	4.9g	48.5g	44.9g	34.5g	1.7g	6g

Sweet & sour prawns — PAGE 138

ENERGY	FAT	SAT FAT	PROTEIN	CARBS	SUGARS	SALT	FIBRE
452kcal	2.4g	0.1g	29.2g	76.6g	22.8g	1.8g	7.3g

Thai-style fish curry — PAGE 140

ENERGY	FAT	SAT FAT	PROTEIN	CARBS	SUGARS	SALT	FIBRE
447kcal	11.6g	5.7g	32.4g	53.6g	6.8g	0.6g	5.4g

Green veg megamix — PAGE 142

ENERGY	FAT	SAT FAT	PROTEIN	CARBS	SUGARS	SALT	FIBRE
302kcal	8.1g	1.1g	26.8g	34.8g	20.6g	1.4g	17.7g

Tahini mushroom noodles — PAGE 144

ENERGY	FAT	SAT FAT	PROTEIN	CARBS	SUGARS	SALT	FIBRE
445kcal	17.8g	2.2g	23.2g	47.1g	6.8g	1.8g	10.4g

Charred Mexican salad — PAGE 146

ENERGY	FAT	SAT FAT	PROTEIN	CARBS	SUGARS	SALT	FIBRE
423kcal	21.6g	5.9g	17.3g	39.8g	20.8g	0.5g	15.8g

Tasty salmon couscous — PAGE 148

ENERGY	FAT	SAT FAT	PROTEIN	CARBS	SUGARS	SALT	FIBRE
587kcal	18.1g	3.7g	44.3g	65.1g	6.7g	0.8g	7.4g

Crispy pork noodle broth — PAGE 150

ENERGY	FAT	SAT FAT	PROTEIN	CARBS	SUGARS	SALT	FIBRE
558kcal	24.6g	5.5g	38.6g	44g	2.4g	1.3g	7.6g

Silken tofu & black beans — PAGE 152

ENERGY	FAT	SAT FAT	PROTEIN	CARBS	SUGARS	SALT	FIBRE
435kcal	22.1g	3.3g	28.8g	26.2g	10.1g	0.9g	15.1g

Chicken fajitas — PAGE 154

ENERGY	FAT	SAT FAT	PROTEIN	CARBS	SUGARS	SALT	FIBRE
538kcal	15.8g	4.5g	46.1g	52.4g	24.4g	1.3g	8.3g

Seared tuna kimchi bowl — PAGE 156

ENERGY	FAT	SAT FAT	PROTEIN	CARBS	SUGARS	SALT	FIBRE
533kcal	15.4g	3.8g	48.8g	48.8g	9.2g	1.8g	12.7g

Lemon tahini chicken & grains — PAGE 158

ENERGY	FAT	SAT FAT	PROTEIN	CARBS	SUGARS	SALT	FIBRE
577kcal	15.4g	3.3g	54g	49.9g	5.4g	1.1g	15.9g

Golden chicken, peppers & rice — PAGE 160

ENERGY	FAT	SAT FAT	PROTEIN	CARBS	SUGARS	SALT	FIBRE
581kcal	22.2g	5.2g	49.4g	45.2g	6.2g	1.8g	10.7g

Crispy black bean beef — PAGE 162

ENERGY	FAT	SAT FAT	PROTEIN	CARBS	SUGARS	SALT	FIBRE
600kcal	19.4g	5.9g	47g	58.9g	10.9g	1.4g	8.8g

Chicken cup salad — PAGE 164

ENERGY	FAT	SAT FAT	PROTEIN	CARBS	SUGARS	SALT	FIBRE
406kcal	4g	1.1g	41g	52.1g	28.6g	0.9g	6.4g

Steak & sticky aubergine salad — PAGE 166

ENERGY	FAT	SAT FAT	PROTEIN	CARBS	SUGARS	SALT	FIBRE
459kcal	13.9g	5.8g	28.9g	55.7g	8.8g	1.2g	7.1g

Chicken balls & rainbow broth — PAGE 168

ENERGY	FAT	SAT FAT	PROTEIN	CARBS	SUGARS	SALT	FIBRE
279kcal	5.9g	1.1g	22.9g	26.1g	5.1g	1.3g	4.7g

Spinach & lentil fritter salad — PAGE 170

ENERGY	FAT	SAT FAT	PROTEIN	CARBS	SUGARS	SALT	FIBRE
505kcal	21.3g	6g	30.2g	50.6g	6.7g	1.7g	3.4g

Seared salmon rice — PAGE 174

ENERGY	FAT	SAT FAT	PROTEIN	CARBS	SUGARS	SALT	FIBRE
562kcal	23.7g	4.9g	40.9g	45.1g	7g	1.6g	9.8g

Chicken in milk — PAGE 176

ENERGY	FAT	SAT FAT	PROTEIN	CARBS	SUGARS	SALT	FIBRE
592kcal	12g	5.5g	58.7g	64.4g	22.2g	1.7g	4.7g

Crispy steamy parcels — PAGE 178

ENERGY	FAT	SAT FAT	PROTEIN	CARBS	SUGARS	SALT	FIBRE
420kcal	8.7g	1.3g	20g	55.2g	15.6g	1.8g	4.3g

Peasto chicken salad — PAGE 180

ENERGY	FAT	SAT FAT	PROTEIN	CARBS	SUGARS	SALT	FIBRE
515kcal	23.8g	5.9g	56.7g	19.8g	6.1g	1.1g	10.2g

Chicken & berry grain bowl — PAGE 182

ENERGY	FAT	SAT FAT	PROTEIN	CARBS	SUGARS	SALT	FIBRE
595kcal	12.7g	4.7g	55.8g	63.3g	11.2g	1.3g	16.6g

Crab spaghetti — PAGE 184

ENERGY	FAT	SAT FAT	PROTEIN	CARBS	SUGARS	SALT	FIBRE
514kcal	12.8g	1.9g	35.3g	70.1g	17.4g	0.9g	14.4g

Vibrant veg & creamy bean salad — PAGE 186

ENERGY	FAT	SAT FAT	PROTEIN	CARBS	SUGARS	SALT	FIBRE
596kcal	31.5g	6g	20.5g	56.8g	12.2g	0.9g	10.1g

Fish in crazy water — PAGE 188

ENERGY	FAT	SAT FAT	PROTEIN	CARBS	SUGARS	SALT	FIBRE
561kcal	20.3g	2.8g	44.8g	47.1g	6.4g	0.7g	15.9g

Super-green orecchiette — PAGE 190

ENERGY	FAT	SAT FAT	PROTEIN	CARBS	SUGARS	SALT	FIBRE
547kcal	16g	5.5g	28.4g	76.3g	5.7g	1.2g	11.4g

Fish parcels & tomato orzo — PAGE 192

ENERGY	FAT	SAT FAT	PROTEIN	CARBS	SUGARS	SALT	FIBRE
430kcal	4.8g	1.9g	37.3g	61.9g	8.5g	0.8g	4.3g

Silky aubergine flavour fest — PAGE 194

ENERGY	FAT	SAT FAT	PROTEIN	CARBS	SUGARS	SALT	FIBRE
495kcal	16.9g	3.3g	21.4g	68.9g	23.6g	1.8g	22.2g

Gochujang tomato noodle soup — PAGE 196

ENERGY	FAT	SAT FAT	PROTEIN	CARBS	SUGARS	SALT	FIBRE
377kcal	10.1g	1.4g	12.1g	60.2g	15.5g	0.7g	6.7g

Roasted veg & chickpea smash — PAGE 198

ENERGY	FAT	SAT FAT	PROTEIN	CARBS	SUGARS	SALT	FIBRE
484kcal	21.4g	4.4g	19.2g	55.6g	36.4g	0.9g	17.9g

Mushroom stew — PAGE 200

ENERGY	FAT	SAT FAT	PROTEIN	CARBS	SUGARS	SALT	FIBRE
580kcal	9.8g	1.4g	34.1g	87.5g	12.7g	1.5g	19.5g

Chicken curry & chapati — PAGE 202

ENERGY	FAT	SAT FAT	PROTEIN	CARBS	SUGARS	SALT	FIBRE
587kcal	18g	6g	51g	57.8g	12.8g	1g	12.3g

Roasted Mediterranean veg — PAGE 204

ENERGY	FAT	SAT FAT	PROTEIN	CARBS	SUGARS	SALT	FIBRE
329kcal	13.9g	2g	6.3g	47.9g	27.1g	0.6g	12.4g

Harissa tuna bean parcels — PAGE 206

ENERGY	FAT	SAT FAT	PROTEIN	CARBS	SUGARS	SALT	FIBRE
526kcal	7.4g	1.3g	31.1g	83.8g	21.9g	1.6g	16.6g

Aubergine involtini — PAGE 208

ENERGY	FAT	SAT FAT	PROTEIN	CARBS	SUGARS	SALT	FIBRE
396kcal	14.7g	5.5g	23.7g	46.8g	23.7g	1.5g	19.2g

Chicken, bean & rice bake — PAGE 210

ENERGY	FAT	SAT FAT	PROTEIN	CARBS	SUGARS	SALT	FIBRE
585kcal	22g	5.6g	32.5g	59.4g	13.3g	1g	16.4g

Veggie curry traybake — PAGE 212

ENERGY	FAT	SAT FAT	PROTEIN	CARBS	SUGARS	SALT	FIBRE
217kcal	11.1g	6g	7.1g	23.9g	15.3g	1.2g	9g

Chicken & mushroom hotpot — PAGE 214

ENERGY	FAT	SAT FAT	PROTEIN	CARBS	SUGARS	SALT	FIBRE
600kcal	16.3g	5.2g	30.7g	83.7g	21.5g	1.6g	12.3g

Spring soup & ricotta toasts — PAGE 218

ENERGY	FAT	SAT FAT	PROTEIN	CARBS	SUGARS	SALT	FIBRE
396kcal	20.1g	5.3g	19.9g	33.3g	6.3g	0.9g	12.5g

Spiced lamb & lentil soup — PAGE 220

ENERGY	FAT	SAT FAT	PROTEIN	CARBS	SUGARS	SALT	FIBRE
550kcal	15g	5.2g	38.2g	68.2g	12.3g	1.8g	9.7g

Golden hasselback salmon — PAGE 222

ENERGY	FAT	SAT FAT	PROTEIN	CARBS	SUGARS	SALT	FIBRE
529kcal	25.1g	4.6g	44.6g	30.6g	7.1g	1.1g	7.4g

Healthy fish & chips — PAGE 224

ENERGY	FAT	SAT FAT	PROTEIN	CARBS	SUGARS	SALT	FIBRE
586kcal	9.2g	2g	41.6g	84.9g	14.8g	1.8g	15.6g

Fish filo parcel & beans — PAGE 226

ENERGY	FAT	SAT FAT	PROTEIN	CARBS	SUGARS	SALT	FIBRE
465kcal	11.9g	3g	42.5g	46.3g	8.1g	1.6g	12.9g

Fish pie soup & eggs on toast — PAGE 228

ENERGY	FAT	SAT FAT	PROTEIN	CARBS	SUGARS	SALT	FIBRE
435kcal	13.7g	4.7g	29.4g	50.6g	12.7g	1.8g	5.3g

Crispy steamed veggie buns — PAGE 230

ENERGY	FAT	SAT FAT	PROTEIN	CARBS	SUGARS	SALT	FIBRE
600kcal	9.9g	2.2g	19.6g	117.6g	15.6g	1.8g	8.9g

Comforting chickpea soup — PAGE 232

ENERGY	FAT	SAT FAT	PROTEIN	CARBS	SUGARS	SALT	FIBRE
442kcal	16g	5.9g	20.4g	56.3g	13.9g	0.5g	12.8g

Winter squash & borlotti soup — PAGE 234

ENERGY	FAT	SAT FAT	PROTEIN	CARBS	SUGARS	SALT	FIBRE
454kcal	11.1g	2.4g	21.9g	69.1g	20.1g	1.8g	19.8g

Fragrant veggie filo tart — PAGE 236

ENERGY	FAT	SAT FAT	PROTEIN	CARBS	SUGARS	SALT	FIBRE
475kcal	15.6g	5.5g	15.9g	72.6g	24.8g	1.8g	10.6g

Mushroom riso soup — PAGE 238

ENERGY	FAT	SAT FAT	PROTEIN	CARBS	SUGARS	SALT	FIBRE
554kcal	22.1g	5.1g	14g	79.6g	9.8g	1.4g	6.9g

Sumptuous squash risotto — PAGE 240

ENERGY	FAT	SAT FAT	PROTEIN	CARBS	SUGARS	SALT	FIBRE
588kcal	13.3g	4.3g	16.6g	107.5g	22.5g	1.6g	7.6g

Happy fish pie — PAGE 242

ENERGY	FAT	SAT FAT	PROTEIN	CARBS	SUGARS	SALT	FIBRE
481kcal	13.4g	5.2g	42.8g	50.4g	10.4g	0.8g	6g

Meatball traybake — PAGE 244

ENERGY	FAT	SAT FAT	PROTEIN	CARBS	SUGARS	SALT	FIBRE
441kcal	18.1g	5.3g	33g	36.4g	19.7g	1.3g	13.3g

Hearty veg casserole — PAGE 246

ENERGY	FAT	SAT FAT	PROTEIN	CARBS	SUGARS	SALT	FIBRE
318kcal	7.2g	2.4g	11.4g	56g	35.2g	0.9g	12g

Chipotle chicken & bean soup — PAGE 248

ENERGY	FAT	SAT FAT	PROTEIN	CARBS	SUGARS	SALT	FIBRE
460kcal	19.6g	5g	31.6g	41g	19.2g	1.2g	13.2g

Roast chicken & sticky spuds — PAGE 250

ENERGY	FAT	SAT FAT	PROTEIN	CARBS	SUGARS	SALT	FIBRE
400kcal	15.6g	3.5g	14.2g	54.7g	11.2g	1.4g	9g

Beef & borlotti bean ragù — PAGE 25

ENERGY	FAT	SAT FAT	PROTEIN	CARBS	SUGARS	SALT	FIBRE
371kcal	17.4g	6g	25.6g	29.6g	15.6g	0.8g	11.4g

Cheat's soft-service ice cream — PAGE 25

ENERGY	FAT	SAT FAT	PROTEIN	CARBS	SUGARS	SALT	FIBRE
143kcal	5.8g	2.1g	3.4g	20.7g	19.1g	0g	3.9g

Blackberry smoothie lollies — PAGE 26

ENERGY	FAT	SAT FAT	PROTEIN	CARBS	SUGARS	SALT	FIBRE
92kcal	4.3g	2g	3.6g	9.9g	9.5g	0g	1g

Hot carrot cup cakes PAGE 262

ENERGY	FAT	SAT FAT	PROTEIN	CARBS	SUGARS	SALT	FIBRE
230kcal	8.3g	1.6g	8.3g	30.6g	11.8g	0.4g	2.3g

Chocolate orange pots PAGE 264

ENERGY	FAT	SAT FAT	PROTEIN	CARBS	SUGARS	SALT	FIBRE
142kcal	6.6g	1.8g	8.4g	13.1g	12.2g	0g	0.3g

Tahini pretzel yoghurt bark PAGE 266

ENERGY	FAT	SAT FAT	PROTEIN	CARBS	SUGARS	SALT	FIBRE
93kcal	4.2g	2g	2.4g	11.3g	9.2g	0.1g	0.7g

Fizzy berry jellies PAGE 268

ENERGY	FAT	SAT FAT	PROTEIN	CARBS	SUGARS	SALT	FIBRE
217kcal	3g	1.3g	9.4g	39.4g	27.4g	0.1g	6.2g

Choccy fro-yo sandwiches PAGE 270

ENERGY	FAT	SAT FAT	PROTEIN	CARBS	SUGARS	SALT	FIBRE
100kcal	4.6g	2g	3.1g	12.3g	4.8g	0.3g	1.2g

Oaty balls: Almond, apricot & choc PAGE 272

ENERGY	FAT	SAT FAT	PROTEIN	CARBS	SUGARS	SALT	FIBRE
63kcal	3.7g	1.2g	1.7g	6.4g	3.1g	0g	1.4g

Oaty balls: Mango, coconut & vanilla PAGE 272

ENERGY	FAT	SAT FAT	PROTEIN	CARBS	SUGARS	SALT	FIBRE
94kcal	4.2g	1.4g	1.8g	12.9g	7.7g	0.9g	0g

Strawberry filo tarts PAGE 274

ENERGY	FAT	SAT FAT	PROTEIN	CARBS	SUGARS	SALT	FIBRE
243kcal	8.6g	1.4g	7.6g	34.4g	9.3g	0.2g	4g

Blueberry muffins PAGE 276

ENERGY	FAT	SAT FAT	PROTEIN	CARBS	SUGARS	SALT	FIBRE
200kcal	9.4g	1.9g	4.8g	25.8g	9.5g	0.4g	1.5g

Mini protein bars PAGE 278

ENERGY	FAT	SAT FAT	PROTEIN	CARBS	SUGARS	SALT	FIBRE
173kcal	8.6g	2.5g	5.1g	19.4g	6.9g	0.1g	3.8g

Banana & almond cake PAGE 280

ENERGY	FAT	SAT FAT	PROTEIN	CARBS	SUGARS	SALT	FIBRE
216kcal	13.9g	1.6g	6.5g	19.3g	13.9g	0.2g	3.3g

Morning kickstarter PAGE 286

ENERGY	FAT	SAT FAT	PROTEIN	CARBS	SUGARS	SALT	FIBRE
14kcal	0.4g	0.1g	0.6g	2g	0.4g	0g	0.8g

Green goddess smoothie PAGE 288

ENERGY	FAT	SAT FAT	PROTEIN	CARBS	SUGARS	SALT	FIBRE
171kcal	10.8g	1.9g	3.8g	16.1g	13.1g	0.1g	2g

Merry berry smoothie PAGE 289

ENERGY	FAT	SAT FAT	PROTEIN	CARBS	SUGARS	SALT	FIBRE
217kcal	8.8g	1g	7.3g	27.7g	6.3g	0g	10.5g

Post-workout protein smoothie PAGE 290

ENERGY	FAT	SAT FAT	PROTEIN	CARBS	SUGARS	SALT	FIBRE
374kcal	5.6g	2.5g	25.1g	59.4g	36.5g	0.8g	3.5g

Matcha & kefir smoothie PAGE 291

ENERGY	FAT	SAT FAT	PROTEIN	CARBS	SUGARS	SALT	FIBRE
40kcal	2.1g	0.2g	1.8g	1.8g	0.3g	0.2g	1.8g

Whipped coffee PAGE 292

ENERGY	FAT	SAT FAT	PROTEIN	CARBS	SUGARS	SALT	FIBRE
107kcal	3.4g	2.1g	7g	13.2g	13.2g	0.2g	0g

Gennaro's coffee PAGE 293

ENERGY	FAT	SAT FAT	PROTEIN	CARBS	SUGARS	SALT	FIBRE
1kcal	0g	0g	0.1g	0.1g	0g	0g	0.2g

A big happy

I mentioned in the introduction to this book that I now have more than 25 years of publishing under my belt, and that's something that I've never taken for granted. Writing cookbooks, sharing inspiration and arming readers with food knowledge is something I love to do, and I remain ever so grateful that this is such a big part of my day job. Over the years, I've been supported by a great many people in the creation of my books, and many of those people you'll see the names of year after year on these thanks pages. I'm lucky enough to have an amazing core team that have been with me for most of the journey, but to also have new faces constantly joining the ranks, bringing with them fresh influences and ideas. I've always believed that it's the people you surround yourself with that are key to your success, and to the people listed here, and those that have helped me along the way, I extend a sincere and heartfelt thank you to each and every one of you.

The true backbone of my team, and the people that help me to live and breathe food, from educating me about new trends and ingredients, to helping me develop, test and finesse recipes, are my food team. At the heart of that team is Ginny Rolfe, my food sister, and the best in the business. Surrounded by a wonderfully talented bunch, including Joss Herd, Anna Helm Baxter, Rachel Young, Ben Slater, my sidekick Hugo Harrison and Sharon Sharpe, this is a group of people that I love to work with on a daily basis. Their lives are organized by Laura McLeish and Rebecca Wheeldon, so thank you, ladies, for that! Big love, as always, to the one and only Pete Begg, and the ever-young Bobby Sebire, two old-timers that are integral to what I do. We also work with some very special freelancers, and on this book that's Isla Murray, Maddie Rix, Fran Paling, Eliot Bourke and Johnny Guselli.

Stepping up and really leading the charge on the nutrition front with grace and patience is my Senior Nutritionist Rozzie Batchelar. And keeping things in check when it comes to food safety, standards, farming and ethics: Lucinda Cobb.

Supporting me on the words, and making sure everything is as clear as can be, is my Editor-in-Chief Rebecca Verity. In turn, she's supported by brilliant Jade 'pie barm pey wet' Melling, the rock of testing, Ruth Tebby, and the rest of the lovely editorial team.

Bringing the design vibes, and helping me to personify health in the look and feel of these pages, is my stylish Creative Director James Verity, supported by lovely Davina Mistry and the rest of the brilliant design team.

Making my recipes come to life with optimism and clarity is my dear chum, photographer Lord David Loftus, and his stoic sidekick Richard Bowyer. And on the portraits, Paul Stuart has utilized his degree very well again, supported by his main man Henry Hewitt.

thank you

Over at my publishers, the illustrious Penguin Random House, there is an army of people to thank, each with their own talent and specialism. I don't have space to give you that detail here, but I'm sure you can hunt it out if you're interested. To the main man, and a dear friend and kind fellow, Mr Tom Weldon, thank you. To the ever-enchanting Louise Moore, Elizabeth Smith, Clare Parker, Tom Troughton, Rebecca Ogden, Juliette Butler, Katherine Tibbals, Lee Motley, Sarah Fraser and Nick Lowndes. To Christina Ellicott, Bronwen Davies, Kelly Mason, Emma Carter, Hannah Padgham, Chris Wyatt and Tracy Orchard. To Chantal Noel, Anjali Nathani, Kate Reiners, Tyra Burr, Joanna Whitehead, Agnes Watters, Lee-Anne Williams, Jessica Meredeen, Danielle Appleton, Grace Dellar, Sally Hargrave, Stuart Anderson, Anna Curvis, Akua Akowuah, Caroline Newbury, Richard Rowlands and Carrie Anderson. And to the legend that is Annie Lee, as well as Alex Newby, Jill Cole and Ruth Ellis.

Back at JO HQ, there is a mighty team of dedicated people that make walking into our offices a complete joy. They work across such a multitude of projects, and do so with continued enthusiasm and energy. Name-checking those that directly worked on the book, a big thank you to the marketing team, particularly Rosalind Godber and Clare Duffy. To comms slay queens Tamsyn Zeitsman and Lydia Waller. To Rich Herd and the VPU, to Letitia Becher and her social crew, to Pamela Lovelock, Therese MacDermott and my rock John Dewar, and to Timiko Cranwell and the legal team. Special shout-outs are needed for three strong and brilliant women, my Deputy Louise Holland, Media MD Zoe Collins, and my EA Ali Solway.

Love, respect and appreciation for my loyal team of office testers, who take these recipes home to cook in their own kitchens, and send me useful feedback that helps me make those recipes even better for you.

On the TV front, there is a cracking series to accompany this book, and I know you're going to love it. Thank you to all the brilliant crew that worked on that, but in particular my HQ heroes Sean Moxhay, Sam Beddoes and Katie Millard. Big love to Katy Hall and Niall Downing, and to Emma Kozlowski, Renzo Luzardo, Emma Parkin and Prarthana Peterarulthas. Tobie Tripp, talented musical composer and friend, thank you as ever. I continue to have lots of love for the team at Channel 4, and at Fremantle. Thank you guys for all you do.

To Julia Bell and Lima O'Donnell, I'm ever so grateful for you, as always.

And to the people that truly make me happy, meaning you're all ever so good for my health. All my love goes to my gorgeous wife Jools, my five beautiful children, who I'm ever so proud of, Poppy, Daisy, Petal, Buddy and River. To my Mum and Dad, my inspiration and my grounding, to the rest of the fam and, of course, the one, the only, the don, Mr Gennaro Contaldo.

Index

Recipes marked V are suitable for vegetarians; in some instances you'll need to swap in a vegetarian alternative to cheese such as Parmesan.

A

almond, apricot & choc oaty fridge balls	V	272
almond butter		
5-minute tasty toppers	V	36
merry berry smoothie	V	289
almonds		
almond, apricot & choc oaty fridge balls	V	272
banana & almond cake	V	280
berry cheesecake oats	V	49
carrot gazpacho	V	104
cherry Bakewell overnight oats	V	48
speedy kedgeree		74
anchovies		
5-minute tasty toppers		36
crispy bean & anchovy eggs		112
golden hasselback salmon		222
apples		
5-minute tasty toppers	V	36
box grater fruit salad	V	38
cheat's bircher muesli	V	34
creamy walnut coleslaw	V	76
crispy mackerel buns		126
mothership overnight oats	V	46–9
smashed salad	V	114
speedy stuffed apple	V	44
apricots		
almond, apricot & choc oaty fridge balls	V	272
fragrant veggie filo tart	V	236
granola fruit cups	V	66
harissa tuna bean parcels		206
hearty veg casserole	V	246
hot carrot cup cakes	V	262
roasted veg & chickpea smash	V	198
artichoke hearts: spring soup & ricotta toasts	V	218
asparagus		
crab spaghetti		184
fluffy spring veg omelette	V	102
green veg megamix	V	142
peasto chicken salad		180
sesame miso shred salad	V	96
speedy silky omelette	V	84
steak & sticky aubergine salad		166
super-green stir-fry	V	132
aubergines		
aubergine involtini	V	208
fragrant veggie filo tart	V	236
roasted Mediterranean veg	V	204
silky aubergine flavour fest	V	194
steak & sticky aubergine salad		166
veggie curry traybake	V	212
avocados		
5-minute tasty toppers		36
avo & black bean omelette	V	122
black bean houmous salad wrap	V	98
charred Mexican salad	V	146
chipotle chicken & bean soup		248
chopped rainbow salad	V	90
crispy sardine & avo wrap		88
green goddess smoothie	V	288
vibrant veg & creamy bean salad	V	186

B

baby corn		
super-green stir-fry	V	132
sweet & sour prawns		138
balsamic vinegar		
cheesy beans on toast	V	62
golden cheese & jammy berries		52
pea & feta egg warm salad	V	106
roasted Mediterranean veg	V	204
strawberry filo tarts	V	274
warm lentil salad	V	78
bananas		
5-minute tasty toppers	V	36
banana & almond cake	V	280
blackberry smoothie lollies	V	260
blueberry muffins	V	276
box grater fruit salad	V	38
cheat's soft-serve ice cream	V	258
extraordinary brekkie smush-in	V	56
frosty porridge	V	40
green goddess smoothie	V	288
hot carrot cup cakes	V	262
mini protein bars	V	278
mothership overnight oats	V	46–9
nutty banana oats	V	34
post-workout protein smoothie	V	290
speedy stuffed apple	V	44
batch-it-up protein rolls	V	68
beans		
aubergine involtini	V	208
avo & black bean omelette	V	122
beef & borlotti bean ragù		252–5
black bean houmous salad wrap	V	98
charred Mexican salad	V	146
cheesy beans on toast	V	
chicken & mushroom hotpot		214
chicken, bean & rice bake		210
chicken curry & chapati	V	202
chipotle chicken & bean soup		248
crispy bean & anchovy eggs		112
crispy black bean beef		162
crispy pork noodle broth		150
easy egg & bean filo twists	V	64
fish filo parcel & beans		226
fish in crazy water		188
green veg megamix	V	142
harissa tuna bean parcels		206
lemon tahini chicken & grains		158
meatball traybake		244
mushroom stew		200
peasto chicken salad		180
sardines on toast & tomato salad		94
silken tofu & black beans	V	152
smashed flatbread burger		130
soy eggs & crispy mackerel rice		108

speedy silky omelette	V	84	Bombay mix			
spring soup & ricotta toasts	V	218	curried egg & rice pots	V	118	
tahini mushroom noodles	V	144	easy prawn curry		134	
tasty salmon couscous		148	silky aubergine flavour fest	V	194	
Thai-style fish curry		140	borlotti beans			
vibrant veg & creamy bean salad	V	186	aubergine involtini	V	208	
winter squash & borlotti soup	V	234	beef & borlotti bean ragù		252–5	
beansprouts			winter squash & borlotti soup	V	234	
mushroom stew		200	box grater fruit salad	V	38	
super-green stir-fry	V	132	bread			
beef			5-minute tasty toppers	V		
beef & borlotti bean ragù		252–5	batch-it-up protein rolls	V	68	
crispy black bean beef		162	beef & borlotti bean ragù		252–5	
meatball traybake		244	carrot gazpacho	V	104	
smashed flatbread burger		130	cheesy beans on toast	V		
steak & sticky aubergine salad		166	chicken curry & chapati	V	202	
beetroot			crispy mackerel buns		126	
boiled egg fridge stash	V	101	extraordinary brekkie smush-in	V	56	
salmon, beet & potato salad		92	fish in crazy water		188	
smashed salad	V	114	fish pie soup & eggs on toast		228	
berries			fluffy spring veg omelette	V	102	
5-minute tasty toppers	V	36	golden cheese & jammy berries		52	
berry cheesecake overnight oats	V	49	sardines on toast & tomato salad		94	
blackberry smoothie lollies	V	260	smashed flatbread burger		130	
blueberry muffins	V	276	smoked salmon & rye omelette		42	
cheat's soft-serve ice cream	V	258	spinach & lentil fritter salad	V	170	
cheesy beans on toast	V		spring soup & ricotta toasts	V	218	
chicken & berry grain bowl		182	super-green orecchiette	V	190	
choccy fro-yo sandwiches	V	270	vibrant veg & creamy bean salad	V	186	
chocolate orange pots	V	264	winter squash & borlotti soup	V	234	
extraordinary brekkie smush-in	V	56	see also tortillas			
fizzy berry jellies		268	broad beans			
fresh infused waters	V	285	peasto chicken salad		180	
frosty porridge	V	40	seared tuna kimchi bowl		156	
golden cheese & jammy berries		52	soy eggs & crispy mackerel rice		108	
merry berry smoothie	V	289	spring soup & ricotta toasts	V	218	
peach melba overnight oats	V	48	tasty salmon couscous		148	
pink Shredded Wheat	V	34	broccoli			
spinach & lentil fritter salad	V	170	golden chicken, peppers & rice		160	
strawberry filo tarts	V	274	green veg megamix	V	142	
vibrant veg & creamy bean salad	V	186	happy fish pie		242	
berry cheesecake overnight oats	V	49	lemon tahini chicken & grains		158	
bircher muesli, cheat's	V	34	roasted veg & chickpea smash	V	198	
black bean houmous salad wrap	V	98	soy eggs & crispy mackerel rice		108	
black bean sauce			super-green orecchiette	V	190	
crispy black bean beef		162	super-green stir-fry	V	132	
silken tofu & black beans	V	152	tuna & broccoli pasta		120	
black beans			Brussels sprouts			
avo & black bean omelette	V	122	green veg megamix	V	142	
black bean houmous salad wrap	V	98	roasted veg & chickpea smash	V	198	
charred Mexican salad	V	146	butter beans			
mushroom stew		200	cheesy beans on toast	V	62	
silken tofu & black beans	V	152	chicken curry & chapati	V	202	
blackberries			chipotle chicken & bean soup		248	
5-minute tasty toppers	V	36	crispy bean & anchovy eggs		112	
blackberry smoothie lollies	V	260	vibrant veg & creamy bean salad	V	186	
blueberries			butternut squash see squash			
berry cheesecake overnight oats	V	49				
blueberry muffins	V	276	**c**			
chicken & berry grain bowl		182				
fizzy berry jellies		268	cabbage			
fresh infused waters	V	285	boiled egg fridge stash	V	101	
vibrant veg & creamy bean salad	V	186	charred Mexican salad	V	146	
boiled egg fridge stash	V	101	creamy walnut coleslaw	V	76	

crispy sardine & avo wrap		88	
green veg megamix	V	142	
sesame miso shred salad	V	96	
sweet & sour prawns		138	
cake: banana & almond cake	V	280	
cannellini beans			
chicken & mushroom hotpot		214	
chicken, bean & rice bake		210	
fish filo parcel & beans		226	
fish in crazy water		188	
harissa tuna bean parcels		206	
lemon tahini chicken & grains		158	
meatball traybake		244	
sardines on toast & tomato salad		94	
smashed flatbread burger		130	
speedy silky omelette	V	84	
capers			
aubergine involtini	V	208	
tuna & broccoli pasta		120	
carrots			
5-minute tasty toppers	V	36	
beef & borlotti bean ragù		252–5	
carrot & sweet potato fritters	V	124	
carrot gazpacho	V	104	
chicken & mushroom hotpot		214	
chipotle chicken & bean soup		248	
creamy walnut coleslaw	V	76	
crispy mackerel buns		126	
crispy steamed veggie buns	V	230	
curried fried eggs & grain salad	V	82	
fish pie soup & eggs on toast		228	
gochujang tomato noodle soup	V	196	
harissa tuna bean parcels		206	
harissa tuna platter		80	
herby chickpea & feta salad	V	116	
hot carrot cup cakes	V	262	
meatball traybake		244	
mushroom riso soup	V	238	
mushroom stew		200	
roasted veg & chickpea smash	V	198	
seared tuna kimchi bowl		156	
sesame miso shred salad	V	96	
smashed salad	V	114	
spiced lamb & lentil soup		220	
winter squash & borlotti soup	V	234	
cashew nut butter: green goddess smoothie	V	288	
cashew nuts			
crispy steamed veggie buns	V	230	
super-green stir-fry	V	132	
cauliflower			
chicken in milk		176	
comforting chickpea soup	V	232	
roasted veg & chickpea smash	V	198	
veggie curry traybake	V	212	
celeriac			
creamy walnut coleslaw	V	76	
roast chicken & sticky spuds		250	
celery			
beef & borlotti bean ragù		252–5	
carrot gazpacho	V	104	
chicken, bean & rice bake		210	
chipotle chicken & bean soup		248	
mushroom riso soup	V	238	
sumptuous squash risotto	V	240	
winter squash & borlotti soup	V	234	
cereal, super-charged	V	34	
chapatis: chicken curry & chapati		202	
chard: roast chicken & sticky spuds		250	
charred Mexican salad	V	146	
cheat's bircher muesli	V	34	
cheat's soft-serve ice cream	V	258	
cheese			
5-minute tasty toppers	V	36	
aubergine involtini	V	208	
black bean houmous salad wrap	V	98	
carrot & sweet potato fritters	V	124	
carrot gazpacho	V	104	
charred Mexican salad	V	146	
cheesy beans on toast	V	62	
chicken & berry grain bowl		182	
chickpea arrabbiata	V	110	
crispy bean & anchovy eggs		112	
easy egg & bean filo twists	V	64	
fish parcels & tomato orzo		192	
fragrant veggie filo tart	V	236	
golden cheese & jammy berries	V	52	
golden chicken, peppers & rice		160	
happy fish pie		242	
hearty veg casserole	V	246	
herby chickpea & feta salad	V	116	
meatball traybake		244	
mushroom riso soup	V	238	
one-cup pancakes	V	58–61	
pea & feta egg warm salad	V	106	
peasto chicken salad		180	
smashed flatbread burger		130	
smashed salad	V	114	
speedy silky omelette	V	84	
spinach & lentil fritter salad	V	170	
spring soup & ricotta toasts	V	218	
sumptuous squash risotto	V	240	
super-green orecchiette	V	190	
vibrant veg & creamy bean salad	V	186	
warm lentil salad	V	78	
winter squash & borlotti soup	V	234	
see also cottage cheese			
cheesy beans on toast	V	62	
cherries			
cherry Bakewell overnight oats	V	48	
chocolate orange pots	V	264	
chestnuts: sumptuous squash risotto	V	240	
chia seeds			
cheat's bircher muesli	V	34	
merry berry smoothie	V	289	
mini protein bars	V	278	
chicken			
chicken & berry grain bowl		182	
chicken & mushroom hotpot		214	
chicken balls & rainbow broth		168	
chicken, bean & rice bake		210	
chicken cup salad		164	
chicken curry & chapati		202	
chicken fajitas		154	
chicken in milk		176	
chipotle chicken & bean soup		248	
creamy peanut chicken		136	
golden chicken, peppers & rice		160	
lemon tahini chicken & grains		158	

peasto chicken salad		180
roast chicken & sticky spuds		250
chickpeas		
carrot & sweet potato fritters	V	124
chickpea arrabbiata	V	110
chopped rainbow salad	V	90
comforting chickpea soup	V	232
curried egg & rice pots	V	118
easy prawn curry		134
golden hasselback salmon		222
healthy fish & chips		224
herby chickpea & feta salad	V	116
roasted veg & chickpea smash	V	198
silky aubergine flavour fest	V	194
chillies		
cheesy beans on toast	V	62
chicken balls & rainbow broth		168
chickpea arrabbiata	V	110
crispy black bean beef		162
crispy sardine & avo wrap		88
curried fried eggs & grain salad	V	82
dukkah poached eggs	V	54
fish in crazy water		188
fish parcels & tomato orzo		192
herby chickpea & feta salad	V	116
sardines on toast & tomato salad		94
sesame miso shred salad	V	96
silken tofu & black beans	V	152
soy eggs & crispy mackerel rice		108
super-green stir-fry	V	132
tasty salmon couscous		148
Thai-style fish curry		140
tuna & broccoli pasta		120
chipotle chicken & bean soup		248
choccy fro-yo sandwiches	V	270
chocolate		
almond, apricot & choc oaty fridge balls	V	272
blackberry smoothie lollies	V	260
choccy fro-yo sandwiches	V	270
chocolate orange pots	V	264
fizzy berry jellies		268
mini protein bars	V	278
tahini pretzel yoghurt bark	V	266
chopped rainbow salad	V	90
clementine: harissa tuna platter		80
cocoa powder		
almond, apricot & choc oaty fridge balls	V	272
chocolate orange pots	V	264
extraordinary brekkie smush-in	V	56
nutty banana oats	V	34
post-workout protein smoothie	V	290
speedy stuffed apple	V	44
tiramisù overnight oats	V	49
coconut cream: comforting chickpea soup	V	232
coconut, creamed: easy prawn curry		134
coconut, desiccated		
5-minute tasty toppers	V	36
blackberry smoothie lollies	V	260
chicken curry & chapati	V	202
mango, coconut & vanilla oaty fridge balls	V	272
piña colada muesli	V	34
coconut milk		
Thai-style fish curry		140
veggie curry traybake	V	212
coconut water: green goddess smoothie	V	288
coffee		
Gennaro's coffee	V	293
tiramisù overnight oats	V	49
whipped coffee	V	292
comforting chickpea soup	V	232
cottage cheese		
5-minute tasty toppers	V	36
avo & black bean omelette	V	122
batch-it-up protein rolls	V	68
crispy sardine & avo wrap		88
fluffy spring veg omelette	V	102
peasto chicken salad		180
post-workout protein smoothie	V	290
smoked salmon & rye omelette		42
sumptuous squash risotto	V	240
super-green orecchiette	V	190
courgettes		
fish in crazy water		188
fish parcels & tomato orzo		192
hearty veg casserole	V	246
herby chickpea & feta salad	V	116
roasted Mediterranean veg	V	204
tasty salmon couscous		148
couscous		
fragrant veggie filo tart	V	236
golden hasselback salmon		222
herby chickpea & feta salad	V	116
tasty salmon couscous		148
crab spaghetti		184
cranberries: merry berry smoothie	V	289
cream cheese: tasty topper	V	36
creamy peanut chicken		136
creamy walnut coleslaw	V	76
crispy bean & anchovy eggs		112
crispy black bean beef		162
crispy mackerel buns		126
crispy pork noodle broth		150
crispy sardine & avo wrap		88
crispy steamed veggie buns	V	230
crispy steamy parcels		178
cucumber		
carrot gazpacho	V	104
charred Mexican salad	V	146
chopped rainbow salad	V	90
crispy bean & anchovy eggs		112
crispy pork noodle broth		150
harissa tuna bean parcels		206
prawn cocktail for one		72
salmon, beet & potato salad		92
seared tuna kimchi bowl		156
smashed salad	V	114
steak & sticky aubergine salad		166
curried egg & rice pots	V	118
curried fried eggs & grain salad	V	82
curry		
chicken curry & chapati		202
easy prawn curry		134
Thai-style fish curry		140
veggie curry traybake	V	212
curry paste		
chicken curry & chapati		202
comforting chickpea soup	V	232
easy prawn curry		134

healthy fish & chips		224
speedy kedgeree		74
Thai-style fish curry		140
veggie curry traybake	V	212
curry powder		
curried egg & rice pots	V	118
curried fried eggs & grain salad	V	82
spiced lamb & lentil soup		220

D

dates		
box grater fruit salad	V	38
chocolate orange pots	V	264
extraordinary brekkie smush-in	V	56
mini protein bars	V	278
nutty banana oats	V	34
oaty fridge balls: 2 tasty ways	V	272
post-workout protein smoothie	V	290
speedy stuffed apple	V	44
tahini pretzel yoghurt bark	V	266
dukkah		
5-minute tasty toppers	V	36
black bean houmous salad wrap	V	98
dukkah poached eggs	V	54

E

easy egg & bean filo twists	V	64
easy prawn curry		134
edamame beans		
crispy black bean beef		162
crispy pork noodle broth		150
green veg megamix	V	142
soy eggs & crispy mackerel rice		108
tahini mushroom noodles	V	144
Thai-style fish curry		140
eggs		
avo & black bean omelette	V	122
banana & almond cake	V	280
batch-it-up protein rolls	V	68
blueberry muffins	V	276
boiled egg fridge stash	V	101
carrot & sweet potato fritters	V	124
crispy bean & anchovy eggs		112
curried egg & rice pots	V	118
curried fried eggs & grain salad	V	82
dukkah poached eggs	V	54
easy egg & bean filo twists	V	64
fish pie soup & eggs on toast		228
fluffy spring veg omelette	V	102
happy fish pie		242
hot carrot cup cakes	V	262
one-cup pancakes	V	58–61
pea & feta egg warm salad	V	106
seared salmon rice		174
smoked salmon & rye omelette		42
soy eggs & crispy mackerel rice		108
speedy kedgeree		74
speedy silky omelette	V	84
spicy tofu & sweet pepper eggs	V	50
spinach & lentil fritter salad	V	170
elderflower cordial: fizzy berry jellies		268
extraordinary brekkie smush-in	V	56

F

fennel		
fragrant veggie filo tart	V	236
harissa tuna platter		80
hearty veg casserole	V	246
meatball traybake		244
sardines on toast & tomato salad		94
vibrant veg & creamy bean salad	V	186
feta cheese		
black bean houmous salad wrap	V	98
carrot & sweet potato fritters	V	124
carrot gazpacho	V	104
charred Mexican salad	V	146
chicken & berry grain bowl		182
crispy bean & anchovy eggs		112
fragrant veggie filo tart	V	236
golden chicken, peppers & rice		160
hearty veg casserole	V	246
herby chickpea & feta salad	V	116
meatball traybake		244
one-cup pancakes	V	58–61
pea & feta egg warm salad	V	106
smashed salad	V	114
filo pastry		
beef & borlotti bean ragù		252–5
easy egg & bean filo twists	V	64
fish filo parcel & beans		226
fragrant veggie filo tart	V	236
harissa tuna bean parcels		206
fish		
5-minute tasty toppers		36
crispy bean & anchovy eggs		112
crispy mackerel buns		126
crispy sardine & avo wrap		88
fish filo parcel & beans		226
fish in crazy water		188
fish parcels & tomato orzo		192
fish pie soup & eggs on toast		228
freeze your fish		173
golden hasselback salmon		222
happy fish pie		242
harissa tuna bean parcels		206
harissa tuna platter		80
healthy fish & chips		224
salmon, beet & potato salad		92
sardines on toast & tomato salad		94
seared salmon rice		174
seared tuna kimchi bowl		156
smoked salmon & rye omelette		42
soy eggs & crispy mackerel rice		108
speedy kedgeree		74
tasty salmon couscous		148
Thai-style fish curry		140
tuna & broccoli pasta		120
5-minute tasty toppers	V	36
fizzy berry jellies		268
flaxseed, milled: blackberry smoothie lollies	V	260
fluffy spring veg omelette	V	102
fragrant veggie filo tart	V	236
fresh infused waters	V	284–5
frosty porridge	V	40

fruit
    box grater fruit salad 38
    granola fruit cups V 66
    one-cup pancakes V 58–61
        see also specific fruit

G

gazpacho, carrot V 104
Gennaro's coffee V 293
gherkins
    crispy mackerel buns 126
    healthy fish & chips 224
ginger
    chicken cup salad 164
    chicken curry & chapati V 202
    choccy fro-yo sandwiches V 270
    comforting chickpea soup V 232
    creamy peanut chicken 136
    crispy black bean beef 162
    crispy steamed veggie buns V 230
    fresh infused waters V 284
    hot carrot cup cakes V 262
    mushroom stew 200
    silken tofu & black beans V 152
    soy eggs & crispy mackerel rice 108
    steak & sticky aubergine salad 166
    super-green stir-fry V 132
ginger, ground
    granola fruit cups V 66
    morning kickstarter V 286
ginger, pickled
    chicken balls & rainbow broth 168
    crispy steamy parcels 178
    seared salmon rice 174
    Thai-style fish curry 140
gnocchi
    beef & borlotti bean ragù 252–5
    chicken & mushroom hotpot 214
goat's cheese
    spinach & lentil fritter salad V 170
    vibrant veg & creamy bean salad V 186
gochujang paste
    gochujang tomato noodle soup V 196
    mushroom stew 200
    steak & sticky aubergine salad 166
golden cheese & jammy berries V 52
golden chicken, peppers & rice 160
golden hasselback salmon 222
grains
    chicken & berry grain bowl 182
    curried fried eggs & grain salad V 82
    lemon tahini chicken & grains 158
    pea & feta egg warm salad V 106
granola fruit cups V 66
grapes: carrot gazpacho V 104
green goddess smoothie V 288
green veg megamix V 142

H

halloumi
    cheesy beans on toast V 62
    golden cheese & jammy berries V 52

happy fish pie 242
haricot beans: easy egg & bean filo twists 64
harissa paste
    5-minute tasty toppers V 36
    chicken, bean & rice bake 210
    easy egg & bean filo twists V 64
    fluffy spring veg omelette V 102
    golden chicken, peppers & rice 160
    golden hasselback salmon 222
    harissa tuna bean parcels 206
    harissa tuna platter 80
    roasted veg & chickpea smash V 198
hazelnuts: chocolate orange pots V 264
healthy fish & chips 224
hearty veg casserole V 246
herby chickpea & feta salad V 116
hoisin sauce
    crispy steamed veggie buns V 230
    green veg megamix V 142
honey
    5-minute tasty toppers V 36
    blueberry muffins V 276
    cheat's soft-serve ice cream V 258
    cheesy beans on toast V
    chicken fajitas 154
    frosty porridge V 40
    golden cheese & jammy berries 52
    tahini pretzel yoghurt bark V 266
    whipped coffee V 292
horseradish: crispy mackerel buns 126
hot carrot cup cakes V 262
hot-smoked trout: speedy kedgeree 74
houmous
    5-minute tasty toppers V 36
    black bean houmous salad wrap V 98
    carrot & sweet potato fritters V 124
    golden chicken, peppers & rice 160

I

ice cream: cheat's soft-serve ice cream V 258

J

jalapeños
    avo & black bean omelette V 122
    charred Mexican salad V 146
    prawn cocktail for one 72

K

kale: golden chicken, peppers & rice 160
kefir
    matcha & kefir smoothie V 291
    whipped coffee V 292
kimchi: seared tuna kimchi bowl 156

L

lamb: spiced lamb & lentil soup 220
leeks
    fish pie soup & eggs on toast 228
    happy fish pie 242
    spring soup & ricotta toasts V 218

lemon tahini chicken & grains		158
lemons		
5-minute tasty toppers		36
aubergine involtini	V	208
carrot & sweet potato fritters	V	124
chicken & berry grain bowl		182
chicken, bean & rice bake		210
chicken in milk		176
crab spaghetti		184
crispy bean & anchovy eggs		112
crispy mackerel buns		126
curried egg & rice pots	V	118
curried fried eggs & grain salad	V	82
dukkah poached eggs	V	54
fish filo parcel & beans		226
fish in crazy water		188
fish parcels & tomato orzo		192
fluffy spring veg omelette	V	102
freeze your fish		173
fresh infused waters	V	285
Gennaro's coffee	V	293
golden chicken, peppers & rice		160
golden hasselback salmon		222
green veg megamix	V	142
happy fish pie		242
harissa tuna bean parcels		206
harissa tuna platter		80
healthy fish & chips		224
herby chickpea & feta salad	V	116
lemon tahini chicken & grains		158
meatball traybake		244
morning kickstarter	V	286
mushroom riso soup	V	238
peasto chicken salad		180
prawn cocktail for one		72
roast chicken & sticky spuds		250
roasted veg & chickpea smash	V	198
salmon, beet & potato salad		92
seared salmon rice		174
seared tuna kimchi bowl		156
silky aubergine flavour fest	V	194
smoked salmon & rye omelette		42
speedy kedgeree		74
spicy tofu & sweet pepper eggs	V	50
spring soup & ricotta toasts	V	218
super-green orecchiette	V	190
tasty salmon couscous		148
tuna & broccoli pasta		120
veggie curry traybake	V	212
warm lentil salad	V	78
lentils		
chicken & berry grain bowl		182
spiced lamb & lentil soup		220
spinach & lentil fritter salad	V	170
warm lentil salad	V	78
lettuce		
chicken cup salad		164
chopped rainbow salad	V	90
curried fried eggs & grain salad	V	82
prawn cocktail for one		72
tahini mushroom noodles	V	144
warm lentil salad	V	78
lime pickle		
spiced lamb & lentil soup		220

veggie curry traybake	V	212
limes		
black bean houmous salad wrap	V	98
box grater fruit salad	V	38
charred Mexican salad	V	146
chicken balls & rainbow broth		168
chicken cup salad		164
chipotle chicken & bean soup		248
chopped rainbow salad	V	90
creamy peanut chicken		136
crispy sardine & avo wrap		88
crispy steamy parcels		178
fresh infused waters	V	285
green goddess smoothie	V	288
piña colada muesli	V	34
prawn & noodle salad		86
sesame miso shred salad	V	96
steak & sticky aubergine salad		166
sweet & sour prawns		138
tahini mushroom noodles	V	144
Thai-style fish curry		140
lollies, blackberry smoothie	V	260

M

mackerel		
5-minute tasty toppers		36
crispy mackerel buns		126
soy eggs & crispy mackerel rice		108
mangetout		
crispy black bean beef		162
green veg megamix	V	142
prawn & noodle salad		86
super-green stir-fry	V	132
sweet & sour prawns		138
mango		
box grater fruit salad	V	38
chicken cup salad		164
easy prawn curry		134
frosty porridge	V	40
prawn cocktail for one		72
mango chutney		
curried egg & rice pots	V	118
curried fried eggs & grain salad	V	82
silky aubergine flavour fest	V	194
mango, dried		
chopped rainbow salad	V	90
creamy peanut chicken		136
mango, coconut & vanilla oaty fridge balls	V	272
maple syrup		
banana & almond cake	V	280
granola fruit cups	V	66
mini protein bars	V	278
Marmite: batch-it-up protein rolls	V	68
matcha & kefir smoothie	V	291
meatball traybake		244
melon: box grater fruit salad	V	38
merry berry smoothie	V	289
milk		
cereal, super-charged	V	34
chicken & mushroom hotpot		214
chicken in milk		176
crispy steamed veggie buns	V	230
happy fish pie		242

merry berry smoothie	V	289	
mothership overnight oats	V	46	
one-cup pancakes	V	58–61	
post-workout protein smoothie	V	290	
mini protein bars	V	278	
miso			
chicken balls & rainbow broth		168	
crispy pork noodle broth		150	
sesame miso shred salad	V	96	
morning kickstarter	V	286	
mothership overnight oats	V	46–9	
mozzarella: warm lentil salad	V	78	
muesli			
cheat's bircher	V	34	
piña colada	V	34	
muffins, blueberry	V	276	
mushrooms			
chicken & mushroom hotpot		214	
chicken in milk		176	
chipotle chicken & bean soup		248	
crispy black bean beef		162	
crispy pork noodle broth		150	
mushroom riso soup	V	238	
mushroom stew	V	200	
spicy tofu & sweet pepper eggs	V	50	
super-green stir-fry	V	132	
tahini mushroom noodles	V	144	
winter squash & borlotti soup	V	234	
mustard			
chicken fajitas		154	
chicken in milk		176	
creamy walnut coleslaw	V	76	
fish filo parcel & beans		226	
fish pie soup & eggs on toast		228	
green veg megamix	V	142	
happy fish pie		242	
roast chicken & sticky spuds		250	
salmon, beet & potato salad		92	
spinach & lentil fritter salad	V	170	
vibrant veg & creamy bean salad	V	186	
warm lentil salad	V	78	

N

noodles			
chicken cup salad		164	
chicken in milk		176	
crispy black bean beef		162	
crispy pork noodle broth		150	
prawn & noodle salad		86	
steak & sticky aubergine salad		166	
sweet & sour prawns		138	
tahini mushroom noodles	V	144	
Thai-style fish curry		140	
nut butter			
5-minute tasty toppers	V	36	
granola fruit cups	V	66	
nuts			
5-minute tasty toppers	V	36	
almond, apricot & choc oaty fridge balls	V	272	
banana & almond cake	V	280	
batch-it-up protein rolls	V	68	
berry cheesecake overnight oats	V	49	
box grater fruit salad	V	38	

carrot gazpacho	V	104	
cherry Bakewell overnight oats	V	48	
chocolate orange pots	V	264	
creamy walnut coleslaw	V	76	
crispy steamed veggie buns	V	230	
granola fruit cups	V	66	
hot carrot cup cakes	V	262	
nutty banana oats	V	34	
peasto chicken salad		180	
pink Shredded Wheat	V	34	
silken tofu & black beans	V	152	
speedy kedgeree		74	
speedy stuffed apple	V	44	
spinach & lentil fritter salad	V	170	
strawberry filo tarts	V	274	
super-green stir-fry	V	132	
veggie curry traybake	V	212	
vibrant veg & creamy bean salad	V	186	
nutty banana oats	V	34	

O

oatcakes			
choccy fro-yo sandwiches	V	270	
harissa tuna platter		80	
oats			
blueberry muffins	V	276	
cheat's bircher muesli	V	34	
frosty porridge		40	
granola fruit cups	V	66	
merry berry smoothie	V	289	
mini protein bars	V	278	
mothership overnight oats	V	46–9	
nutty banana oats	V	34	
oaty fridge balls: 2 tasty ways	V	272	
post-workout protein smoothie	V	290	
oaty fridge balls: 2 tasty ways	V	272	
olives			
lemon tahini chicken & grains		158	
sardines on toast & tomato salad		94	
speedy silky omelette	V	84	
omelettes			
avo & black bean omelette	V	122	
fluffy spring veg omelette	V	102	
smoked salmon & rye omelette		42	
speedy silky omelette	V	84	
one-cup pancakes	V	58–61	
onions			
beef & borlotti bean ragù		252	
chicken & mushroom hotpot		214	
chicken, bean & rice bake		210	
chicken cup salad		164	
chicken curry & chapati	V	202	
chicken fajitas		154	
chipotle chicken & bean soup		248	
chopped rainbow salad	V	90	
comforting chickpea soup	V	232	
crab spaghetti		184	
creamy walnut coleslaw	V	76	
crispy bean & anchovy eggs		112	
easy prawn curry		134	
fish pie soup & eggs on toast		228	
fragrant veggie filo tart	V	236	
gochujang tomato noodle soup	V	196	

hearty veg casserole	V	246
meatball traybake		244
mushroom riso soup	V	238
roast chicken & sticky spuds		250
roasted Mediterranean veg	V	204
roasted veg & chickpea smash	V	198
sardines on toast & tomato salad		94
silken tofu & black beans	V	152
speedy kedgeree		74
spiced lamb & lentil soup		220
sumptuous squash risotto	V	240
veggie curry traybake	V	212
warm lentil salad	V	78
oranges		
cherry Bakewell overnight oats	V	48
chocolate orange pots	V	264
fizzy berry jellies		268
granola fruit cups	V	66
hot carrot cup cakes	V	262
strawberry filo tarts	V	274
super-green stir-fry	V	132
orzo: fish parcels & tomato orzo		192

P

pak choi		
green veg megamix	V	142
silken tofu & black beans	V	152
pancakes, one-cup	V	58–61
paneer cheese		
cheesy beans on toast	V	62
golden cheese & jammy berries	V	52
parsnips: beef & borlotti bean ragù		252–5
passata: chickpea arrabbiata	V	110
pasta		
chickpea arrabbiata	V	110
crab spaghetti		184
fish parcels & tomato orzo		192
super-green orecchiette	V	190
tuna & broccoli pasta		120
pea & feta egg warm salad	V	106
peaches		
box grater fruit salad	V	38
granola fruit cups	V	66
peach melba overnight oats	V	48
prawn & noodle salad		86
peanut & sesame chilli oil		
crispy pork noodle broth		150
prawn & noodle salad		86
spicy tofu & sweet pepper eggs	V	50
peanut butter		
cheat's soft-serve ice cream	V	258
creamy peanut chicken		136
extraordinary brekkie smush-in	V	56
mini protein bars	V	278
peanuts		
crispy steamed veggie buns	V	230
nutty banana oats	V	34
silken tofu & black beans	V	152
veggie curry traybake	V	212
pears		
box grater fruit salad	V	38
creamy walnut coleslaw	V	76

peas		
chicken & berry grain bowl		182
fish in crazy water		188
healthy fish & chips		224
pea & feta egg warm salad	V	106
peasto chicken salad		180
seared salmon rice		174
soy eggs & crispy mackerel rice		108
speedy kedgeree		74
spiced lamb & lentil soup		220
spring soup & ricotta toasts	V	218
super-green orecchiette	V	190
super-green stir-fry	V	132
peasto chicken salad		180
peppers		
5-minute tasty toppers	V	36
beef & borlotti bean ragù		252–5
charred Mexican salad	V	146
chicken, bean & rice bake		210
chicken fajitas		154
chopped rainbow salad	V	90
creamy peanut chicken		136
easy egg & bean filo twists	V	64
fish parcels & tomato orzo		192
golden chicken, peppers & rice		160
lemon tahini chicken & grains		158
meatball traybake		244
pea & feta egg warm salad	V	106
roasted Mediterranean veg	V	204
roasted veg & chickpea smash	V	198
sardines on toast & tomato salad		94
seared salmon rice		174
sesame miso shred salad	V	96
smashed salad	V	114
spicy tofu & sweet pepper eggs	V	50
pesto: smashed flatbread burger		130
pies		
beef & borlotti bean ragù		252–5
fish pie soup & eggs on toast		228
happy fish pie		242
piña colada muesli	V	34
pine nuts: peasto chicken salad		180
pineapple		
piña colada muesli	V	34
sweet & sour prawns		138
pink Shredded Wheat	V	34
pistachio nuts		
5-minute tasty toppers	V	36
strawberry filo tarts	V	274
pomegranate seeds		
chopped rainbow salad	V	90
silky aubergine flavour fest	V	194
poppadoms		
silky aubergine flavour fest	V	194
spiced lamb & lentil soup		220
pork		
crispy pork noodle broth		150
meatball traybake		244
smashed flatbread burger		130
porridge, frosty	V	40
post-workout protein smoothie	V	290
potatoes		
comforting chickpea soup	V	232
fish pie soup & eggs on toast		228

happy fish pie			242
hearty veg casserole	V		246
roast chicken & sticky spuds			250
salmon, beet & potato salad			92
prawns			
crispy steamy parcels			178
easy prawn curry			134
prawn & noodle salad			86
prawn cocktail for one			72
sweet & sour prawns			138
pretzels: tahini pretzel yoghurt bark	V		266

R

radishes			
black bean houmous salad wrap	V		98
chopped rainbow salad	V		90
smashed salad	V		114
tahini mushroom noodles	V		144
ras el hanout			
carrot & sweet potato fritters	V		124
chicken & berry grain bowl			182
fragrant veggie filo tart	V		236
hearty veg casserole	V		246
raspberries			
5-minute tasty toppers	V		36
choccy fro-yo sandwiches	V		270
chocolate orange pots	V		264
extraordinary brekkie smush-in	V		56
fizzy berry jellies			268
fresh infused waters	V		285
peach melba overnight oats	V		48
pink Shredded Wheat	V		34
spinach & lentil fritter salad	V		170
rice			
chicken balls & rainbow broth			168
chicken, bean & rice bake			210
curried egg & rice pots	V		118
easy prawn curry			134
golden chicken, peppers & rice			160
mushroom riso soup	V		238
seared salmon rice			174
seared tuna kimchi bowl			156
soy eggs & crispy mackerel rice			108
speedy kedgeree			74
sumptuous squash risotto	V		240
rice paper wrappers: crispy steamy parcels			178
ricotta cheese			
5-minute tasty toppers	V		36
aubergine involtini	V		208
spring soup & ricotta toasts	V		218
roast chicken & sticky spuds			250
roasted Mediterranean veg	V		204
roasted veg & chickpea smash	V		198
rocket: chickpea arrabbiata	V		110

S

salads			
black bean houmous salad wrap	V		98
charred Mexican salad	V		146
chicken & berry grain bowl			182
chicken cup salad			164
chopped rainbow salad	V		90
curried fried eggs & grain salad	V		82
harissa tuna platter			80
herby chickpea & feta salad	V		116
pea & feta egg warm salad	V		106
peasto chicken salad			180
prawn & noodle salad			86
prawn cocktail for one			72
salmon, beet & potato salad			92
sardines on toast & tomato salad			94
sesame miso shred salad	V		96
smashed salad	V		114
spinach & lentil fritter salad	V		170
steak & sticky aubergine salad			166
vibrant veg & creamy bean salad	V		186
warm lentil salad	V		78
salads, fruit: box grater fruit salad	V		38
salmon			
golden hasselback salmon			222
salmon, beet & potato salad			92
seared salmon rice			174
speedy kedgeree			74
tasty salmon couscous			148
sardines			
crispy sardine & avo wrap			88
sardines on toast & tomato salad			94
seared salmon rice			174
seared tuna kimchi bowl			156
seeds			
batch-it-up protein rolls	V		68
blackberry smoothie lollies	V		260
box grater fruit salad	V		38
crispy steamy parcels			178
easy egg & bean filo twists	V		64
extraordinary brekkie smush-in	V		56
frosty porridge	V		40
granola fruit cups	V		66
merry berry smoothie	V		289
mini protein bars	V		278
seared salmon rice			174
seared tuna kimchi bowl			156
sesame miso shred salad	V		96
smashed salad	V		114
speedy stuffed apple	V		44
sesame miso shred salad	V		96
sesame seeds			
crispy steamy parcels			178
easy egg & bean filo twists	V		64
seared salmon rice			174
seared tuna kimchi bowl			156
sesame miso shred salad	V		96
silken tofu & black beans	V		152
silky aubergine flavour fest	V		194
smashed flatbread burger			130
smashed salad	V		114
smoked salmon			
smoked salmon & rye omelette			42
speedy kedgeree			74
smoothies			
blackberry smoothie lollies	V		260
green goddess smoothie	V		288
matcha & kefir smoothie	V		291
merry berry smoothie	V		289
post-workout protein smoothie	V		290
soda water: fizzy berry jellies			268

soups
    carrot gazpacho — V — 104
    chicken balls & rainbow broth — 168
    chipotle chicken & bean soup — 248
    comforting chickpea soup — V — 232
    crispy pork noodle broth — 150
    fish pie soup & eggs on toast — 228
    gochujang tomato noodle soup — V — 196
    mushroom riso soup — V — 238
    spiced lamb & lentil soup — 220
    spring soup & ricotta toasts — V — 218
    winter squash & borlotti soup — V — 234
soured cream
    berry cheesecake overnight oats — V — 49
    fish pie soup & eggs on toast — 228
soy sauce
    creamy peanut chicken — 136
    crispy steamy parcels — 178
    prawn & noodle salad — 86
    seared salmon rice — 174
    seared tuna kimchi bowl — 156
    soy eggs & crispy mackerel rice — 108
    spicy tofu & sweet pepper eggs — V — 50
    super-green stir-fry — V — 132
    sweet & sour prawns — 138
    tahini mushroom noodles — V — 144
speedy kedgeree — 74
speedy silky omelette — V — 84
speedy stuffed apple — V — 44
spiced lamb & lentil soup — 220
spicy tofu & sweet pepper eggs — V — 50
spinach
    carrot & sweet potato fritters — V — 124
    chicken in milk — 176
    crispy steamed veggie buns — V — 230
    curried egg & rice pots — V — 118
    fish filo parcel & beans — 226
    fluffy spring veg omelette — V — 102
    green goddess smoothie — V — 288
    pea & feta egg warm salad — V — 106
    roast chicken & sticky spuds — 250
    smoked salmon & rye omelette — 42
    speedy kedgeree — 74
    spinach & lentil fritter salad — V — 170
    super-green orecchiette — V — 190
    vibrant veg & creamy bean salad — V — 186
sponge fingers: fizzy berry jellies — 268
spring onions
    avo & black bean omelette — V — 122
    charred Mexican salad — V — 146
    crispy mackerel buns — 126
    crispy pork noodle broth — 150
    crispy steamed veggie buns — V — 230
    easy egg & bean filo twists — V — 64
    fluffy spring veg omelette — V — 102
    harissa tuna platter — 80
    mushroom stew — 200
    salmon, beet & potato salad — 92
    seared salmon rice — 174
    soy eggs & crispy mackerel rice — 108
    tasty salmon couscous — 148
spring soup & ricotta toasts — V — 218
squash
    chicken, bean & rice bake — 210
    hearty veg casserole — V — 246
    roasted Mediterranean veg — V — 204
    sumptuous squash risotto — V — 240
    winter squash & borlotti soup — V — 234
steak & sticky aubergine salad — 166
strawberries
    cheat's soft-serve ice cream — V — 258
    chocolate orange pots — V — 264
    fizzy berry jellies — 268
    golden cheese & jammy berries — V — 52
    pink Shredded Wheat — V — 34
    strawberry filo tarts — V — 274
sugar snap peas
    creamy peanut chicken — 136
    sesame miso shred salad — V — 96
    sweet & sour prawns — 138
    Thai-style fish curry — 140
sumptuous squash risotto — V — 240
super-green orecchiette — 190
super-green stir-fry — V — 132
sweet & sour prawns — 138
sweet chilli dipping sauce
    chicken cup salad — 164
    crispy steamy parcels — 178
    sweet & sour prawns — 138
sweet potatoes
    carrot & sweet potato fritters — V — 124
    dukkah poached eggs — V — 54
    healthy fish & chips — 224
    roasted Mediterranean veg — V — 204
sweetcorn
    charred Mexican salad — V — 146
    chicken & mushroom hotpot — 214
    prawn cocktail for one — 72

T

tahini
    black bean houmous salad wrap — V — 98
    carrot & sweet potato fritters — V — 124
    cheat's soft-serve ice cream — V — 258
    crispy pork noodle broth — 150
    lemon tahini chicken & grains — 158
    sesame miso shred salad — V — 96
    tahini mushroom noodles — V — 144
    tahini pretzel yoghurt bark — V — 266
tapenade: tuna & broccoli pasta — 120
tarts
    fragrant veggie filo tart — V — 236
    strawberry filo tarts — V — 274
tasty salmon couscous — 148
Thai-style fish curry — 140
tiramisù overnight oats — V — 49
tofu
    chocolate orange pots — V — 264
    gochujang tomato noodle soup — V — 196
    mushroom stew — 200
    silken tofu & black beans — V — 152
    spicy tofu & sweet pepper eggs — V — 50
tomato purée: east egg & bean filo twists — V — 64
tomatoes
    5-minute tasty toppers — 36
    aubergine involtini — V — 208
    avo & black bean omelette — V — 122

beef & borlotti bean ragù		252–5	
black bean houmous salad wrap	V	98	
carrot gazpacho	V	104	
charred Mexican salad	V	146	
cheesy beans on toast	V	62	
chicken curry & chapati	V	202	
chicken fajitas		154	
chipotle chicken & bean soup		248	
chopped rainbow salad	V	90	
comforting chickpea soup	V	232	
crab spaghetti		184	
crispy bean & anchovy eggs		112	
crispy sardine & avo wrap		88	
dukkah poached eggs	V	54	
easy prawn curry		134	
fish filo parcel & beans		226	
fish in crazy water		188	
fish parcels & tomato orzo		192	
fragrant veggie filo tart	V	236	
gochujang tomato noodle soup	V	196	
golden hasselback salmon		222	
hearty veg casserole	V	246	
herby chickpea & feta salad	V	116	
meatball traybake		244	
prawn & noodle salad		86	
roasted Mediterranean veg	V	204	
roasted veg & chickpea smash	V	198	
sardines on toast & tomato salad		94	
smashed flatbread burger		130	
speedy silky omelette	V	84	
tasty salmon couscous		148	
tuna & broccoli pasta		120	
veggie curry traybake	V	212	
warm lentil salad	V	78	
tortillas			
avo & black bean omelette	V	122	
black bean houmous salad wrap	V	98	
chicken fajitas		154	
crispy sardine & avo wrap		88	
trout			
fish filo parcel & beans		226	
speedy kedgeree		74	
tuna			
harissa tuna bean parcels		206	
harissa tuna platter		80	
seared tuna kimchi bowl		156	
tuna & broccoli pasta		120	

v

vegetables			
chicken balls & rainbow broth		168	
crispy steamy parcels		178	
golden hasselback salmon		222	
one-cup pancakes	V	58–61	
sweet & sour prawns		138	
see also specific vegetables			
veggie curry traybake	V	212	

w

walnuts			
5-minute tasty toppers	V	36	
creamy walnut coleslaw	V	76	
hot carrot cup cakes	V	262	
speedy stuffed apple	V	44	
spinach & lentil fritter salad	V	170	
vibrant veg & creamy bean salad	V	186	
warm lentil salad	V	78	
water chestnuts			
crispy black bean beef		162	
crispy steamed veggie buns	V	230	
crispy steamy parcels		178	
mushroom stew		200	
whipped coffee	V	292	
winter squash & borlotti soup	V	234	
Worcestershire sauce: prawn cocktail for one		72	

y

yoghurt			
5-minute tasty toppers	V	36	
banana & almond cake	V	280	
blackberry smoothie lollies	V	260	
blueberry muffins	V	276	
box grater fruit salad	V	38	
cheat's soft-serve ice cream	V	258	
chicken, bean & rice bake		210	
chicken curry & chapati	V	202	
chicken fajitas		154	
choccy fro-yo sandwiches	V	270	
chocolate orange pots	V	264	
creamy walnut coleslaw	V	76	
crispy mackerel buns		126	
curried egg & rice pots	V	118	
curried fried eggs & grain salad	V	82	
extraordinary brekkie smush-in	V	56	
fish filo parcel & beans		226	
fizzy berry jellies		268	
frosty porridge	V	40	
golden hasselback salmon		222	
granola fruit cups	V	66	
harissa tuna bean parcels		206	
harissa tuna platter		80	
hot carrot cup cakes	V	262	
mothership overnight oats	V	46–9	
peach melba overnight oats	V	48	
prawn cocktail for one		72	
roast chicken & sticky spuds		250	
roasted veg & chickpea smash	V	198	
salmon, beet & potato salad		92	
seared tuna kimchi bowl		156	
silky aubergine flavour fest	V	194	
speedy kedgeree		74	
speedy stuffed apple	V	44	
strawberry filo tarts	V	274	
tahini pretzel yoghurt bark	V	266	
tasty salmon couscous		148	
tiramisù overnight oats	V	49	

For a quick reference list of all the vegetarian, vegan, dairy-free and gluten-free recipes in this book, visit:

jamieoliver.com/EatYourselfHealthy/special-diets

The Jamie Oliver collection

1. The Naked Chef *1999*
2. The Return of the Naked Chef *2000*
3. Happy Days with the Naked Chef *2001*
4. Jamie's Kitchen *2002*
5. Jamie's Dinners *2004*
6. Jamie's Italy *2005*
7. Cook with Jamie *2006*
8. Jamie at Home *2007*
9. Jamie's Ministry of Food *2008*
10. Jamie's America *2009*
11. Jamie Does . . . *2010*
12. Jamie's 30-Minute Meals *2010*
13. Jamie's Great Britain *2011*
14. Jamie's 15-Minute Meals *2012*
15. Save with Jamie *2013*
16. Jamie's Comfort Food *2014*
17. Everyday Super Food *2015*
18. Super Food Family Classics *2016*
19. Jamie Oliver's Christmas Cookbook *2016*
20. 5 Ingredients – Quick & Easy Food *2017*
21. Jamie Cooks Italy *2018*
22. Jamie's Friday Night Feast Cookbook *2018*
23. Veg *2019*
24. 7 Ways *2020*
25. Together *2021*
26. ONE *2022*
27. 5 Ingredients Mediterranean *2023*
28. Simply Jamie *2024*
29. Easy Air Fryer *2025*
30. Eat Yourself Healthy *2025*

Hungry for more?

For handy nutrition advice, as well as videos, features, hints, tricks and tips on all sorts of different subjects, loads of brilliant recipes, plus much more, check out

JAMIEOLIVER.COM **#EATYOURSELFHEALTHY**

PENGUIN MICHAEL JOSEPH

UK | USA | CANADA | IRELAND | AUSTRALIA | INDIA | NEW ZEALAND | SOUTH AFRICA

Penguin Michael Joseph is part of the Penguin Random House group of companies whose addresses can be found at global.penguinrandomhouse.com

Penguin Michael Joseph, Penguin Random House UK, One Embassy Gardens, 8 Viaduct Gardens, London SW11 7BW

penguin.co.uk

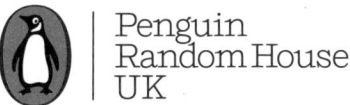

First published 2025

001

Copyright © Jamie Oliver, 2025

Recipe photography copyright © Jamie Oliver Enterprises Limited, 2025

© 2007 P22 Underground Pro Demi. All Rights Reserved, P22 Type Foundry, Inc.

The moral right of the author has been asserted

Food photography by David Loftus / Portrait photography by Paul Stuart

Michael Mosley portrait © Andrew Crowley/Telegraph Media Group Holdings Ltd

Design by Jamie Oliver Limited

Penguin Random House values and supports copyright. Copyright fuels creativity, encourages diverse voices, promotes freedom of expression and supports a vibrant culture. Thank you for purchasing an authorized edition of this book and for respecting intellectual property laws by not reproducing, scanning or distributing any part of it by any means without permission. You are supporting authors and enabling Penguin Random House to continue to publish books for everyone. No part of this book may be used or reproduced in any manner for the purpose of training artificial intelligence technologies or systems. In accordance with Article 4(3) of the DSM Directive 2019/790, Penguin Random House expressly reserves this work from the text and data mining exception

Colour reproduction by Altaimage Ltd

Printed in Germany by Mohn Media

The authorized representative in the EEA is Penguin Random House Ireland, Morrison Chambers, 32 Nassau Street, Dublin D02 YH68

A CIP catalogue record for this book is available from the British Library

ISBN: 978–0–241–65783–6

Penguin Random House is committed to a sustainable future for our business, our readers and our planet. This book is made from Forest Stewardship Council® certified paper

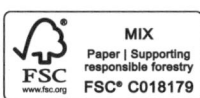

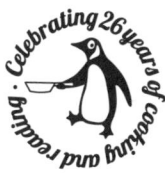

Big love

Thank you for buying my cookbook! Each purchase supports my Ministry of Food Foundation, which is on a mission to teach 1 million people to cook by 2030. In secondary schools, we offer the 10 Skills Food Education programme; in local communities, we support partners with cooking lessons; and in the workplace, we teach a Learn to Cook in 12 Hours course, all with the aim of helping people lead healthier, happier lives.

FIND OUT MORE: JAMIEOLIVER.COM/MOF

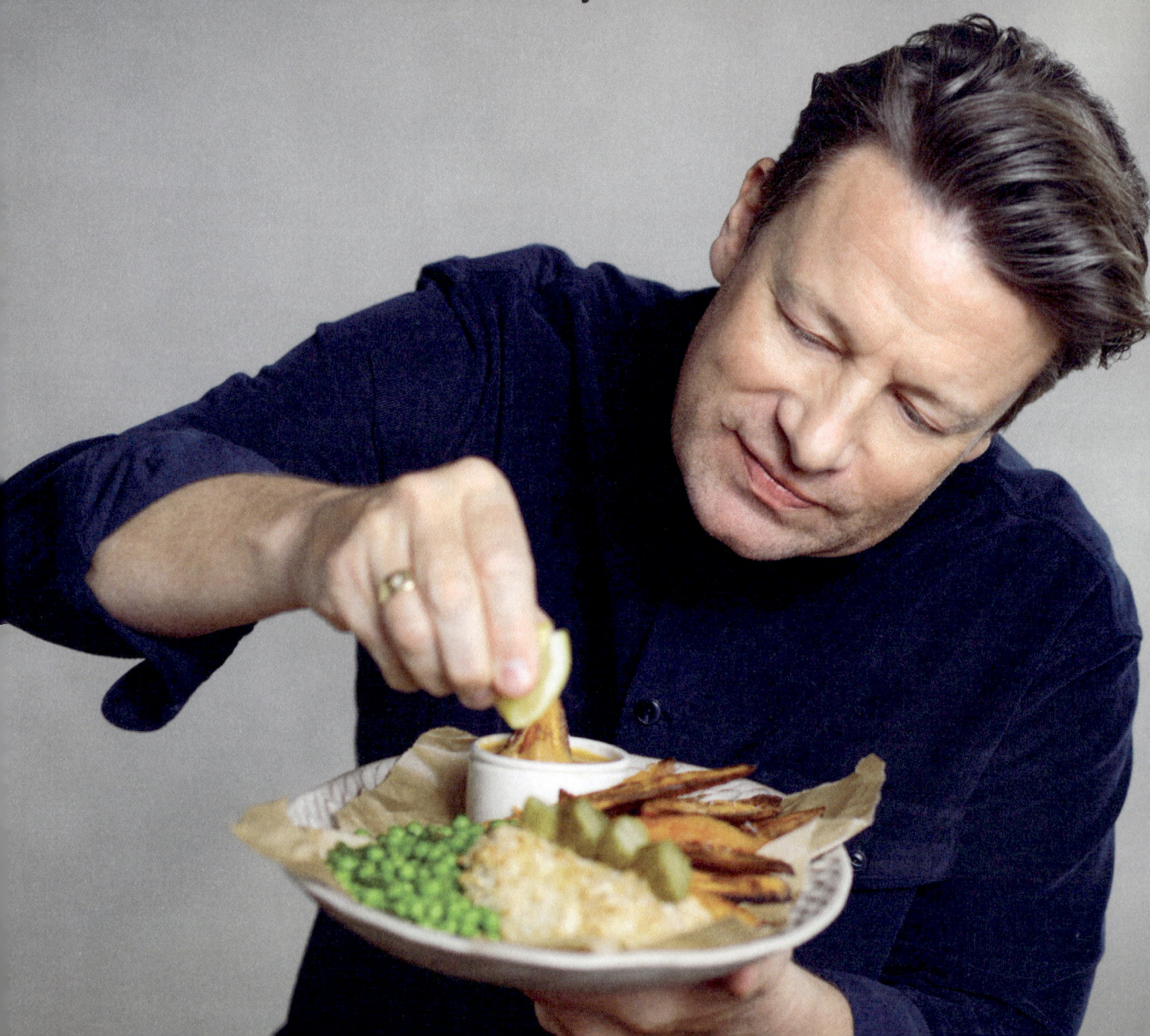

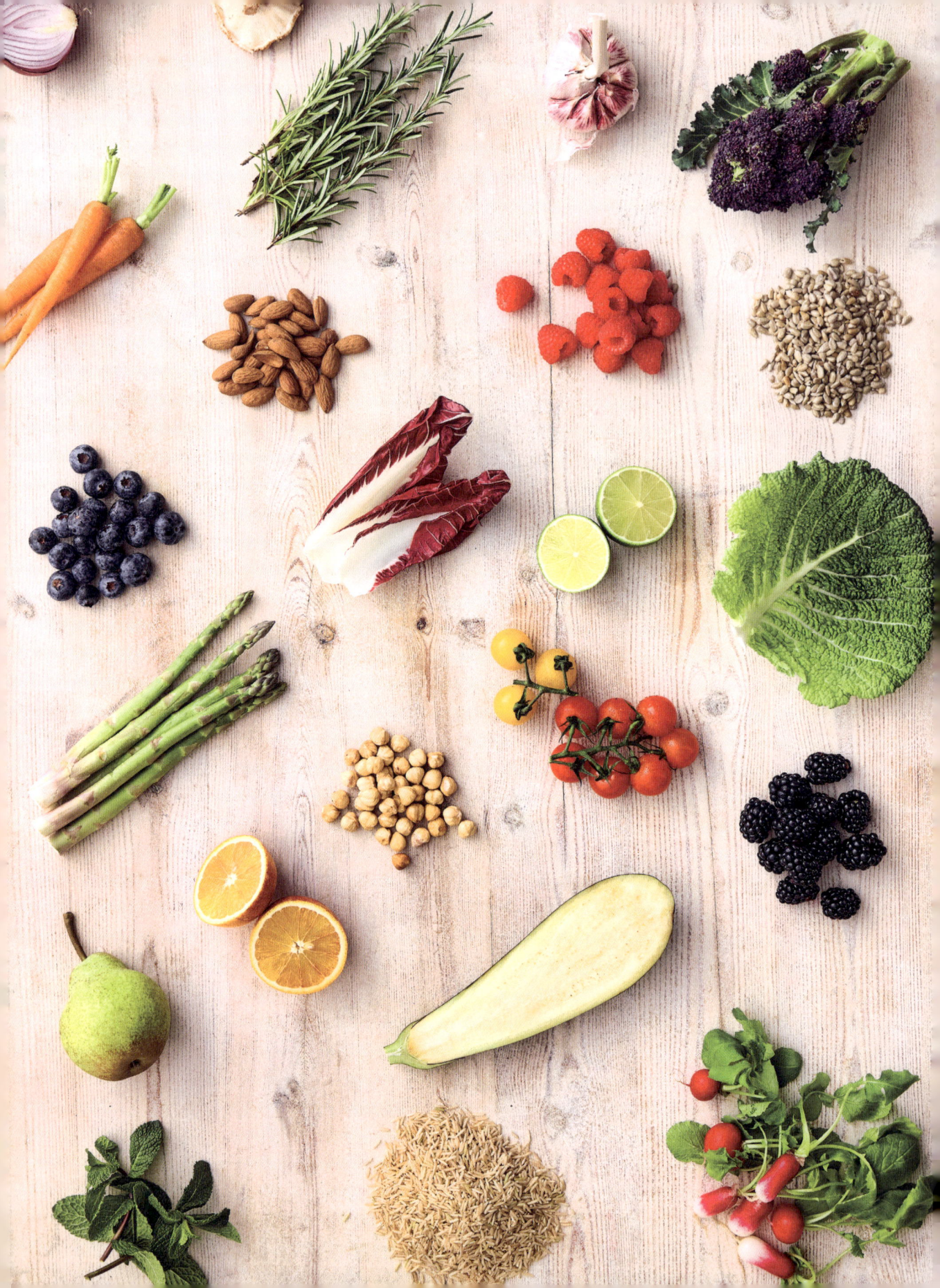